Quality of Life

To
Tessa and Emma Fayers
and
Christine Machin

Quality of Life

Assessment, Analysis and Interpretation

PETER M. FAYERS

Medical Research Council Clinical Trials Unit, London, UK
and Unit of Applied Clinical Research,
Norwegian University of Science and Technology,
Trondheim, Norway

and

DAVID MACHIN

NMRC Clinical Trials & Epidemiology Research Unit, Singapore
and School of Health and Related Research,
University of Sheffield, UK

JOHN WILEY & SONS, LTD
Chichester • New York • Weinheim • Brisbane • Singapore • Toronto

Other Wiley Editorial Offices

John Wiley & Sons, Inc., 605 Third Avenue,
New York, NY 10158-0012, USA

WILEY-VCH Verlag GmbH, Pappelallee 3,
D-69469 Weinheim, Germany

John Wiley & Sons Australia, 33 Park Road, Milton,
Queensland 4064, Australia

John Wiley & Sons (Asia) Pte Ltd, 2 Clementi Loop #02-01,
Jin Xing Distripark, Singapore 129809

John Wiley & Sons (Canada) Ltd, 22 Worcester Road,
Rexdale, Ontario M9W 1L1, Canada

Library of Congress Cataloging-in-Publication Data

Fayers, Peter M.
    Quality of life : assessment, analysis, and interpretation / Peter M. Fayers and David Machin.
        p. cm.
    Includes bibliographical references and index.
    ISBN 0-471-96861-7 (cased : alk. paper)
    1. Quality of life—research. 2. Outcome assessment (Health Care).
    3. Health—Research—Methodology. I. Machin, David. II. Title.
    [DNLM: 1. Research—methods. 2. Outcome Assessment (Health Care). 3. Quality of
    Life. W 20.5 F283q 2000]
    R852.F39 2000
    362.1′07′2—dc21   00-022183

British Library Cataloguing in Publication Data

A catalogue record for this book is available from the British Library

ISBN 0-471-96861-7

Typeset in 10/12pt Times by Mayhew Typesetting, Rhayader, Powys
Printed and bound in Great Britain by Biddles Ltd, Guildford and King's Lynn
This book is printed on acid-free paper responsibly manufactured from sustainable forestation, in
which at least two trees are planted for each one used for paper production.

Contents

Preface

Measurement of quality of life has grown to become a standard endpoint in many randomised controlled trials and other clinical studies. In part, this is a consequence of the realisation that many treatments for chronic diseases frequently fail to cure, and that there may be limited benefits gained at the expense of taking toxic or unpleasant therapy. Sometimes therapeutic benefits may be outweighed by quality of life considerations. In studies of palliative therapy, quality of life may become the principal or only endpoint of consideration. In part, it is also a recognition that patients should have a say in the choice of their therapy, and that patients place greater emphasis upon non-clinical aspects of treatment than healthcare professionals did in the past. Nowadays, many patients and patient-support groups demand that they should be given full information about the consequences of their disease and its therapy, including impact upon aspects of quality of life, and that they should be allowed to express their opinions. The term *quality of life* has become a catch-phrase, and patients, investigators, funding bodies and ethical review committees often insist that, where appropriate, quality of life should be assessed as an endpoint for clinical trials.

The assessment, analysis and interpretation of quality of life relies upon a variety of psychometric and statistical methods, many of which may be less familiar than the other techniques used in medical research. Our objective is to explain these techniques in a non-technical way. We have assumed some familiarity with basic statistical ideas, but we have avoided detailed statistical theory. Instead, we have tried to write a practical guide that covers a wide range of methods. We emphasise the use of simple techniques in a variety of situations by using numerous examples, taken both from the literature and from our own experience. A number of these inevitably arise from our own particular field of interest—cancer clinical trials. This is also perhaps justifiable in that much of the pioneering work on quality of life assessment occurred in cancer, and cancer still remains the disease area that is associated with the largest number of quality of life instruments and the most publications. However, the issues that arise are common to quality of life assessment in general.

ACKNOWLEDGEMENTS

We would like to say a general thank you to all those with whom we have worked on aspects of quality of life over the years; especially, past and present members of the EORTC Quality of Life Study Group, and colleagues from the former MRC Cancer Therapy Committee Working Parties. Particular thanks go to Stein Kaasa of the Norwegian University of Science and Technology at Trondheim who permitted PMF to work on this book whilst on sabbatical and whose ideas greatly influenced our thinking about quality of life, and to Kristin Bjordal of the Radium Hospital, Oslo, who made extensive input and comments on many chapters and provided quality of life data that we used in examples. Finn Wisløff, for the Nordic Myeloma Study Group, very kindly allowed us to make extensive use their QoL data for many examples. We are grateful to the National Medical Research Council of Singapore for providing funds and facilities to enable us to complete this work. We also thank Dr Julian Thumboo, Tan Tock Seng Hospital, Singapore, for valuable comments on several chapters. Several chapters, and Chapter 7 in particular, were strongly influenced by manuals and guidelines published by the EORTC Quality of Life Study Group.

Peter Fayers and David Machin
January 2000

A Introduction

1 Introduction

A key methodology for the evaluation of therapies is the randomised controlled trial (RCT). These clinical trials have traditionally considered relatively objective clinical outcome measures, such as cure, biological response to treatment, or survival. More recently, investigators and patients alike have argued that subjective indicators should also be considered. These subjective indicators are often regarded as indicators of quality of life. They comprise a variety of measurement scales such as emotional functioning (including anxiety and depression), physical functioning, social functioning, pain, fatigue, other symptoms and toxicity. A large number of questionnaires or *instruments* have been developed for quality of life assessment and they have been used in a wide variety of circumstances. This book is concerned with the development, analysis and interpretation of data from these quality of life instruments.

1.1 WHAT IS QUALITY OF LIFE?

Quality of life (QoL) is an ill-defined term. The World Health Organization (WHO, 1948) has declared health to be "a state of complete physical, mental and social well-being, and not merely the absence of disease". Many other definitions of both "health" and "quality of life" have been attempted, often linking the two and, for QoL, frequently emphasising components of happiness and satisfaction with life. In the absence of any universally accepted definition, some investigators argue that most people, in the western world at least, are familiar with the expression "quality of life" and have an intuitive understanding of what it comprises.

However, it is clear that QoL means different things to different people, and takes on different meanings according to the area of application. To a town planner, for example, it might represent access to green space and other facilities. In the context of clinical trials we are rarely interested in QoL in such a broad sense, but are concerned only with evaluating those aspects that are affected by disease or treatment for disease. This may sometimes be extended to include indirect consequences of disease such as unemployment or financial difficulties. To distinguish between QoL in its more general sense and the requirements of clinical medicine and clinical trials, the term "health-related quality of life" (HRQoL) is frequently used in order to remove ambiguity.

Health-related QoL is still a loose definition. What aspects of QoL should be included? It is generally agreed that the relevant aspects may vary from study to study, but can include general health, physical functioning, physical symptoms and toxicity, emotional functioning, cognitive functioning, role functioning, social well-being and functioning, sexual functioning, and existential issues. In the absence of any agreed formal definition of QoL, most investigators circumvent the issues by describing what *they* mean by QoL, and then letting the items (questions) in their questionnaire speak for themselves. Thus some questionnaires focus upon the relatively objective signs such as patient-reported toxicity, and in effect define the relevant aspects of QoL as being, for their purposes, limited to treatment toxicity. Other investigators argue that what matters most is the impact of toxicity, and therefore their questionnaires place greater emphasis upon psychological aspects such as anxiety and depression. Yet others try to allow for spiritual issues, ability to cope with illness, and satisfaction with life.

Some QoL instruments focus upon a single concept, such as emotional functioning. Other instruments regard these individual concepts as aspects or *dimensions* of QoL, and therefore include items relating to several concepts. Although there is disagreement about what components should be evaluated, most investigators agree that a number of the above dimensions should be included in QoL questionnaires, and that QoL is a multidimensional construct. Because there are so many potential dimensions, it is impractical to try to assess all these concepts simultaneously in one instrument. Most instruments intended for health-status assessment include at least some items that focus upon physical, emotional and social functioning. For example, if emotional functioning is accepted as being one aspect of QoL that should be investigated, then several questions could evaluate anxiety, tension, irritability, depression, and so on. Thus instruments may contain many items. Although a single "global" question, such as "How would you rate your overall quality of life?", is a useful adjunct to multi-item instruments, global questions are often regarded as too vague and non-specific to be used on their own. Most of the general questionnaires that we describe include one or more global questions alongside a number of other items covering specific issues. Some instruments place greater emphasis upon the concept of global questions, and the EuroQol questionnaire (Appendix E4) asks a parsimonious five questions before using a single global question that enquires about "your health". Even more extreme is the Perceived Adjustment to Chronic Illness Scale (PACIS) described by Hürny *et al.* (1993). This instrument consists of a single, carefully-phrased question that is a global indicator of coping and adjustment: "How much effort does it cost you to cope with your illness?" This takes responses ranging between "No effort at all" and "A great deal of effort".

One unifying and non-controversial theme throughout all the approaches is that the concepts forming these dimensions can be assessed only by *subjective measures*, and that they should be evaluated by *asking the patient*. "Proxy" assessments, by a relative or other close observer, are usually employed only if the patient is unable to make a coherent response—for example, some patients who are very young or very old, severely ill, or have mental impairment. Furthermore, many of these individual concepts—such as emotional functioning and fatigue—lack a formal, agreed definition that is universally understood by patients. In many cases the problem is compounded by language differences and some concepts do not readily translate to other tongues. There are also cultural differences regarding the importance of the issues. Single-item questions on these aspects of QoL, as for global questions about overall QoL, are likely to be ambiguous and unreliable. Therefore it is usual to develop questionnaires that consist of multi-item measurement scales for each concept.

This book accepts a broad definition of "quality of life", and therefore discusses the design, application and use of single- and multi-item, subjective, measurement scales. Furthermore, although we are predominantly concerned with health-related QoL, in this book we use the briefer and more common abbreviation, QoL, as a synonym for HRQoL.

1.2 HISTORICAL DEVELOPMENT

One of the earliest references that impinges upon a definition of QoL appears in the Nichomachean Ethics, when Aristotle (384–322BC) noted that "Both the multitude and persons of refinement . . . conceive 'the good life' or 'doing well' to be the same thing as 'being happy'. But what constitutes happiness is a matter of dispute . . . some say one thing and some another, indeed very often the same man says different things at different times: when he falls sick he thinks health is happiness, when he is poor, wealth." The Greek ευδαιμονια is commonly translated as "happiness" although Harris Rackham, the translator that we cite, noted in 1926 that a more accurate rendering would embrace "well-being", with Aristotle denoting by ευδαιμονια both a state of feeling and a kind of activity. In modern parlance, this is assuredly quality of life. Although the term "quality of life" did not exist in the Greek language of 2000 years ago, Aristotle clearly appreciated that QoL not only means different things to different people but also varies according to a person's current situation. "Quality of life" was rarely mentioned until the 20th century, although one early commentator on the subject noted that happiness could be sacrificed for QoL: "Life at its noblest leaves mere happiness far behind; and indeed cannot endure it. . . . Happiness is not the object of life: life has no object: it is an end in itself; and courage consists in the readiness to sacrifice happiness for an intenser quality of life." (George Bernard Shaw, 1900). It would appear that by this time "quality of life" had become a familiar term that did not require further explanation. Specific mention of QoL in relation to patients' health came much later. The influential WHO 1948 definition of health cited above was one of the earliest statements recognising and stressing the importance of the three dimensions—physical, mental and social—in the context of disease.

One of the first instruments that broadened the assessment of patients beyond physiological and clinical examination was the Karnofsky Performance Scale proposed in 1947 for use in clinical settings. This is a simple scale ranging from 0 for "dead" to 100 indicating "normal, no complaints, no evidence of disease". Health-care staff make the assessment. Over the years, it has led to a number of other scales for functional ability, physical functioning, and "activities of daily living" (ADL), such as the Barthel Index. Although these questionnaires are still sometimes described as QoL instruments, they capture only one aspect of it and provide an inadequate representation of patients' overall well-being and QoL.

The next generation of questionnaires, in the late 1970s and early 1980s, that quantified health status were used for the general evaluation of health. These instruments focused on physical functioning, physical and psychological symptoms, impact of illness, perceived distress, and life satisfaction. Examples of such instruments include the Sickness Impact Profile and the Nottingham Health Profile. Although these instruments are frequently described as QoL questionnaires, their authors neither designed them nor claimed them as QoL instruments.

Meanwhile, Priestman and Baum (1976) were adapting linear analogue self-assessment (LASA) methods to assess QoL in breast cancer patients. The LASA approach, which is also sometimes called a visual analogue scale (VAS), provides a 10-cm line, with the ends labelled with words describing the extremes of a condition. The patient is asked to mark the point along the line that corresponds with their feelings. An example of a LASA scale is contained in the EuroQol (Appendix E4). Priestman and Baum measured a variety of subjective effects, including well-being, mood, anxiety, activity, pain, social activities and the patient's opinion as to "Is the treatment helping?"

Much of the development of QoL instruments has built upon these early attempts, although newer instruments emphasise more strongly the subjective aspects such as emotional, role, social and cognitive functioning. Frequently, one or more general or global questions concerning overall QoL are included. However, despite a shift to the inclusion of psychological and social aspects, these instruments continue to link QoL to the functional capacity. Thus, if a patient is unable to achieve full physical, psychological or social functioning, it is assumed that their QoL is poorer. Although this may in general seem a reasonable assumption, it can lead to theoretical problems. In particular, many forms of functioning, especially physical functioning, may be regarded as *causal* variables that can be expected to change or affect a patient's QoL, but do not necessarily reflect the true level of their QoL (see Chapter 2). For example, a patient may have a poor QoL irrespective of whether their physical functioning is impaired; this might arise because of other factors such as pain. Therefore scales measuring functional status assess only whether there are problems that *may* cause distress to the patient or impair their QoL; these scales do not necessarily indicate the patient's QoL. Despite these reservations, most instruments continue to focus on health status, functional status, and checklists of symptoms. For clinical purposes this may be logical since, when comparing treatments, the clinician is most concerned with the differences in the symptoms and side-effects due to the various therapies, and the impact of these differences upon QoL.

A number of other theoretical models for QoL have been proposed. The *expectations* model of Calman (1984) suggested that individuals have aims and goals in life, and QoL is a measure of the difference between the hopes and expectations of the individual and the individual's present experience. It is concerned with the difference between perceived goals and actual goals. The gap may be narrowed by improving the function of a patient or by modifying their expectations. Instruments such as the Schedule for Evaluation of Individual Quality of Life (SEIQoL) and the Patient Generated Index (PGI), described in Section 1.6, use Calman's expectations model as a conceptual basis and provide the facility to incorporate personal values.

The *needs* model relates QoL to the ability and capacity of patients to satisfy certain human needs. QoL is at its highest when all needs are fulfilled, and at its lowest when few needs are satisfied. "Needs" include such aspects as identity, status, self-esteem, affection, love, security, enjoyment, creativity, food, sleep, pain avoidance, activity, etc. Hunt and McKenna (1992) have used this model to generate several QoL measures. Somewhat related is the *reintegration to normal living* model that has also been regarded as an approach to assessing QoL. Reintegration means the ability to do what one has to do or wants to do, but it does not mean being free of disease or symptoms.

Other definitions or indicators of QoL that have been suggested are *personal well-being* and *satisfaction with life*. The *impact of illness on social, emotional, occupational and family domains* emphasises the illness aspect. The *existential* approach notes that preferences are not fixed and are both individual and vary over time—as was recognised so long ago by Aristotle. Having a "positive approach to life" can give life high quality, regardless of the medical condition. Therefore it can be important to assess existential beliefs and also *coping*. A patient's perception of their QoL can be altered by influencing their existential beliefs or by helping them to cope better. The existential model of QoL leads to the inclusion of such items as pleasure in life, and positive outlook to life.

Patient-preference measures differ from other models of QoL in that they explicitly incorporate "weights" that reflect the importance that patients attach to specific dimensions. Different states and dimensions are compared against each other, to establish a ranking in terms of their value or in terms of patients' preferences of one state over another. These and other *utility measure* approaches to QoL assessment are derived from decision-making theory, and are frequently employed in economic evaluation of treatments.

Thus there is continuing philosophical debate about the meaning of QoL, and about what should be measured. Perhaps the simplest and most pragmatic view is that all of these concepts reflect issues that are of fundamental importance to patients' well-being. They are all worth investigating and quantifying.

1.3 WHY MEASURE QUALITY OF LIFE?

There are several reasons why QoL assessments may be included in RCTs, and it is important to distinguish between them as the nature of the measurements, and the questionnaires that are employed, will depend upon the objectives of the trial. Perhaps the most obvious reason is in order to compare the study treatments, in which case it is important to identify those aspects of QoL that may be affected by the therapy. These include both benefits, as may be sought in palliative trials that are expected to improve QoL, and negative changes, such as toxicity and side-effects of therapy.

CLINICAL TRIALS OF TREATMENT WITH CURATIVE INTENT

Many clinical trial organisations have now introduced the assessment of QoL as being a standard part of new trials. An obvious reason for the emphasis towards QoL as an important endpoint is that treatment of fatal diseases can, and often does, result in limited gains in cure or prolonged survival. With some notable exceptions, little improvement has been seen in patients with major cancer diagnoses, HIV or AIDS. At the same time therapeutic interventions in these diseases frequently cause serious side-effects and functional impairment.

There are numerous examples in which QoL assessments have had an unexpectedly important role in the interpretation and conclusions of RCTs, and it is perhaps surprising that it has taken so long for the relevance of QoL assessment to be appreciated. For example, one of the earlier randomised trials to include QoL assessment was by Coates *et al.* (1987) who reported that, contrary to their initial expectations, continuous as opposed to intermittent chemotherapy for advanced breast cancer not only prolonged survival but most importantly resulted in superior QoL.

Similarly, other RCTs recognised that QoL may be the principal outcome of interest. For example, an RCT comparing three anti-hypertensive therapies conducted by Croog *et al.* (1986) demonstrated major differences in QoL, and the cancer chemotherapy trial of Buccheri *et al.* (1989) suggested that small treatment benefits may be more than outweighed by the poorer QoL and cost of therapy. In extreme cases, the cure might be worse than the disease.

Example from the literature

Testa *et al.* (1993) describe an RCT evaluating hypertensive therapy in men. Two angiotensin-converting-enzyme inhibitors, captopril and enalapril, were compared. In total, 379 active men with mild to moderate hypertension, aged 55 to 79, were randomised between the treatment arms. QoL was one of the main outcome measures. Several QoL scales were used, including an Overall QoL scale based on a mean score from 11 subscales.

In order to interpret the magnitude of the differences in QoL that were observed, stressful life events that produced an equivalent change in QoL scores were considered, and the responses to the Overall QoL scale were re-calibrated accordingly (see Chapter 16). Overall QoL scores shifted positively for captopril by 0.11 units, and negatively for enalapril by 0.11. Negative shifts of 0.11 corresponded to those encountered when there was "major change in work responsibility", "in-law troubles" or "mortgage foreclosure". On the basis of these investigations, a clinically important change was deemed to be one between 0.1 and 0.2.

It was concluded that, although the therapies were indistinguishable in terms of clinical assessments of efficacy and safety, they produced substantial and different changes in QoL.

CLINICAL TRIALS OF TREATMENT WITH PALLIATIVE INTENT

One consequence of ageing societies is the corresponding increased prevalence of chronic diseases. The treatment outcome in such diseases cannot be cure, but must relate to improvement of the well-being of patients thus treated. The aim is to palliate symptoms, or to prolong the time without symptoms. Traditionally, clinical and not QoL outcomes have been the principal endpoints. For example, in an RCT of therapy for advanced oesophageal cancer, absence of dysphagia might have been the main outcome measure indicating success of therapy. Nowadays, in trials of palliative care, QoL is more frequently chosen as the outcome measure of choice. Symptom relief is now recognised as but one aspect of palliative intervention and comprehensive assessment of QoL is often as important as evaluation of symptoms.

Example from the literature

Bonkovsky *et al.* (1999) used the Medical Outcomes Study (MOS) SF-36 and additional items, to evaluate the benefit of therapy with interferon for patients with chronic hepatitis C. It was expected that most patients would have a normal life span. It had been shown that patients with hepatitis C have a clinically and socially important reduction in QoL, although it was unclear whether this results from the disease or its associated comorbidity.

The RCT recruited 642 patients, and an additional 750 healthy controls provided a baseline assessment. Patients had lower scores than the controls on all eight SF-36 scales, and these differences were considered clinically and socially relevant.

Between the randomised groups, those who sustained virological response to interferon experienced improvements in five of the eight SF-36 scales, and these improvements were clinically important and worthwhile. However, only 15% of patients obtained sustained virological response from the 24 weeks of interferon.

Example from the literature

Fatigue, lethargy, anorexia, nausea and weakness are common in patients with advanced cancer. It had been suggested that progestagens, including megestrol acetate (MA), might have a useful function for palliative treatment of advanced endocrine-insensitive tumours. Beller *et al.* (1997) reported a double-blind RCT of 240 patients randomised to 12 weeks of high- or low-dose MA, or to matching placebo. Nutritional status was recorded, and QoL was measured using six linear analogue self-assessment (LASA) scales, at randomisation and after four, eight and twelve weeks.

Patients receiving MA reported substantially better appetite, mood and overall QoL than patients receiving placebo, with a larger benefit being seen for the higher dose. Table 1.1 shows the average change from the baseline at time of randomisation. No statistically significant differences were observed in the nutritional status measurements. Side-effects of therapy were minor and did not differ across treatments.

The authors concluded that high-dose MA provides useful palliation for patients with endocrine-insensitive advanced cancer. It improves appetite, mood and overall quality of life in these patients, although not through a direct effect on nutritional status.

IMPROVING SYMPTOM RELIEF, CARE, OR REHABILITATION

Traditionally medicine has tended to concentrate upon symptom relief as an outcome measure. Studies using QoL instruments may reveal other issues that are equally or more important to patients. For example, in advanced oesophageal cancer, it has been found that many patients say that fatigue has a far greater impact upon their QoL than dyspnoea. Such a finding is contrary to traditional teaching, but has been replicated in various cancers.

Table 1.1   Average difference in QoL between baseline and subsequent weeks (Based on Beller *et al.*, 1997)

LASA scores	Placebo	Low-dose MA	High-dose MA	*p*-value (trend)
Physical well-being	5.8	6.5	13.9	0.13
Mood	−4.1	0.4	10.2	0.001
Pain	−5.3	−6.9	1.9	0.13
Nausea/vomiting	−1.4	8.7	7.2	0.08
Appetite	9.7	17.0	31.3	0.0001
Overall QoL	−2.7	2.8	13.1	0.001
Combined QoL measure	−2.1	2.4	12.3	0.001

Example from the literature

Smets *et al.* (1998) used the Multidimensional Fatigue Inventory (MFI-20, Appendix E14) to assess fatigue in 250 patients who were receiving radiotherapy with curative intent for various cancers. Patients rated their fatigue at two-weekly intervals during treatment and within two weeks after completion of radiotherapy.

There was a gradual increase in fatigue during radiotherapy and a decrease after completion of treatment. After treatment, 46% of the patients reported fatigue as being among the three symptoms causing most distress, and 40% reported having been tired throughout the treatment period.

Smets *et al.* concluded that there is a need to give preparatory information to new patients who are at risk of fatigue, and interventions including exercise and psychotherapy may be beneficial. They also suggested that their results might be underestimates because the oldest and most tired patients were more inclined to refuse participation.

Rehabilitation programmes, too, have traditionally concentrated upon physical aspects of health, functioning and ability to perform activities of daily living; these physical aspects were most frequently evaluated by healthcare workers or other observers. Increasingly, patient-completed QoL assessment is now perceived as essential to the evaluation of successful rehabilitation. Problems revealed by questioning patients can lead to modifications and improvement in the programme, or alternatively may show that some methods offer little benefit.

Example from the literature

Results from several small trials had suggested that group therapy, counselling, relaxation therapy and psychoeducation might have a role in the rehabilitation of patients following acute myocardial infarction. Jones and West (1996) reported an RCT that examined the impact of psychological rehabilitation after myocardial infarction. In this trial, 2328 patients were randomised between policies of no-intervention and intervention consisting of comprehensive rehabilitation with psychological therapy and opportunities for group and individual counselling. Patients were assessed both by interview and by questionnaires for anxiety and depression, state anxiety, expectations of future life, psychological well-being, sexual activity and functional disability.

At six months, 34% of patients receiving intervention had clinically significant levels of anxiety, compared with 32% of no-intervention patients. In both groups, 19% had clinically significant levels of depression. Differences for other domains were also minimal.

The authors concluded that rehabilitation programmes based upon psychological therapy, counselling, relaxation training, and stress management seem to offer little objective benefit to myocardial infarction patients.

FACILITATING COMMUNICATION WITH PATIENTS

Another reason for assessing QoL is to establish information about the range of problems that affect patients. In this case, the investigator may be less interested in whether there are treatment differences, and might even anticipate that both study arms will experience similar levels of some aspects of QoL. The aim is to collect information in a form that can be communicated to future patients, enabling them to anticipate and understand the consequences of their illness and its treatment. Patients themselves often express the wish for more emphasis upon research into QoL issues, and seek insight into the concomitants of their disease and its treatment.

Example from the literature

The Dartmouth COOP, a primary-care research network, developed nine pictorial charts to measure patient function and QoL in a busy office practice (Nelson *et al.*, 1990). Each chart has a five-point scale, is illustrated, and can be self- or office-staff administered. The charts are used to measure patients' overall physical functioning, emotional problems, daily activities, social activities, pain, overall health and QoL. The QoL item is presented as a ladder, and was later used in the QOLIE-89 instrument (Appendix E10, question 49).

Nelson *et al.* report results for over 2000 patients in four diverse clinical settings. Most clinicians and patients reported that the charts were easy to use and provided a valuable tool. For nearly half of the patients in whom the charts uncovered new information, changes in clinical management were initiated as a consequence.

It was concluded that the COOP Charts are practical, reliable, valid, sensitive to the effects of disease and useful for measuring patient function quickly.

PATIENT PREFERENCES

Not only does a patient's self-assessment often differ substantially from the judgement of their doctor or other healthcare staff, but patients' preferences also seem to differ from those of other people. Many patients accept toxic chemotherapy for the prospect of minimal benefit in terms of probability of cure or prolongation of life, contrary to the expectations of medical staff. Therefore QoL should be measured from the patient's perspective, using a patient-completed questionnaire.

Example from the literature

Slevin *et al.* (1990) asked 106 consecutive patients with solid tumours to complete questionnaires about their willingness to receive chemotherapy. They were told that the more-intensive regimen was likely to have considerable side-effects and drawbacks, such as severe nausea and vomiting, hair loss, frequent tiredness and weakness, frequent use of drips and needles, admission to hospital, decreased sexual interest, and possible infertility. They were given different scenarios, such as (a) small (1%) chance of cure, (b) no cure, but chance of prolonging life by three months, and (c) 1% chance of symptom relief only. All patients knew they were about to commence chemotherapy, and thus considered the questions seriously. Cancer nurses, general practitioners, radiotherapists, oncologists and sociodemographically matched controls were asked the same questions.

Table 1.2 shows the percentage of respondents that would accept chemotherapy under each scenario. There are major and consistent differences between the opinions of patients and the others, and also between the different healthcare staff.

Slevin *et al.* comment that patients appear to regard a minute chance of possible benefit as worthwhile, whatever the cost. They conclude: "It may be that the only people who can evaluate such life and death decisions are those faced with them."

Table 1.2 Percentage of respondents willing to accept intensive and mild chemotherapy with a minimum chance of effectiveness (Based on Slevin *et al.*, 1990)

	Controls	Cancer nurses	General practitioners	Radio-therapists	Oncologists	**Cancer patients**
Number	100	303	790	88	60	**100**
Cure (1%)						
Intensive regimen	19	13	12	4	20	**53**
Mild regimen	35	39	44	27	52	**67**
Prolonging life by 3 months						
Intensive regimen	10	6	3	0	10	**42**
Mild regimen	25	25	27	13	45	**53**
Relief of symptoms (1%)						
Intensive regimen	10	6	2	0	7	**43**
Mild regimen	19	26	21	2	11	**59**

These results have been closely replicated by others. For example, Lindley *et al.* (1998) examined QoL in 86 breast cancer patients, using the SF-36 and the Functional Living Index—Cancer (FLIC). They noted that "the majority of patients indicated a willingness to accept six months of chemotherapy for small to modest potential benefit".

LATE PROBLEMS OF PSYCHOSOCIAL ADAPTATION

Cured patients and long-term survivors may have continuing problems long after their treatment is completed. These late problems may be overlooked, and QoL reported in such patients often gives results that are contrary to expectations.

Example from the literature

Bjordal *et al.* (1994b), in a study of long-term survivors from a trial of radiotherapy for head and neck cancer, unexpectedly found that the hypofractionated patients reported slightly better QoL than those who received conventional therapy. Hypofractionated patients had slightly better EORTC QLQ-C30 mean scores for role, social and emotional function and better overall QoL (Table 1.3), and reported less fatigue. However, both groups reported high levels of symptoms 7–11 years after their radiotherapy, such as dryness in the mouth and mucus production, and high levels of psychological distress (30% being clinical "cases").

The authors concluded that clinicians need to be aware of these problems, and some patients would benefit from social support or medication. It was proposed that the GHQ-20 could facilitate the screening for patients whose psychological distress might be treated.

Table 1.3 Quality of life in head and neck cancer patients 7–11 years after curative treatment (Based on Bjordal *et al.*, 1994b, and Bjordal and Kaasa, 1995)

	Conventional radiotherapy (*n*=103)	Hypofractionated radiotherapy (*n*=101)	*p*-value
EORTC QLQ-C30 function scales (mean scores)			
Physical function	74	79	NS
Role function	72	83	0.03
Social function	73	83	0.02
Emotional function	77	84	0.02
Cognitive function	80	83	NS
Overall QoL	61	69	0.04
EORTC QLQ-C30 symptom scales (mean scores)			
Pain	19	15	NS
Fatigue	32	25	0.04
Emesis	6	5	NS
GHQ scores			
Mean score	20.8	19.7	NS
Cases	31%	32%	NS

MEDICAL DECISION-MAKING

QoL can be a predictor of treatment success and several studies have found that factors such as overall QoL, physical well-being, mood, and pain are of prognostic importance. For example, in cancer patients, pre-treatment assessments of QoL have been shown to be strongly predictive of survival. On this basis, it is possible to argue, as do Coates *et al.* (1993), for the routine assessment of QoL in therapy trials.

It is not clear in these circumstances whether QoL scores reflect an early perception by the patient of disease progression, or whether QoL status in some way influences the course of disease. If the former, level of QoL is merely predictive of outcome. If it affects outcome, there could be potential to use improvement in QoL as an active form of therapy. Whatever the nature of the association, these findings underline the importance of evaluating QoL and using it when making medical decisions. Similar results have been observed in various disease areas. For example, Jenkins (1992) observes that preoperative QoL partially predicts the recovery process in heart surgery patients. Changes in QoL scores during treatment have also been shown to have prognostic value.

Example from the literature

Coates *et al.* (1997) showed that patients' self-assessment of QoL is an important prognostic factor of survival in advanced cancer patients. Adult patients with advanced malignancy from 12 institutions in 10 countries completed the EORTC QLQ-C30 questionnaire. Baseline patient and disease characteristics were recorded.

Follow-up information was obtained on 656 patients, of whom 411 had died. In addition to age and performance status, the QLQ-C30 global QoL scale and the scales of physical, role, emotional, cognitive and social function were each predictive of subsequent survival duration. Table 1.4 shows the association of survival with the scores for overall physical condition (Q29) and overall quality of life (Q30). In this table, items Q29 and Q30 were each divided about their respective medians, and the hazard ratios show that patients with high scores were less likely to die than those below the median. For example, the hazard ratio of 0.89 for Q29 indicates that the rate of death in patients with high scores was only 89% of the death rate in those with low scores.

Coates *et al.* concluded that QoL scores carry prognostic information independent of other recorded factors.

Table 1.4 Prognostic significance for survival of two single-item QoL scores in patients with cancer, after allowing for performance status and age (Based on Coates *et al.*, 1997)

QoL variable	Hazard ratio	95% confidence interval	*p*-value
Physical condition (Q29)	0.89	0.82–0.96	0.003
Overall QoL (Q30)	0.87	0.80–0.94	0.001

1.4 WHICH CLINICAL TRIALS SHOULD ASSESS QoL?

It would be inappropriate to suggest that *all* RCTs, even in cancer, HIV or chronic diseases, should make a formal assessment of QoL. Clearly there are situations where such information is not relevant. For example, when evaluating a potentially curative treatment that is not very likely to have adverse side-effects, or if the treatments and side-effects are similar in the various study arms, it might be unnecessary to make such assessment. However, many trial groups now insist that the investigators should at least consider the QoL implications and should positively justify *not* including the assessment of QoL.

When is QoL assessment a relevant endpoint? Gotay and Moore (1992) have proposed the following classification of trials for QoL purposes:

1. QoL may be the main endpoint. This is frequently true in palliative care, or when patients are seriously ill with incurable disease.
2. Treatments may be expected to be equivalent in efficacy, and a new treatment would be deemed preferable if it confers QoL benefits.
3. A new treatment may show a small benefit in cure rates or survival advantage but this might be offset by QoL deterioration.
4. Treatments may differ considerably in their short-term efficacy, but if the overall failure rate is high then QoL issues should be considered.

Furthermore, despite the optimism of those who launch trials that seek a survival breakthrough, all too often completed trials show a limited survival advantage. Thus in these cases the relevance of QoL assessment has to be considered, since any gain in therapeutic efficacy would have to be weighed against possible negative effects pertaining to QoL.

1.5 HOW TO MEASURE QUALITY OF LIFE

ASK THE PATIENT

Observers are poor judges of patients' opinions. Many studies have shown that independent assessments by either healthcare professionals or patients' relatives differ from the responses obtained when patients complete self-reported question- naires. In some conditions observers appear to consistently overestimate QoL scores, in others underestimate; there is general agreement that patients' opinions vary considerably from the expectations of both staff and relatives. It has been suggested that observers tend to underestimate the impact of psychological aspects and tend to emphasise the importance of the more obvious symptoms. The impacts of pain, nausea and vomiting have all been reported as being underestimated. "Expected" symptoms and toxicity tend to be accepted and hence ignored by clinical staff. Studies of nausea and vomiting in cancer patients receiving chemo- therapy have found that doctors assume these symptoms are likely to occur and, as a consequence, often report only the more severe events. However, the patients that were reported as having no problems may assert that they suffered quite a lot of vomiting (Fayers, 1991).

Observers frequently misjudge the absolute levels of both symptoms and general QoL. In addition, the patients' willingness to trade QoL for possible cure may be misjudged. Many patients are willing to accept unpleasant or toxic therapy for seemingly modest benefits in terms of cure, although a few patients will refuse treatment even when there is a high chance of substantial gain. Physicians and nurses are more likely to say that they would be unwilling to accept the therapy for such small potential benefit. When patients with cancer choose between two treatments, if they believe their disease is likely to be cured they may be willing to accept a treatment that adversely affects their QoL.

Observers, including health professionals, may tend to base their opinions of overall QoL upon physical signs such as symptoms and toxicity. However, in many disease areas, conventional clinical outcomes have been shown to be poorly correlated with patients' assessment of QoL. Thus, for example, in patients with asthma, Juniper *et al.* (1993) observed that correlations between clinical assessments and how patients felt and functioned in day-to-day activities were only modest.

Example from the literature

An early investigation conducted by Jachuk *et al.* (1982) into QoL concerned the effect of hypotensive drugs. Seventy-five patients with controlled hypertension each completed a questionnaire, as did a relative and doctor. A global, summary question was included, about whether there was an overall improvement, no change, or deterioration.

As Table 1.5 shows, whilst the physicians assessed all patients as having improved, approximately half the patients thought there was no change or deterioration, and all but one patient was assessed by their relatives as having deteriorated. Patients attributed their deterioration as due to decline in energy, general activity, sexual inactivity, and irritability. Physicians, focusing upon control of hypertension, largely ignored these factors. Relatives commonly thought there was moderate or severe impairment of memory, energy, activity, and increase in hypochondria, irritability and worry.

Table 1.5 Results of overall assessments of QoL by 75 patients with controlled hypertension, their attending physicians, and the patients' relatives (Based on Jachuk *et al.*, 1982)

	Improved	No change	Worse	Total
Physician	75	0	0	75
Patient	36	32	7	75
Relative	1	0	74	75

1.6 INSTRUMENTS

A large number of instruments have been developed for QoL assessment and we provide a range of examples to illustrate some of the approaches used. Those reproduced (in the Appendix) have been chosen on grounds of variety, to show particular features, and because these particular instruments are amongst the most widely used in clinical trials.

The aims and content of each instrument are described, together with an outline of the scoring procedures and any constructed multi-item scales. Most of the instruments use fairly simple forms of scoring, and the following basic procedure is usually used.

First, the successive levels of each categorical item are numbered increasingly. For example, a common scheme with four-category items is to grade responses such as "not at all", "a little", "quite a bit" and "very much" as being 0 to 3 respectively or, if preferred, 1 to 4; as it makes no difference after standardising the final scores. Second, when a scale contains multiple items, these are usually summed. Thus a 4-item scale, with items scored 0 to 3, would yield a working score ranging from 0 to 12. Finally, the working score is usually standardised to range of 0 to 100, and called the *scale score*. This enables different scales, possibly with different numbers of items and/or where the items have different numbers of categories, to be compared. In our example this would be achieved by multiplying by 100/12. We term this procedure the *standard scoring method*.

GENERIC INSTRUMENTS

Some instruments are intended for general use, irrespective of the illness or condition of the patient. These *generic* questionnaires may often be applicable to healthy people, too. Some of the earliest ones were developed initially with population surveys in mind, although they were later applied in clinical trial settings.

There are many instruments that measure physical impairment, disability or handicap. Although commonly described as QoL scales, these instruments are better called "measures of health status" because they focus on physical symptoms. They emphasise the measurement of general health, and make the implicit assumption that poorer health indicates poorer QoL. One weakness about this form of assessment is that different patients may react differently to similar levels of impairment. Many of the earlier questionnaires to some degree adopt this approach. We illustrate two of the more influential instruments, the Sickness Impact Profile (SIP) and the Nottingham Health Profile (NHP). Some scales specifically address activities of daily living, and we describe the Barthel questionnaire.

Few of the early instruments had scales that examine the subjective non-physical aspects of QoL, such as emotional, social and existential issues. Newer instruments, however, emphasise these subjective aspects strongly, and also commonly include one or more questions that explicitly enquire about overall QoL. We illustrate this approach by the Medical Outcomes Study 36-Item Short Form (SF-36). More recently, some brief instruments that place even less emphasis upon physical functioning have been developed. Two such instruments are the EuroQol, that is intended to be suitable for use with cost-utility analysis, and the SEIQoL, which allows patients to choose those aspects of QoL that they consider most important to themselves.

Sickness Impact Profile (SIP)

The SIP of Bergner *et al.* (1981) is a measure of perceived health status, as measured by its impact upon behaviour. Appendix E1 shows an extract of SIP—the full questionnaire takes 16 pages. It was designed for assessing new treatments and for evaluating health levels in the population, and is applicable across a wide range of types and severities of illness. The SIP consists of 136 items, and takes about 20–30 minutes to complete. The items describe everyday activities, and the respondents have to mark those activities they can accomplish and those statements they agree with. It may be either interviewer- or self-administered. Twelve main areas of dysfunction are covered but there is no global question about overall health or QoL. It has been shown that the SIP is sensitive even to minor changes in morbidity. However, in line with its original design objectives, it emphasises the impact of health upon activities and behaviour, including social functioning, rather than on feelings and perceptions—although there are some items relating to emotional well-being.

The items are negatively worded, representing dysfunction. Data from a number of field studies were compared against assessments made by healthcare professionals and students, leading to "scale values". These scale values are used as weights when summing the individual items to obtain the scale score. The standard scoring method is used for each of the twelve dysfunction scales. Two higher order dimensions, summarising physical and psychosocial domains respectively, are recognised and these are scored in a similar manner.

Nottingham Health Profile (NHP)

The NHP of Hunt *et al.* (1981) measures emotional, social and physical distress (Appendix E2). The NHP was influenced by the SIP, but asks about feelings and emotions directly rather than by changes in behaviour. Thus although the authors did not develop or claim it to be a QoL instrument, it does emphasise subjective aspects of health assessment. It was based upon the perceptions and the issues that were mentioned when patients were interviewed. When it was developed, the idea of asking patients about their feelings was a novel concept.

The version 2 contains 38 items in six sections, covering sleep, pain, emotional reactions, social isolation, physical mobility and energy level. Each question takes a yes/no answer. As with the SIP, each item reflects departures from normal and items are weighted to reflect their importance. Earlier versions included seven statements about areas of life that may be affected by health, with the respondent indicating whether there has been any impact in those areas. These statements were less applicable to the elderly, unemployed, disabled or those on low income than were the other items, and are usually omitted. The NHP forms a *profile* of six scores corresponding to the different sections of the questionnaire, and there is no single summary index.

The NHP is short compared to the SIP, and is easy to complete. The wording is simple and easily understood. It is often used in population studies of general health evaluation, and has been used in medical and non-medical settings. It is also frequently used in clinical trials, although it was not designed for that purpose. However, it tends to emphasise severe disease states and is perhaps less sensitive to minor—yet important—changes and differences in health state. The NHP assesses whether there are any health problems, but is not sufficiently specific to identify particular problems. Some items do not apply to hospitalised patients, and the developers do not recommend it for these patients. Its simplicity, whilst being for many purposes an advantage, also means that it does not provide suitable coverage for the conditions that apply to patients in many clinical trials.

Medical Outcomes Study 36-Item Short Form (SF-36)

The SF-36 developed by Ware *et al.* (1993) evaluates general health status, and was intended to fill a gap between the much more lengthy questionnaires and other relatively coarse single-item measures (Appendix E3). It is designed to provide assessments involving generic health concepts that are not specific to any age, disease or treatment group. Emphasis is placed upon physical, social and emotional functioning. The SF-36 has become the most widely used of the general health status measures. It can be either self-assessed or administered by a trained interviewer.

As the name implies, there are 36 questions addressing eight health concepts (a simpler 12-question form, the SF-12, is also available). There are two summary measures, physical health and mental health. Physical health is divided into scales for physical functioning (10 items), role-physical (4), bodily pain (2) and general health (5). Mental health comprises scales for vitality (4 items), social functioning (2), role-emotional (3) and mental health (5). In addition, there is a general health transition question, which asks: "Compared to one year ago, how would you rate your general health now?" There is also a global question about the respondent's perception of their health: "In general, would you say your health is: (excellent, very good, good, fair, poor)?" Most questions refer to the past four weeks, although some relate to the present. A few questions, such as those for "role-physical", take yes/no responses, while some, such as the physical functioning items, have three categories (limited a lot, limited a little, not limited at all), and other items have five or six categories for responses.

The designers of the SF-36 selected, standardised and tested the items so that they can be scored using the standard scoring method.

Most of the items appear broadly sensible. However, the physical functioning scale, in common with many similar scales, poses questions about interpretation. Questions ask whether your health limits you in "vigorous activities, such as running, lifting heavy objects, participating in strenuous sports" or in "walking more than a mile". It is not clear how those who never participate in such activities should respond—their health may be severely impaired, and yet they should respond "No, not limited at all" and will therefore receive a score indicating better functioning than might be expected. Some of the alternative questionnaires therefore restrict physical functioning questions to activities that are expected to be applicable to everyone, whilst others such as the Rotterdam Symptom Checklist (described below) stress that the questions are hypothetical.

EuroQol (EQ-5D)

The EuroQol of Brooks *et al.* (1996) is another general-purpose instrument, this time emphasising both simplicity and the multi-country aspects (Appendix E4). It takes about two minutes to complete, but aims to capture physical, mental and social functioning, and is intended to be applicable over a wide range of health interventions. The EuroQol group, acknowledging its simplicity, recommend that it should be used alongside other instruments.

Five dimensions of QoL are recognised: mobility, self-care, usual activities, pain/discomfort and anxiety/depression. Each of these is addressed by a simple three-category response scale. The principal EuroQol question is represented by a 20-cm vertical VAS, scored from 0 to 100, on which the respondent should mark "your own health state today", ranging from best imaginable health state to the worst imaginable health state. A single index is generated for all health states. Perhaps because of its simplicity, the EuroQol has been less frequently used as the outcome measure for clinical trials. It has been used most widely for general healthcare evaluation, including cost-utility evaluation.

Schedule for Evaluation of Individual Quality of Life (SEIQoL) and the Patient Generated Index (PGI)

The SEIQoL (Hickey *et al.*, 1996) and the PGI (Ruta *et al.*, 1994) are examples of instruments that were developed to assess QoL from the individual's perspective. The respondents can nominate areas of life that are particularly important to them, and the current level of functioning in each of these areas is evaluated.

The procedure is as follows. First, the patient is invited to nominate the five most important aspects of their quality of life. Most patients readily list five areas, but if they find it difficult a standard list of prompts is used. Second, the patient is asked to score each nominated item or aspect, according to its severity. The third and final stage is to provide relative weights for the importance of each item.

The two instruments differ in the way they implement the second and third stages. For the second stage, the PGI (Appendix E5) invites the patient to score their chosen items using scales from 0, "the worst you could imagine," to 10, "exactly as you would like to be". The SEIQoL offers a vertical visual analogue scale for each of their chosen areas, and patients are asked to rate themselves on the scale between "as good as can possibly be" to "as bad as can possibly be". Each SEIQoL scale generates a score between 0 and 100. At the third stage, the PGI asks patients to "spend" a total of ten imaginary points to improve areas of their life. The SEIQoL provides patients with a plastic disk that consists of five overlapping segments; each segment can be rotated around the central pivot, allowing its exposed size to be adjusted relative to the other segments. The patient is asked "How do the five areas compare in importance to each other?" This procedure generates five weights that sum to 100%. For both instruments, the investigator calculates a score by multiplying the individual's self rating in each of their chosen areas by the relative weight that they assigned to it, and summing the products over the five areas.

Both the SEIQoL and the PGI recognise that sometimes seemingly trivial problems may be of major significance to certain patients, whilst other issues that are thought by observers to be important may in fact be considered unimportant.

DISEASE-SPECIFIC INSTRUMENTS

Generic instruments, intended to cover a wide range of conditions, have the advantage that scores from patients with various diseases may be compared against each other and against the general population. On the other hand, these instruments fail to focus on the issues of particular concern to patients with disease, and may often lack the sensitivity to detect differences that arise as a consequence of treatment policies that are compared in clinical trials. This has led to the development of disease-specific questionnaires. We describe three contrasting questionnaires that are used in a single disease area—cancer—and a very different style of questionnaire that is widely used in epilepsy.

European Organization for Research and Treatment of Cancer (EORTC) QLQ-C30

The EORTC QLQ-C30 is a cancer-specific 30-item questionnaire (Aaronson *et al.*, 1993); see Appendix E6. The QLQ-C30 questionnaire was designed to be multi-dimensional in structure, appropriate for self-administration and hence brief and easy to complete, applicable across a range of cultural settings, and suitable for use in clinical trials of cancer therapy. It incorporates five functional scales (physical, role, cognitive, emotional, and social), three symptom scales (fatigue, pain, and nausea and vomiting), a global health-status/QoL scale, and a number of single items assessing additional symptoms commonly reported by cancer patients (dyspnoea, loss of appetite, insomnia, constipation, and diarrhoea) and perceived financial impact of the disease.

In the QLQ-C30 version 3.0 all items have response categories with four levels, from "not at all" to "very much", except the two items for overall physical condition and overall QoL, which use seven-point items ranging from "very poor" to "excellent". The standard scoring method is used. High scale scores represent high response levels, with high functional scale scores representing high/healthy levels of functioning, and high scores for symptom scales/items representing high levels of symptomatology/problems (Fayers *et al.*, 1999).

The QLQ-C30 is available in a range of languages and has been widely used in multinational cancer clinical trials. It has been found to be sensitive to differences between patients, treatment effects, and changes over time.

EORTC Disease- or Treatment-Specific Modules

The EORTC QLQ-C30 is an example of an instrument that is designed to be modular, with the core questionnaire evaluating those aspects of QoL that are likely to be relevant to a wide range of cancer patients. For each cancer site particular issues are often important, such as specific disease-related symptoms or aspects of morbidity that are consequences of specific forms of therapy. The QLQ-H&N35, described by Bjordal *et al.* (1999), is one of several modules that address additional issues (Appendix E7). This supplements the core QLQ-C30 with an additional 35 items for patients with head and neck cancer.

Functional Assessment of Cancer Therapy—General (FACT-G)

The Functional Assessment of Chronic Illness Therapy (FACIT) Measurement System is a collection of QoL questionnaires targeting chronic illnesses. The core questionnaire, or FACT-G, was developed by Cella *et al.* (1993) and is a widely used cancer-specific instrument (Appendix E8). Similar to the EORTC QLQ-C30, the FACIT questionnaires adopt a modular approach and so a number of supplementary modules specific to a tumour type, treatment or condition are available. Non-cancer-specific FACIT questionnaires are also available for other diseases such as HIV infection and multiple sclerosis.

The FACT-G version 4 contains 27 items arranged in subscales covering four dimensions of QoL: physical well-being, social/family well-being, emotional well-being, and functional well-being. Items are rated from 0 to 4. The items are labelled from "not at all" to "very much", which is the same as for the QLQ-C30 but with the addition of a central "somewhat". Some items are phrased negatively, and should be reverse-scored. Subscale scores are derived by summing item responses, and a total score is derived by summing the subscale scores. Version 3 included an additional item after each subscale, enabling patients to weight each domain on an 11-point scale from "not at all" to "very much so". These questions were of the form: "Looking at the above 7 questions, how much would you say your PHYSICAL WELL-BEING affects your quality of life?" A similar set of items is optional for version 4.

Individual questions are phrased in the first person ("I have a lack of energy"), as compared with the QLQ-C30 that asks questions in the second person ("Have you felt weak?"). Both questionnaires relate to the past week, and both make similar claims regarding validity and sensitivity.

Rotterdam Symptom Checklist (RSCL)

The RSCL (de Haes *et al.*, 1996) is another instrument that is intended for measuring the QoL of cancer patients (Appendix E9). The RSCL has been used extensively in European cancer clinical trials. It covers broadly similar ground to the EORTC QLQ-C30, and has a similar number of questions. It not only contains questions relating to general psychological distress, but also, as its name implies, places greater emphasis upon the symptoms and side-effects that are commonly experienced by cancer patients.

There are two features that are worthy of special note. Firstly, the RSCL has an introductory text explaining "for all symptoms mentioned, indicate to what extent you have been bothered by it, . . .". This is in contrast to the QLQ-C30 and most other instruments, which merely enquire about the presence of symptoms. Thus one patient might have "a little" stomach ache but, when asked if it bothers them, might respond "not at all"; another might respond that the same ache bothers them "quite a bit". What is less clear is whether most patients read the questionnaire with sufficient care to appreciate the subtle significance of the instructions. The second feature relates to the activities-of-daily-living scale. Here, too, there are explicit instructions, stating: "We do not want to know whether you actually do these, but only whether you are able to perform them presently." Thus a patient might not "go shopping", but is requested to indicate whether they could if they wanted to. This is in marked contrast with the equivalent scale on the SF-36 that not only asks about actual functioning but also includes some strenuous tasks that are perhaps less likely to be applicable to the chronically ill.

The RSCL consists of 30 questions on four-point scales ("not at all", "a little", "quite a bit", "very much"), a question about activity level, and a global question about "your quality of life during the past week" with seven categories. There are two main scales, physical symptom distress and psychological distress, in addition to the scales for activity level and overall valuation. The standard scoring method is used.

Quality of Life in Epilepsy (QOLIE-89)

In contrast with the previous examples, the QOLIE-89 is a 13-page, 89-item questionnaire aimed at patients with epilepsy (Devinsky *et al.*, 1995); Appendix E10 shows extracts. It is based upon a number of other instruments, in particular the SF-36, with additional items from other sources. It contains five questions concerning worry about seizures, and questions about specific "bothersome" epilepsy-related limitations such as driving restrictions. Shorter versions with 31 and 10 items are available. The QOLIE-89 contains 17 multi-item scales that tap into a number of health concepts, including: overall QoL, emotional well-being, role limitations owing to emotional support, social support, social isolation, energy/fatigue, seizure worry, health discouragement, attention/concentration, language, memory, physical function, health perceptions. An overall score is derived by weighting and summing the scale scores. There are also four composite scores representing issues related to epilepsy, cognition, mental health and physical health.

The QOLIE-89 has been developed and tested upon adults. Epilepsy is a serious problem for younger patients too, but children and adolescents experience very different problems from adults. Adolescents may be particularly concerned about problems of forming relationships with friends of the opposite sex, and anxious about possibilities of marriage and their dependence upon parents. Children may feel excluded from school or other activities, and may be teased by other children. Very young children may be unable to complete the questionnaire alone, and parents or others will have to assist. Thus QoL questionnaires intended for adults are unlikely to be satisfactory for younger age groups. One example of a generic QoL questionnaire that has been used for children with epilepsy is the 16D. Apajasalo *et al.* (1996) reported results in young adolescents aged 12–15, comparing normal children against patients with epilepsy.

One interesting feature of the QOLIE-89 is that there are five questions about general QoL issues. Questions 1, 2, 3, 49 and 89 use various formats to enquire about health perceptions, overall QoL, overall health and change in health.

Paediatric Asthma Quality of Life Questionnaire (PAQLQ)

The PAQLQ developed by Juniper *et al.* (1996) has been designed to measure the problems that children between the ages of 7 and 17 experience as a result of asthma; extracts from the self-administered version are shown in Appendix E11. The PAQLQ has 23 items relating to three dimensions, namely symptoms, activity limitations and emotional function. Items are scored from 1 to 7. Three of the activity questions are "individualised" with the children identifying important activities at the beginning of the study. There is a global question, in which children are asked to think about all the activities they did in the past week, and to indicate how much they were bothered by their asthma during these activities. The items reflecting each dimension are averaged, forming three summary scales that take values between 1 and 7.

Parents often have a poor perception of their child's health-related QoL, and so it is important to ask the children themselves about their experiences. Since children may have difficulty in completing the self-administered questionnaire, Juniper *et al.* (1996) suggest using the interviewer-administered version, administered by a trained interviewer who has experience of working with children. Children may be strongly influenced by adults and by their surroundings, and so detailed guidelines and interviewing tips are provided. The PAQLQ has been tested in children aged between 7 and 17 years, and has demonstrated good measurement properties in this age group.

INSTRUMENTS FOR SPECIFIC ASPECTS OF QOL

The instruments described above purport to measure general QoL, and include at least one general question about overall QoL or health. In many trials this may be adequate for treatment comparison, but sometimes the investigators will wish to explore particular issues in greater depth. We describe four instruments that are widely used in clinical trials to explore anxiety and depression, physical functioning, pain, and fatigue. These domains of QoL are particularly important to patients with chronic or advanced diseases. Many other instruments are available, both for these areas and others. Additional examples are coping (Hürney *et al.*, 1993), satisfaction (Baker and Intagliata, 1982), existential beliefs (Salmon, Mauzi and Valori, 1996) and self-esteem (Rosenberg, 1965). Since these questionnaires evaluate specific aspects of QoL, in order for a patient assessment to be called "quality of life" these instruments would normally be used in conjunction with more general questionnaires.

Hospital Anxiety and Depression Scale (HADS)

The HADS was developed by Zigmond and Snaith (1983), and was initially intended as a clinical screening tool to detect anxiety and depression (Appendix E12). It has become widely used in clinical trials for a wide range of conditions, including arthritis, bowel dysfunction, cancer, dental phobia, osteoporosis, and stroke. The HADS consists of 14 questions that are completed by the patients. Each question uses a four-point scale. Seven of these questions were designed to address anxiety, and the other seven depression. The HADS deliberately excludes items that may be associated with emotional or physical impairment, such as dizziness and headaches; it emphasises the psychological signs or consequences of anxiety and depression.

Two particular features of the HADS are interesting from the point of view of scale design. The questions addressing anxiety and depression alternate (odd and even items, respectively), and half of the questions are worded positively and half negatively (for example, "I feel cheerful" and "I get sudden feelings of panic").

Each item is scored 0 to 3, where 3 represents the state associated with the most anxiety or depression. The items are summed after suitable ordering, yielding two subscales ranging from 0 to 21. Based upon psychiatric diagnosis, HADS ratings of 11 or more are regarded as definite cases that would normally require therapy; ratings of 7 or less are non-cases; those scoring 8 to 10 are doubtful cases who are usually referred for further psychiatric assessment.

Another widely used instrument is the Beck Depression Inventory (BDI) of Beck *et al.* (1961), which measures existence and severity of depression. It can be either self-rated or administered orally, and emphasises cognitive rather than affective symptoms.

McGill Pain Questionnaire (MPQ)

The MPQ is one of the most widely used tests for the measurement of pain (Melzack, 1975). The full version has 20 main groups of items, each with between two and six adjectives as response categories, such as flickering, quivering, pulsing, throbbing, beating, pounding. It takes 5–15 minutes to complete. Based upon a literature search of terms used to describe pain, the MPQ uses a list of descriptive words that the subject ticks. The words are chosen from three classes of descriptors—sensory (such as temporal, spatial, pressure, thermal), affective (such as tension, fear) and evaluative (such as intensity, experience of pain). There is a six-point intensity scale for present pain, from no pain through to excruciating pain. Three major measures are derived: a pain rating index, using numerical scoring; the number of descriptive words chosen; and the value from the pain intensity scale. Pain-rating index scores can be calculated either across all items or for three major psychological dimensions called sensory–discriminative, motivational–affective, and cognitive–evaluative.

The short version, termed the SF-MPQ (Melzack, 1987), is shown in Appendix E13. It has 15 items that are graded by the respondent from none (0) through to severe (3). There is also a 10-cm VAS, ranging from no pain through to worst possible pain, and the same six-point intensity scale as in the full version. It takes 2 to 5 minutes to complete. Each description carries a weight that corresponds to severity of pain. This leads to a summary score that ranges from 0 (no pain) to 5 (excruciating pain). The SF-MPQ has subscales for affective and sensory components of pain, as well as a total score.

Pain is a complicated and controversial area for assessment, although some of the problems serve to illustrate general issues in QoL assessment. For example, the Zung (1983) self-rating Pain and Distress Scale measures physical and emotional distress caused by pain, rather than severity of pain itself. This recognises that severity of pain, either as indicated by pain stimuli or by the subject's verbal description, may result in different levels of distress in different patients. One level of pain stimulus may produce varying levels of suffering, as determined by reactions and emotions, in different patients. Also, pain thresholds can vary. Another issue to be considered when assessing pain is that analgesics can often control pain very effectively. Should one be making an allowance for increasing dosages of, say, opiates when evaluating levels of pain? In some studies it may be appropriate to measure "uncontrolled pain", in which case one might argue that it is irrelevant to enquire about analgesics. On the other hand, high doses of analgesics can be accompanied by disadvantages.

Multidimensional Fatigue Inventory (MFI)

The MFI of Smets *et al.* (1995) is a 20-item self-report instrument designed to measure fatigue (Appendix E14). It covers five dimensions, each of four items: general fatigue, physical fatigue, mental fatigue, reduced motivation, and reduced activity. There are equal numbers of positively and negatively worded statements, to counter possible response bias, and the respondent must indicate to what extent the particular statement applies to him or her. The five-point items take responses between "yes, that is true" and "no, that is not true", and are scored 1 to 5, where 5 corresponds to highest fatigue. The five scale scores are calculated by simple summation.

Four of the scales appear to be highly correlated, with mental fatigue behaving differently from the others. This suggests that there may be one or two underlying dimensions for fatigue. However, for descriptive purposes, and for a better understanding of what fatigue entails in different populations, the authors suggest that the separate dimensions be retained and that the five scales should not be combined. If a global score is required, the general fatigue scale should be used.

Barthel Index of Disability (BI)

Disability scales were among the earliest attempts to evaluate issues that may be regarded as related to QoL. They are still commonly employed, but mainly as a simple indication of one aspect of the patient's overall QoL. The BI (Mahoney and Barthel, 1965) was developed to measure disability, and is one of the most commonly used of the class of scales known as activities-of-daily-living (ADL) scales. ADL scales focus upon a range of mobility, domestic and self-care tasks, and ignore issues such as pain, emotions and social functioning. The assumption is that a lower ADL score implies a lower QoL.

The BI is used to assess functional dependency before and after treatment, and to indicate the amount of nursing care that is required. It has been used widely for assessing rehabilitation outcome and stroke disability, and has been included in clinical trials. Unlike any of the other scales that we have described, it need not be completed by the patient personally, but is more intended for administration by a nurse, physiotherapist or doctor concerned with the patient's care. It therefore provides an interesting contrast against the subjective self-assessment that has been adopted by many of the more recent measures. The BI examines the ability to perform normal or expected activities. Ten activities are assessed, each with two or three response categories, scored 5, 10 or 15; items are left blank and scored 0 when patients fail to meet the defined criteria. Overall scores range for 0 (highest dependency) to 100 (least dependence). It takes about one minute to assess a patient.

The original BI uses a crude scoring system, since changes in points do not appear to correspond to equivalent changes in all the scales. Also, patients can be at the highest (0) point on the scale and still become more dependent, and can similarly exceed the lowest (100) value. Modified versions of the BI largely overcome these deficiencies. For example, Shah, Vanclay and Cooper (1989) expanded the number of categories and proposed changes to the scoring procedures (Appendix E15). The BI and its modified versions continue to be used widely as a simple method of assessing the effectiveness of rehabilitation outcome.

Many ADL scales exist and the Katz et al. (1963) index is another widely used example. The concept here is that loss of skills occurs in a particular sequence, with complex functions suffering before others. Therefore six items were chosen so as to represent a hierarchical ordering of difficulty. A simplified scoring system is provided, in which the number of activities that require assistance are summed to provide a single score. Thus while 0 indicates no help is required, 6 means that there is dependency for all the listed activities. The Katz index has been used with both children and adults, and for a wide range of conditions. In comparison with the BI, which measures ability, the Katz index measures independence.

Instrumental Activities of Daily Living (IADL) scales include items that reflect ability to live and adapt to the environment. This includes activities such as shopping and travelling, and thus these scales evaluate ability to live independently within the community, as opposed to needing help with basic functions such as dressing and washing oneself. One example is the Functional Activity Questionnaire (FAQ) which was designed for use in community studies of normal ageing and mild senile dementia (Pfeffer *et al.*, 1982).

1.7 CONCLUSIONS

Definitions of QoL are controversial. Different instruments use different definitions, and frequently no specific model for QoL is stated formally. There is a wide range of QoL instruments available, although this range is likely to be reduced once the purpose of evaluating QoL is considered. In a clinical trial setting, the disease area and therapies being evaluated will usually limit the choice. Common features of the instruments are that the patients themselves are asked, there are frequently several subscales, the scales are often based upon multiple items, and the scales represent constructs that cannot be measured directly. In Chapters 2–7 we shall explain methods for constructing such scales. Most importantly, we describe the desirable measurement properties of scales. We show how to "validate" scales, and how to confirm whether an instrument appears to be consistent with the hypothetical model that the designers intended.

2 Principles of Measurement Scales

Summary

The principal methods for developing and validating new questionnaires are introduced, and the different approaches are described. These range from simple global questions to detailed psychometric and clinimetric methods. We review traditional psychometric techniques including summated scales and factor analysis models, as well as psychometric methods that place emphasis upon probabilistic item response models. Whereas psychometric methods lead to scales for QoL that are based upon items reflecting patients' levels of QoL, the clinimetric approach makes use of composite scales that may include symptoms and side-effects of treatment. This chapter contrasts the different methods, which are then explained in detail in subsequent chapters.

2.1 INTRODUCTION

Questionnaires for assessing QoL usually contain multiple questions, although a few may attempt to rely upon a single *global* question such as "Overall, what has your quality of life been like over the last week? (very good, better than average, about average, worse than average, very bad)". Some QoL questionnaires are designed such that all items are combined together; for example items might be averaged, to produce an overall score for QoL. Most instruments, however, recognise that QoL has many dimensions and will attempt to group the items into separate "scales" corresponding to the different dimensions. Thus we explore the relationship between items and scales, and introduce the concepts underlying scales and their measurement.

2.2 SCALES AND ITEMS

Each question on the QoL questionnaire is an expression in words for an *item*. Most QoL instruments consist of many questions, representing many items. Some of these items may aim to measure a simple aspect of QoL, such as a physical symptom. In such cases, sometimes a single item will suffice to encapsulate all that is required. Other QoL concepts may be more complex, and the developers of an instrument might decide that it is preferable to use several questions that can be combined to form a *multi-item scale*.

For example, some drugs may cause vomiting and therefore questions for patients receiving potentially emetic drugs might aim to assess the level of vomiting. This is typically true for cytotoxic chemotherapy that is used as treatment for cancer. Some cancer-specific instruments contain a single question about vomiting. An example is the question "Have you vomited? (not at all, a little, quite a bit, very much)" on the EORTC QLQ-C30. However, a single question about vomiting may be considered too imprecise to measure severity, frequency and duration of vomiting, and usage of anti-emetics. The QLQ-C30 already contained 30 questions, and it was felt undesirable to lengthen it. The developers considered it more important to retain questions about other symptoms and functions rather than add extra items about vomiting. Thus a single question about vomiting and one about nausea was thought adequate for general-purpose assessment of QoL. However, vomiting can sometimes be an outcome of particular interest, in which case studies might benefit from the addition of supplementary questions on this topic.

Symptoms are often conceptually simple. For example, vomiting has a clear definition and there is little controversy about its meaning. Multi-item scales are frequently used when assessing more complex issues. For example, the more psychological dimensions may be less well defined in many people's perception. Even when there is a commonly agreed single definition, it may be misunderstood by the patients who complete the questionnaire. For example, terms such as "anxiety" and "depression" are rather more abstract in nature than most clinical symptoms, and different investigators may adopt differing definitions. Psychological literature distinguishes these two terms, but patients may be less certain of their distinction and may interpret anxiety and depression in many different ways. They may also have widely differing opinions as to the severity intended by "very anxious." Because of the nature of psychological constructs, it is usually impossible to rely upon a single question for the assessment of a patient. Most psychometric tests will contain multiple items addressing each psychological aspect.

QoL instruments commonly contain a mixture of single-item and multi-item scales. A major aspect of scale design is the determination of the number of items that should comprise a particular scale and, if more than one item is appropriate, the assessment of how consistently these items hang together.

2.3 CONSTRUCTS AND LATENT VARIABLES

Some psychological aspects of QoL will have clear, precise and universally agreed definitions. As we have noted, others may be more contentious and may even reflect the opinions of an individual investigator. Many of these psychological aspects are not directly and reliably measurable, and in some cases it may be debatable as to whether the concepts that are being described really do exist as distinct and unique aspects of QoL. These concepts constitute psychological models that may be regarded as convenient representations of QoL issues in patients. They are commonly described as being postulated *constructs*, *latent traits* or *factors*.

These hypothetical constructs that are believed or postulated to exist are represented or measured by *latent variables*. Examples of latent variables are QoL itself, or its constituent components such as anxiety. Thus latent variables are the representations of constructs and are used in models. The aims of numerical methods in QoL research may largely be summarised as testing the adequacy and validity of models based upon postulated constructs, and estimation of the values of the latent variables that comprise those models. The term "factor", apart from its use as a synonym for constructs, is commonly used to denote lower level constructs such as when one construct, for example overall QoL, is decomposed into a number of components or *factors*. Thus, physical functioning, role functioning, social functioning, and emotional functioning are latent variables which are all aspects, or factors, for QoL.

Constructs and latent variables are abstract concepts. Thus Nunnally and Bernstein (1994) have described constructs as "useful fictions", and "something that scientists 'construct' or put together in their own imaginations". They also note that the name given to any one specific construct is no more than a word, and although the name may appear to imply a meaningful set of variables, there is no way to prove that any combination of these variables "measures" the named construct. Since latent variables cannot be measured directly, they are usually assessed by means of multi-item tests or questionnaires. QoL instruments often contain 20 or more questions. Sometimes a single global question is also used—for example, "How would you rate your overall quality of life during the past week?"

In contrast to the (unobserved) latent variables that reflect hypothetical constructs, the so-called *manifest variables* are the observed responses made by patients to questionnaire items.

When a single latent trait, or factor, underlies the data, the construct is described as being *unidimensional*. Many models for QoL assume that it can be represented by a number of lower level factors such as physical functioning, emotional functioning and cognitive functioning. Therefore, QoL is often described as being *multidimensional* in nature.

2.4   INDICATOR VARIABLES AND CAUSAL VARIABLES

The majority of items to be found in personality, intelligence or educational attainment tests and other psychometric assessments are designed to reflect either a level of ability or a state of mind. Such items do not alter or influence the latent construct that they measure. (Although "learning effects" can interfere with the measurement of intelligence or education, appearing to alter the latent construct, they are less important for our discussion of QoL.) The test items are commonly given a variety of descriptive names, including "effect indicators" because they indicate the level of the latent variable; or "manifest response variables" because they are observed responses to items in a test. We shall call them simply *indicator variables*.

However, the symptoms assessed in QoL scales may cause a change in QoL. If a patient acquires serious symptoms their overall QoL is changed by those symptoms. In fact, the reason for including symptoms in QoL instruments is principally because they are believed to affect QoL. Conversely, having a poor QoL does not imply that the patient has specific symptoms. Unlike educational tests, in which a person with highest ability has greatest probability of answering all questions successfully, a patient with poor QoL need not necessarily be suffering from all symptoms. Symptoms and similar items can be called *causal variables* (Fayers and Hand, 1997a). Symptoms and side-effects are good examples of causal variables in relation to overall QoL. Although symptoms are indicator variables for disease, and side-effects are indicator variables for treatment, neither treatment nor disease is the main concern when assessing QoL, and so for this purpose symptoms and side-effects are purely causal. Typical characteristics of causal items are that one on its own may suffice to change the latent variable, and it is unnecessary—and usually rare—that patients must suffer from all items in order to have a poor QoL (Fayers *et al.*, 1997a). For example, few patients will experience all possible symptoms and side-effects, but one serious symptom—such as pain—suffices to reduce overall QoL.

Variables may frequently be partly indicator and partly causal. They may also exchange roles. For example, a patient may experience symptoms, become distressed, and then perceive—and report—the symptoms as being worse than they are. An initially causal variable has acquired additional indicator properties. Another example is the phenomenon of anticipatory nausea and vomiting. Cytotoxic chemotherapy for cancer commonly induces these side-effects. Some cancer patients who have experienced these problems after their initial course of treatment may start vomiting prior to administration of a subsequent course. Again, a variable that might seem to be purely causal has acquired some of the properties of an indicator. The reverse may also apply. A distressed patient may become unable to sleep, so that insomnia is an indicator variable for psychological distress. Continued insomnia, however, may then cause additional anxiety and distress. Thus there will often be uncertainty and ambiguity about the precise role of variables in QoL assessment. Disease or treatment-related symptom clusters are likely to be predominantly causal; it may be less clear whether psychological and other items are mainly causal or indicator in nature.

The terms "causal indicator" and "effect indicator" are widely used in the field of structural equation modelling (Bollen, 1989). They are unfortunate choices of words, since in ordinary speech "cause" and "effect" are commonly regarded as dynamic and opposite. In our context, changes in so-called effect indicators need not be "caused" by the latent variable; they merely reflect its level. In an educational test, correct answers to questions are neither "caused" by high ability, nor cause high ability. Therefore we shall call them indicator variables because they reflect high ability. In statistical terms, a good indicator variable is one that is highly correlated with the latent variable, and no implication of causality need be present. Thus the flavour of an indicator variable is captured by such phrases as "it reflects the latent variable", or "it is a manifestation of the latent variable".

One of the principal consequences of causal variables affecting QoL assessment is that many models assume that the observed items depend solely upon the latent variable. That is, if QoL is "high", high levels of the items should reflect this. Furthermore, if the observed values of the items are correlated, these correlations arise solely because of the effect of the latent variable. These assumptions are clearly untrue for causal variables. Here, the correlations between, say, symptoms arise mainly because of the changing disease patterns. The correlations between a causal variable and QoL as the latent variable are likely to be weak or obscured by the stronger correlations between symptom-clusters.

How can one identify causal variables? Perhaps the easiest method is the "thought test". For example, if we consider vomiting: think of the question "could severe vomiting affect QoL level?" Yes, almost certainly. "Could QoL level affect vomiting?" Possibly, but it is more likely that vomiting is a consequence of the treatment or the disease. Hence, most would conclude, vomiting is likely to be a causal variable.

This distinction between causal variables and indicator variables has become well known in the field of structural equation modelling. However, the implications of this distinction are rarely recognised in clinical scale development, even though these two types of items behave in fundamentally different ways in measurement scales, and have considerable impact upon the design of scales.

Example

The Hospital Anxiety and Depression Scale (HADS) questionnaire is an instrument with a simple latent structure (Appendix E12). Zigmond and Snaith (1983) designed it such that seven questions should relate to anxiety, and seven to depression. The design assumes that "anxiety" and "depression" are meaningful concepts, and that they can be quantified. It is postulated that they are two distinct constructs. It is assumed that anxiety and depression cannot be measured reliably and adequately by single questions such as "How anxious are you? (not at all, a little, quite a bit, very much)", and that multiple questions must be employed. In common with most questionnaires that assess *psychological* aspects of QoL, the HADS items are predominantly indicator variables. If anxious, patients are expected to have high scores for the anxiety items; if depressed, they should score highly on the depression items.

2.5   SINGLE GLOBAL QUESTIONS VERSUS MULTI-ITEM QUESTIONNAIRES

GLOBAL QUESTIONS

As Gill (1995) has commented, "The simplest and most overtly sensible approach to measure QoL is to use global rating scales. These ratings, which have been successfully used to assess pain, self-rated health, and a myriad of other complex clinical phenomena, can allow expression for the disparate values and preferences of individual patients." Investigators can ask patients to give several global ratings, such as one for overall QoL and another for "health-related" QoL or for physical well-being. Global single-item measures allow the subject to define the concept in a way that is personally meaningful, providing a measure that can be responsive to individual differences. Global single-item indicators require that subjects consider all aspects of a phenomenon, ignore aspects that are not relevant to their situations, and differentially weight the other aspects according to their values and ideals in order to provide a single rating. A global single-item measure may be a more valid measure of the concept of interest than a score from a multi-item scale.

Unfortunately, there is considerable disagreement as to whether it is meaningful to ask a patient questions such as "Overall, what would you say your quality of life has been like during the last week? (excellent, very good, good, fair, poor, very poor, extremely poor)." Some authors argue that responses to these global questions are unreliable and difficult to interpret, and that it is better to ask multiple questions about the many aspects of QoL. They suggest that responses to the individual questions can be aggregated to form a summary "global score" that measures overall QoL, using either an unweighted summation that attaches equal importance to all questions, or a weighted summation that uses patients' opinions of the relative importance of questions. Other authors dissent, some maintaining that QoL is a multidimensional construct and that it is meaningless to try to sum the individual items to form a single overall score for QoL.

In practice, as described in the preceding chapter, many instruments include at least one global question in addition to a number of multi-item scales. Often a global question is used for overall QoL, for overall health, or for similar concepts that are assumed to be broadly understood by the majority of patients.

MULTI-ITEM QUESTIONNAIRES

Multi-item scales more commonly focus upon specific aspects of QoL that are perhaps more likely to be unidimensional constructs. Measures from multi-items usually have several advantages over a score estimated from the responses to a single item.

One of the main objections to the use of single items in global questions is that latent variables covering constructs such as QoL, role functioning and emotional functioning, are complex and ill-defined. Different people may have different ideas as to their meaning. Multi-item scales are often used when trying to measure latent variables such as these. Many aspects of scale development have their origins in psychometric testing. For example, from the earliest days it was accepted that intelligence could not be defined and measured using a single-question intelligence test. Thus multiple questions were recognised to be necessary to cover the broad range of aspects of intelligence (such as verbal, spatial, and inductive intelligence). An intelligence test is therefore an example of a multi-item test that attempts to measure a postulated construct. Under the "latent variable model" we assume that the data structure can be divided up into a number of hypothetical constructs, such that each distinct construct is a latent variable representing a unidimensional concept. Since these constructs may be abstract and therefore not directly measurable, they are commonly assessed using multi-item questionnaires.

Psychometric theory also favours multi-item tests because they are usually more reliable and less prone to random measurement errors than single-item measures for assessing attributes such as intelligence, personality or mood. For example, in educational and intelligence tests, multi-item scales reduce the probability of obtaining a high score through either luck or correct-guessing of answers. Another reason for using multi-item tests is that a single item with, for example, a seven-category response scale lacks precision and cannot discriminate between fine degrees of an attribute, since for each patient it can assume only one of the specified response levels. By contrast, tests involving large numbers of items are potentially capable of very fine discrimination.

2.6 SINGLE-ITEM VERSUS MULTI-ITEM SCALES

RELIABITY

A *reliable* test is one that measures something in a consistent, repeatable and reproducible manner. For example, if a patient's QoL were to remain stable over time, a reliable test would be one that would give very similar scores on each measurement occasion. In Chapter 3 we show that *reliability* of a measurement can be measured by the squared ratio of the true-score standard deviation (*SD*) over the observed-score *SD*, and in Chapter 4 we extend the discussion to include multi-item scales. It is often stated that multi-item scales are more reliable than single-item tests. This is a reasonable claim—in some circumstances.

Consider a questionnaire such as the HADS. The anxiety subscale comprises questions that include "I feel tense or 'wound up'", "Worrying thoughts go through my mind" and "I get sudden feelings of panic". A patient with a given level of anxiety will tend to answer positively to all these items. However, there will be variability in the responses, with some patients responding more strongly to one question than another. This patient variability would render a single-item test unreliable. However, by averaging the responses from a large number of questions we effectively reduce the impact of the variability. In statistical terms, the reliability of the scale is increased by including and averaging a number of items, where each item is associated with an independent "random error term". Cronbach's coefficient α is a measure of reliability of multi-item scales (Chapter 4), and can be used to calculate the potential gain of adding extra items to a scale.

Many psychological concepts, for instance depression, are subjective states and difficult to define precisely. If asked a single question such as "Are you depressed?", patients may vary in the perception of their state, and may also be unsure how to classify themselves. Thus a large random error may be associated with global questions. Spector (1992) wrote: "Single items do not produce responses by people that are consistent over time. Single items are notoriously unreliable." On the other hand, as we shall show, estimates of gain in reliability for multi-item scales are based upon conditions that are often inapplicable to the items found in QoL scales. Therefore it does not necessarily follow that increasing the number of items in a QoL scale will increase its overall reliability. A review of published empirical studies has suggested that global questions regarding QoL can possess high reliability (Youngblut and Caspar, 1993). Thus opinions continue to differ as to whether or not single-item global questions are reliable.

PRECISION

Numerical precision concerns the number of digits to which a measurement is made. If a scale has a range from 0 to 100, a measurement made to the nearest 1 is more precise than one rounded to the nearest 10. Precision is important because it indicates the potential ability of the scale to discriminate amongst the respondents.

Single-item global questions are frequently categorical in form, and these offer limited precision. For example, the SF-36 asks "In general, would you say your health is: . . .?" (response categories from 1 = excellent to 5 = poor), while the EORTC QLQ-C30 asks "How would you rate your overall quality of life during the past week?" (response categories from 1 = very poor to 7 = excellent). These questions have a precision that is delimited by the number of valid categories from which the respondent must choose, and the QLQ-C30, with seven categories, potentially offers more precision that the SF-36 with five. Although it might seem tempting to allow a larger number of response categories, this can lead to difficulties in distinguishing shades of meaning for adjacent ones. Offering a large number of categories also leads to unreliability in the sense that, in repeated testing, respondents will not consistently choose the same answer from the closely adjacent possibilities. Scales with a maximum of four or five response categories are often recommended, and it would seem of little value to go beyond seven to nine categories.

Multi-item tests, on the other hand, can have greater precision. For example, if four-point categorical questions are used, and five questions are summed into a summary score, the resultant score would have 20 possible categories of response.

Some single-item assessments attempt to overcome this by using visual analogue scales (VAS) in which a line, typically 10 cm long, is labelled at each end by extreme values. Respondents are invited to mark the line at a distance from the two ends according to their level of QoL. In principal such scales can provide fine discrimination, since the investigator may choose to measure the positions of the response very precisely. In practice, however, there must be doubt as to whether patients can really discriminate between fine differences of position along the line.

VALIDATION

The items of a multi-item scale can be compared against each other, to check whether they are consistent and whether they appear to be measuring the same postulated underlying construct. Psychometric tests of validity are to a large extent based upon an analysis of the inter-item correlation structure. These validation tests cannot be employed on a scale that contains only a single item. It has been argued that the ability to check the internal structure of multi-item scales is an essential feature, and the inability to do the same for single-item measures is their most fundamental problem. Blalock (1982) has pointed out that with a single measure of each variable, one can remain blissfully unaware of the possibility of measurement error, but in no sense will this make the inferences more valid.

This criticism of single-item scales serves merely to indicate the need to adopt suitable methods of validation. Internal validity, as typified by Cronbach's reliability coefficient α (Chapter 4), can only be calculated for multi-item scales, and cannot be explored when there is but a single item. However, insight into properties analogous to internal validity may be obtained by introducing additional, temporary items. During the scale development phase, redundant items could be added to the questionnaire purely for validation purposes; they could be abandoned once the scale is approved for use.

Both single- and multi-item scales can, and should be, investigated for external validity. This places emphasis upon examination of the relationships and correlations with other items and scales, and with external variables such as response to treatment. Assessment of all scales should include evaluation of test–retest reliability, sensitivity and ability to detect expected differences between groups such as treatment or disease, and responsiveness to changes over time (Chapter 3).

SCOPE

QoL, like many constructs, is a complex issue and not easily assessed by a single question. Many patients, when asked "How would you rate your overall quality of life?" may reply, "Well, it depends what you mean by QoL. Of course I've got lots of symptoms, if that's what you mean. But I guess that is to be expected." In other words, the global question oversimplifies the issues and some patients may have difficulty in answering it. They find it more straightforward to describe individual aspects of QoL. This is often advocated as a reason for multi-item questionnaires, and is perhaps the most pertinent argument for caution in the use of global questions. If patients have difficulty understanding or answering a question, their responses must surely be regarded with suspicion.

An investigator who uses multi-item tests can choose items so that the scope and coverage of the questionnaire is made explicit. Areas of interest can be defined by the selective inclusion of items, and the scope of the questionnaire can be widened by including as many questions as are deemed necessary to cover all the topics of interest. Alternatively, the scope can be made more restricted or tightly defined, by excluding unwanted items, either at the questionnaire design stage or during analysis. Multi-item questionnaires allow the investigator greater freedom for creating his or her own definition of QoL—even though this may not correspond to the patient's view of what is meant by "quality of life".

2.7   PSYCHOMETRICS AND ITEM RESPONSE THEORY

The theory of multi-item tests is based upon measurement models that make various assumptions about the nature of the items. These form what is often called *traditional psychometrics*, and are based largely on either summated scales in which the scores on multiple items added together, or linear models such as factor analysis models. In contrast, models that stress the importance of item response models, in which patients with a particular level of ability have a *probability of responding* positively to different questions, are often called *modern psychometrics*.

PARALLEL TESTS

One of the most common models is founded upon the theory of *parallel tests*. This posits that each individual measurement item is a test or a question that reflects the level of the underlying construct. For example, when evaluating anxiety, each question should reflect the underlying level of patients' anxiety. Each item should be distinct from the others, yet will nevertheless be similar and comparable in all important respects. The item responses should differ only as a consequence of random error. Such items are described as being parallel. There are a number of assumptions inherent in this model, of which the most important are:

1. Each of the items (say, x_i for the ith item) is a test that gives an unbiased estimate of the latent variable (θ). That is, on average, the value of each item equals the value of the latent variable plus random variability (the "error term"). Thus $x_i = \theta + e_i$, where e_i is an error term that has, on average, a mean value of zero.

2. The e_i error terms are uncorrelated. That is, any two items (x_i, x_j) should only appear to be correlated because the latent variable varies. If we consider a group of patients with identical level of QoL (constant θ), their x values should be uncorrelated with each other.
3. Each item is assumed to have the same amount of potential error as any other item. That is, $SD(e_i) = SD(e_j)$. This implies that, for a group of patients corresponding to any one particular value of the latent variable, the items x_i and x_j have equal SDs.
4. The error terms are uncorrelated with the latent variable. That is, the correlation between e_i and θ is zero.

The theory of parallel tests underpins the construction of simple summated scales in which the scale score is computed by simply adding together all of the item scores. These scales are often called *Likert summated scales*, after the influential papers by Likert (1932, 1952). The Likert method is most successful when the response scale for each item covers a wide range of scale levels.

However, the constraints of strictly parallel tests have been recognised as being unnecessarily restrictive. Most of the psychometric properties are retained even when the SDs of the error terms are allowed to differ, so that $SD(e_i) \neq SD(e_j)$. Such models are known as *randomly parallel tests*, or *tau-equivalent tests* since τ (tau) is the mathematical symbol that is often used to represent the true score for a test. This implies that the items are still parallel with respect to how much they are influenced by the latent variable, but they may have different error SDs arising from extraneous non-specified factors. Thus in tau-equivalent tests, like parallel tests, the mean value x_i of item i is on average equal to θ.

Much of the early development of psychometric questionnaires was centred upon educational testing, in which examination questions can be carefully designed so as to comply with these exacting demands. For QoL instruments, one might anticipate that some items in a scale might take responses that are on average higher (or lower) than other items in the scale. In psychometric terms, these may be *essentially tau-equivalent tests*, with items having different mean values (that is, a constant bias relative to the latent variable and to each other, so that the mean value of item i is $\theta + k_i$ where k_i is a constant bias for item i). One thing in common with all these models is the assumption that the tests consist of indicator variables that are solely linear functions of the latent variable (with a random error component included). Many of the traditional psychometric methods remain applicable to essentially tau-equivalent tests (Lord and Novick, 1968).

The majority of QoL instruments have been designed upon the principles of parallel tests and summated Likert scales. The related psychometric methods (Chapter 4) to a large extent assume that the scales contain solely indicator variables. The inter-item correlations that exist between causal variables can render these methods inapplicable.

FACTOR MODELS

Parallel tests and Likert summated scales are unidimensional models; that is, they assume that all the items are measuring a single construct, or factor. If an instrument is thought to consist of several multi-item scales, each will have to be analysed separately. By comparison, *factor analysis* is a much more general approach that can model a number of factors simultaneously, using the inter-item correlations and *SD*s to estimate and test the goodness-of-fit of the models. The factor structure models are linear combinations of the observed variables, with the latent variables being estimated by weighted summation that reflects the importance of each of these variables. The basic factor analysis models belong to traditional psychometrics, and they assume that all items are indicator variables such that the inter-item correlations arise through the relationship between these observed variables and the latent variable.

However, when causal variables are present the so-called exploratory factor analysis model breaks down. For example, many symptoms will be correlated because they are related to disease progression or treatment side-effects; these correlations indicate nothing about the relationship between the symptoms and QoL. Structural equation models (SEM) provide generalisations of the factor model, and also include *multiple-indicator multiple cause* (MIMIC) models. These models are able to handle causal variables, but place far greater demands upon the data and do not provide a solution in every circumstance.

ITEM RESPONSE THEORY

Whilst most QoL and other clinical scales have been developed and based upon traditional psychometric theory, with summated scales being particularly common, newer instruments make greater use of so-called modern psychometric theory. This largely centres around item response theory (IRT). For this model, items may have varying "difficulty". It is assumed that patients will have different probabilities of responding positively to each item, according to their level of ability (that is, the level of the latent variable). Whereas traditional methods focus upon measures such as averages, IRT places emphasis upon probabilities of responses.

The design of scales using IRT methods is markedly different from when traditional methods are used. Likert summated scales assume items of broadly similar difficulty, with each item having response categories to reflect severity or degree of response level. In contrast, IRT scales are based upon items of varying difficulty, and frequently each item will have only two response categories, such as "yes" or "no".

IRT models, like factor models, assume that the observed variables reflect the value of the latent variable, and that the item correlations arise solely by virtue of this relationship with the latent variable. Thus it is implicit that all items are indicator variables. This model is inappropriate for symptoms and other causal variables.

2.8 PSYCHOMETRIC VERSUS CLINIMETRIC SCALES

Feinstein (1987) has argued that many clinical scales possess fundamentally different attributes from psychometric scales, and that their development and validation should therefore proceed along separate paths. He proposed the name *clinimetrics* for the domain concerned with construction of clinical indexes. A "good" and useful clinimetric scale may consist of items comprising a variety of symptoms and other clinical indices, and does not necessarily need to satisfy the same requirements that are demanded of other scales. Psychometricians try to measure a *single attribute with multiple items* and use the validation methods described in Chapter 4 to demonstrate that the multiple-component items are all measuring (more or less) the same single attribute (latent variable). Clinicians try to measure *multiple attributes with a single index*, and aim their strategies at choosing and suitably emphasising the most important attributes to be included in the index.

Example

> The Apgar (1953) score is used to assess the health of newborn babies. This index combines five seemingly disparate symptoms related to heart rate, respiratory rate, reflex responses, skin colour and muscle tone, yet provides an effective and well-established predictor of neonatal outcome. Each item is scored 0 to 2, and a sum-score of 7 or more indicates good prognosis.

When a single attribute (latent variable) is being assessed using multiple items, the investigators will often have a model for the structural relationships in mind. Thus, psychometricians usually think in terms of how the latent variable manifests itself in terms of the observed variables. This leads to the use of factor analysis and other techniques for the extraction of scores. On the other hand, the summary indices that clinicians often seek to encapsulate the values from a number of measured attributes may sometimes be completely arbitrary, and are defined rather than modelled. Sometimes various target criteria are employed when developing an index, such as its prognostic or predictive ability for some future outcome such as length of subsequent survival or cure.

When measuring QoL, one might define a hypothetical construct for the latent variable "overall QoL". Using a psychometric model, one would seek indicator variables that are postulated to reflect overall QoL, and would then collect experimental data to explore and test the model, and to determine whether the variables fit the model. Using a clinimetric approach, one could identify those items which patients regard important to good QoL (that is, causal items affecting QoL), and use these to define a summary index. Whereas the psychometric approach emphasises constructing, validating and testing models, the clinimetric approach usually involves defining and developing an index that is "clinically sensible" and has desirable properties for prognosis or prediction.

The distinction between *clinimetric indexes* and *psychometric scales* has far-reaching implications for the assessment of reliability and validity. It is also closely related to the distinction between *causal items* and *indicator items*, and these concepts explain and justify most of the differences between psychometric and clinimetric scales. The greater part of psychometric theory presumes that all of the items in a scale are indicator variables. Clinimetric scales behave differently from psychometric scales principally because they can contain both causal variables and indicator variables.

2.9 SUFFICIENT CAUSES AND NECESSARY CAUSES

In epidemiology the concepts of causal variables have been highly developed. Thus in 1976 Rothman introduced the concept of necessary and sufficient causes. An epidemiological example is infection with mycobacterium tuberculosis (TB). Nothing else can cause TB, and so bacterial infection by this mycobacterium is a *necessary* condition. It is also a sufficient cause for TB because no additional factors are needed; this mycobacterium on its own is *sufficient* to cause TB. Although necessary causes are only infrequently applicable to scale development, the presence of sufficient causes can be of considerable importance. For example, symptoms are examples of causal items that may also sometimes be sufficient causes; a single symptom, such as pain, may be sufficient to cause QoL to become low. If a QoL instrument contains a scale consisting of several symptoms, a high level of symptomatology for one symptom may be sufficient to impair QoL, irrespective of the values of the other symptoms.

This concept of causal variables often being sufficient causes has a number of implications for scale development. The latent variable, QoL, is not equally reflected by all the component items of the scale. There are no grounds to assume that a summated scale will be applicable and, to the contrary, frequently it is unlikely that all the items in a symptom scale will be equally important as determinants of QoL. For example, suppose disease progression can cause severe pain in some patients, but causes severe nutritional problems in others. A high score on either one of these symptoms would suffice to reduce QoL, and the maximum symptom score could be a better predictor of QoL than the mean of the two items. Thus, instead of a simple summated scale that gives equal weight (importance) to each item, other functions, for example maximum scores, may be more appropriate. When items represent causal variables that are also sufficient causes, linear models such as Likert summated scales and weighted sum scores may be unsatisfactory predictors of QoL.

2.10 DISCRIMINATIVE, EVALUATIVE AND PREDICTIVE INSTRUMENTS

Throughout the stages of scale development, validation and evaluation it is important to consider the intended use of the measurement scale. Guyatt, Feeny and Patrick (1993) draw attention to the need to distinguish between discriminative, evaluative and predictive instruments. Some scales are intended to differentiate between people who have a better QoL and those with a worse QoL; these are *discriminative scales*. Other scales are intended to measure how much QoL changes; these are *evaluative scales*. Scales may also be designed to *predict* future outcomes for patients. If an instrument is intended to be discriminative, it may be less important to include symptoms that are common to all patients and unlikely to differ between the various treatment groups. For example, fatigue is not only common for patients with thyroid disease but is also common amongst patients without the disease, and hence it might be considered an unimportant item in a purely discriminative instrument. However, fatigue is indeed an important symptom for people with thyroid disease, and a change in fatigue over time could be a key item for evaluating effects of therapy.

In general, an instrument that is primarily intended to be *evaluative* or *predictive* should be *responsive* to within-patient changes over time. However, if an instrument is intended to be mainly discriminative, patient-to-patient differences are more important than responsiveness. A discriminative instrument should yield consistent measurements when applied repeatedly to a patient whose condition is stable and has not changed; that is, it should provide repeatable, reproducible results. In particular, it should possess high *test–retest* reliability. It should in addition be sensitive to between-patient differences.

Sensitivity, responsiveness and repeatability are important to all instruments (Chapter 3), but when the instrument is intended for specific applications one or the other property may receive greater priority or, alternatively, different standards may be set for acceptability of the instrument. Thus the emphasis will vary according to the primary objectives in developing the instrument.

2.11 MEASURING QOL: INDICATOR OR CAUSAL ITEMS

QoL instruments commonly contain both indicator and causal variables. Whereas the level of QoL is reflected in the values of indicator variables, it is affected by causal variables. However, psychometric methods, which have formed the basis for development and validation for the majority of QoL instruments, is founded upon the assumption that all of the items are indicator variables. The concept of causal variables explains many of the differences between psychometric and clinimetric methods, and why psychometric methods are less appropriate in the context of these variables and the clinimetric approach is often preferable.

The distinction between causal and indicator variables affects all stages of instrument development, from selection of items through validation to scoring and hence analysis. Thus, for example, when selecting items for an instrument, the psychometric approach leads to multiple (parallel) indicator variables for each scale, whilst for causal variables such as symptoms the most important considerations are content validity and breadth of coverage.

Essentially, QoL instruments serve two very different functions, and should be designed accordingly. On the one hand, they serve to alert the clinician about problems concerning symptoms and side-effects, and help in the management of patients. For this purpose, the clinician will often want the results of each symptom reported separately. Where multi-item scales are needed, they are best constructed on clinimetric principles. However, sometimes scale scores have been formed simply by summing disparate symptoms and other physical aspects, even when these cannot form a coherent clinical scale indicating the level of QoL. Such scores may, however, provide a health-related measure of total symptom burden.

On the other hand, QoL instruments are also intended to assess overall QoL and its aspects. For this, indicator variables may be the most effective, and they should be chosen and validated using psychometric techniques. These indicator variables might be expressions of patients' perception of their QoL, or how aspects of their QoL status are impaired or reduced. That is, the indicators should reflect the effects of impairment rather than being items that cause impairment.

It might be thought, therefore, that QoL is best assessed by forming scales consisting solely of indicator variables. However, this is tantamount to arguing that if, for example, a patient who suffers many symptoms can cope with their problems and neither reports nor shows visible outward signs of suffering, then their QoL is fine. This clearly raises philosophical issues regarding perceptions and meaning of "good QoL". Thus most investigators intuitively feel the need to include information about symptoms and functional problems in any assessment of QoL. Equally, clinicians would generally try to relieve symptoms even though patients might claim that they can cope with their problems or disabilities.

An alternative approach to the assessment of overall QoL is simply to ask the patient, and many instruments do contain a global question such as "How would you rate your overall quality of life during the past week?" Gill and Feinstein (1994) advocate that all instruments should contain such questions.

2.12 CONCLUSIONS

The distinction between causal and indicator variables, although rarely recognised, carries far-reaching implications regarding the methods of scale construction and validation, as does the distinction between psychometric and clinimetric methods. The majority of QoL instruments contain a mixture of both types of items.

Most instruments also contain both single and multi-item scales, and the majority of the modern QoL instruments include at least one global question assessing overall reported QoL.

The chapters in Part B explore the ways in which such instruments may be validated and examined for evidence of reliability and sensitivity.

B Developing and Testing Questionnaires

3 Scores and Measurements: Validity, Reliability, Sensitivity

Summary

In this chapter we explore properties that are common to all forms of measures. This includes both single-item measurements, such as the response to a single global question, and summary scores derived from multi-item scales, such as the scores from the summated scales that are used in many QoL instruments. These properties include validity, reliability, sensitivity and responsiveness. This chapter focuses upon those aspects of the properties that apply to single items and summary scale scores. Chapter 4 discusses related techniques that apply to multi-item scales, when the within-scale between-item relationships can be examined.

3.1 INTRODUCTION

All measurements, from blood pressures to QoL assessments, should satisfy basic properties if they are to be clinically useful. These are primarily validity, reliability, repeatability, sensitivity and responsiveness.

Validation of instruments is the process of determining whether there are grounds for believing that the instrument measures what it is intended to measure, and that it is useful for its intended purpose. For example, to what extent is it reasonable to claim that a "quality of life" questionnaire really is assessing QoL? Since we are attempting to measure an ill-defined and unobservable latent variable (QoL), we can only infer that the instrument is valid in so far as it correlates with other observable behaviour. This validation process consists of a number of stages, in which it is hoped to collect convincing evidence that the instrument taps into the intended constructs and that it produces useful measurements reflecting patients' QoL. Validity can be subdivided into three main aspects.

Content validity concerns the extent to which the items are sensible and reflect the intended domain of interest. *Criterion validity* considers whether the scale has empirical association with external criteria such as other established instruments. *Construct validity* examines the theoretical relationship of the items to each other and to the hypothesised scales. Of these three types of validity, construct validity is the most amenable to exploration by numerical analysis. Two aspects of construct validity are *convergent validity* and *discriminant validity*. Some items or scales, such as anxiety and depression, may be expected to be highly correlated, or convergent. Others may be expected to be relatively unrelated, or divergent, and possessing discriminant validity. If a group of patients with a wide range of diagnoses and treatments is included, a very high scale-to-scale correlation could imply low discriminant validity and might suggest that the two scales measure similar things. If scale-to-scale correlations do not correspond roughly to what is expected, the postulated relationships between the constructs are questionable.

Reliability and *repeatability* concern the random variability associated with measurements. Ideally, patients whose QoL status has not changed should make very similar, or repeatable, responses each time they are assessed. If there is considerable random variability, the measurements are unreliable. It would be difficult to know how to interpret the results from individual patients if the measurements are not reliable. Poor reliability can sometimes be a warning that validity might be suspect, and that the measurement is detecting something different from what we intend it to measure.

Sensitivity is the ability of measurements to detect differences between patients or groups of patients. If we can demonstrate that a measurement is sensitive and detects differences believed to exist between groups of patients, such as differences between poor and good prognosis patients, we will be more confident that it is valid and measuring what we believe it to be measuring. Sensitivity is also important in clinical trials since a measurement is of little use if it cannot detect the differences in QoL that may exist between the randomised groups.

Responsiveness is similar to sensitivity, but relates to the ability to detect changes when a patient improves or deteriorates. A measurement has limited use for patient monitoring unless it reflects changes in the patient's condition. A sensitive measurement will usually, but not necessarily, also be responsive to changes.

Validity, reliability, sensitivity and responsiveness are interrelated, yet each is independently important. Assessing validity, in particular, is a complex and never-ending task. In QoL research, scales can never be proved to be valid. Instead, the process of validation consists of accruing more and more evidence that the scales are sensible and that they behave in the manner that is anticipated.

For a discussion of statistical significance and *p*-values, mentioned in this chapter, see Chapters 4 and 14.

3.2   CONTENT VALIDITY

Content validity relates to the adequacy of content of an instrument, in terms of the number and scope of the individual questions that it contains. It makes use of the conceptual definition of the constructs being assessed, and consists of reviewing the instrument to ensure that it appears to be sensible and covers all of the relevant issues. Thus content validation involves the critical examination of the basic structure of the instrument, a review of the procedures used for the development of the questionnaire, and also consideration of the applicability to the intended research question. In order to claim content validity, the design and development of an instrument should follow rigorously defined development procedures.

ITEM COVERAGE AND RELEVANCE

Comprehensive coverage is one of the more important aspects of content validity, and the entire range of relevant issues should be covered by the instrument. An instrument aiming to assess symptomatology, for example, should include items relating to all major relevant symptoms. Otherwise there could be undetected differences between groups of patients. In an extreme case, important side-effects may remain undetected and unreported. Although these side-effects may have a substantial effect upon QoL, a single global question about overall QoL may lack the specificity and sensitivity to detect a group difference.

The extent of item coverage is not amenable to formal statistical testing, and depends largely upon ensuring that the instrument has been developed according to rigorous pre-defined methods. The item generation process should include input from specialists in the disease area, a review of published data and literature, and interviews with patients suffering from the illness. Evidence of having followed formal, documented procedures will tend to support claims regarding the content validity of the instrument.

At the same time, all the items that *are* included should be relevant to the concept being assessed, and any irrelevant items should be excluded. Item relevance is commonly approached by using an expert panel to assess whether individual items are appropriate to the construct being assessed, and also by asking patients their opinion as to the relevance of the questions. Methods of construct validation can also indicate those items that appear to be behaving differently from other items in a scale (see Chapter 4). These items can then be critically reviewed, to decide whether they really do or do not relate to the construct that is being evaluated. Items should also be excluded if they are redundant because they overlap with or duplicate the information contained in other items.

FACE VALIDITY

Face validity involves checking whether items in an instrument appear "on the face of it" to cover the intended topics clearly and unambiguously. Face validity is closely related to content validity, and is often considered to be an aspect of it. The main distinction is that face validity concerns the critical review of an instrument *after* it has been constructed, whilst the greater part of content validation consists of ensuring that comprehensive and thorough development procedures were rigorously followed and documented.

Content validity is optimised by including a wide range of individuals in the development process, and face validity may be maximised in a similar way. Thus when confirming face validity the opinion of experts (such as doctors, nurses, and social scientists) should be sought, and patients should be asked whether the instrument seems sensible. Although investigators describing validation of instruments often state that consensus opinion was sought and that the instrument is believed to have good face validity or content validity, explicit details are often lacking. It is important to describe the composition and functioning of the individuals involved in the development and validation processes.

Example from the literature

Langfitt (1995) compared three QoL instruments for patients with intractable epilepsy. The instruments were the Washington Psychosocial Seizure Inventory

(WPSI), the Epilepsy Surgery Inventory 55 (ESI-55), and the SIP. Two psychologists independently classified each item from the three questionnaires according to its relevance to different QoL domains. A third, independent rater resolved disagreements. Thus, for example, the SIP and WPSI both included 26 questions about social functioning, whereas the ESI-55 only had two (Table 3.1).

The author concluded that the ESI-55 and SIP have a more suitable content for assessment of the broad impact of epilepsy on QoL than the WPSI instrument which focuses on psychological and social adjustment. Langfitt also presented information on reliability and construct validity to support the recommendations.

Table 3.1 Number of items on the ESI-55, SIP and WPSI that are relevant to patients with epilepsy, by QoL domain (Based on Langfitt, 1995)

QoL domains		ESI-55	SIP	WPSI
Physical	Symptoms	2	5	2
	Functional status	10	55	2
	Energy/sleep and rest	4	8	4
Psychological	Social functioning	2	26	26
	Emotional status	6	7	37
	Cognition	5	16	7
	Health perceptions	7	2	3
	General life satisfaction	3	1	10
Role activities		15	16	16
Not classified		1	0	25
Totals		55	136	132

3.3   CRITERION VALIDITY

Criterion validity involves assessing an instrument against the true value, or against some other standard that is accepted as providing an indication of the true values for the measurements. It can be divided into *concurrent validity* and *predictive validity*.

CONCURRENT VALIDITY

Concurrent validity means agreement with the true value. Such a "gold standard" is not available for QoL instruments since they measure postulated constructs that are experimental and subjective. Therefore the most common approach involves comparing new questionnaires against one or more well-established instruments. This may be reasonable if the objective of developing a new instrument is to produce a shorter or simpler questionnaire, in which case the more detailed, established instrument may be believed to set a standard at which to aim. More frequently, the rationale for creating a new instrument is that the investigators believe existing ones to be suboptimal. In this case, the comparison of new against established is of limited value since the latter has, in effect, already been rejected as the gold standard.

Another approach is to use indirect methods of comparison. A detailed interview, using staff trained in interviewing techniques, might yield estimates of the constructs that are perhaps believed to be approximations to a true value.

Example

Anxiety and depression are psychological concepts that have traditionally been assessed by using in-depth interviews to rate their severity and to detect patient "cases" needing psychiatric intervention. If the psychiatric assessment is regarded as an approximation of the true level of these states, it can serve as a criterion against which a patient's self-completed questionnaire is compared. Anxiety and depression are perhaps different from most QoL scales, in that there is (arguably) a clearer definition and better consensus among psychiatrists of the meaning of these terms. On that assumption, it would seem reasonable to regard a brief patient-questionnaire, taking a few minutes to complete, as a convenient method for estimating the "true" values of the detailed interview.

As already mentioned, a new instrument is usually compared against values obtained from other, well-established or lengthier instruments, an in-depth interview, or an observer's assessment. If agreement between the two methods is considered to be poor, the concurrent validity is low. It may be difficult to determine with certainty whether one or both of the methods has low validity, but the low level of agreement serves as an indicator that something may be amiss.

Example from the literature

Zigmond and Snaith (1983) asked 100 patients from a general medical outpatient clinic to complete the HADS questionnaire. Following this, they used a 20-minute psychiatric interview to assess anxiety and depression. A summary of the results is shown in Table 3.2, with patients grouped into three categories according to whether they were psychiatric cases, doubtful cases or non-cases of anxiety and depression.

For diagnosing psychiatric cases, the depression scale gave 1% false positives and 1% false negatives, and the anxiety scale 5% false positives and 1% false negatives.

Table 3.2 HADS questionnaire completed by 100 patients from a general medical outpatient clinic (Based on Zigmond and Snaith, 1983)

HADS score	Depression			Anxiety		
	Non-cases	Doubtful cases	Cases	Non-cases	Doubtful cases	Cases
0–7	57	11	*1*	41	4	*1*
8–10	8	7	3	10	9	1
11–21	*1*	4	8	*5*	15	14

False positives and false negatives are shown in bold italics.

PREDICTIVE VALIDITY

Predictive validity concerns the ability of the instrument to predict future health status, future events, or future test results. For example, it has frequently been reported that overall QoL scores are predictive of subsequent survival time in cancer trials, and that QoL assessment is providing additional prognostic information to supplement the more-objective measures such as tumour stage and extent of disease. The implication is that future health status can serve as a criterion against which the instrument is compared. Thus for purposes of criterion validity, future status is regarded as a better indicator of the current true value of the latent variable than the observed patient responses from the instrument being developed. To make such an assumption, the investigator will have to form a conceptual model of the construct being assessed and its relationship with future outcomes. Therefore predictive validity is more conveniently discussed from the perspective of being an aspect of construct validity.

3.4 CONSTRUCT VALIDITY

Construct validity is one of the most important characteristics of a measurement instrument. It is an assessment of the degree to which an instrument measures the construct that it was designed to measure. The subject of construct validity is a difficult and controversial one. It involves first forming a hypothetical model, describing the constructs being assessed and postulating their relationships. Data are then collected, and an assessment is made as to the degree to which these relationships are confirmed. If the results confirm prior expectations about the constructs, the implication is that the instrument *may* be valid and that we may therefore use it to make inferences about patients.

The "*may* be valid" emphasises the controversial aspect of construct validation. The difficulty is that the criterion, and the construct, is not directly measurable. Hence a formal statistical test cannot be developed. Since assessment of construct validity relies upon expressing opinions about expected relationships amongst the constructs, and confirming that the observed measurements behave as expected, we cannot *prove* that questionnaire items are valid measures for the constructs, nor that the constructs are valid representations of behaviour. All we can do is collect increasing amounts of evidence that the measurements appear to be sensible, and that the postulated constructs behave as anticipated and that there are no grounds for rejecting them. The greater the supporting evidence, the more confident we are that our model is an adequate representation of the constructs that we label QoL.

More formally, construct validity embraces a variety of techniques, all aimed at assessing two things: firstly, whether the theoretical postulated construct appears to be an adequate model; and secondly whether the measurement scale appears to correspond to that postulated construct. Translating this into practical application, construct validation is primarily concerned with checking:

1. *Dimensionality*: do all items in a subscale relate to a single latent variable, or is there evidence that more latent variables are necessary to explain the observed variability?

2. *Homogeneity*: do all the items in a subscale appear to be tapping equally strongly into the same latent variable?
3. *Overlap between latent variables*: do some items from one subscale correlate with other latent variables?

Construct validation is a lengthy and on-going process, of learning more about the construct, making new predictions and then testing them. Each study that supports the theoretical construct serves to strengthen the theory, but a single negative finding may call into question the entire construct.

Mainly, assessment of construct validity makes use of correlations, changes over time, and differences between groups of patients. It involves building and testing conceptual models that express the postulated relationships between the hypothetical domains of QoL and the scales that are being developed to measure these domains.

KNOWN-GROUPS VALIDATION

One of the simpler forms of construct validation is *known-groups validity*. This is based on the principle that certain specified groups of patients may be anticipated to score differently from others, and the instrument should be sensitive to these differences. For example, patients with advanced cancer might be expected to have poorer QoL than those with early disease. A valid scale should show differences, in the predicted direction, between these groups. Known-groups comparisons are therefore a combination of tests for validity and a form of sensitivity or responsiveness assessment. A scale that cannot successfully distinguish between groups with known differences, either because it lacks sensitivity or because it yields results that are contrary to expectations, is hardly likely to be of value for many purposes.

Investigators frequently select patients in whom one may anticipate that there will be substantial differences between the groups. This implies that even a very small-sized study will provide sufficient evidence to confirm that the observed differences are unlikely to be due to chance; what matters most is the magnitude of the differences, not the p-values. Although statistical significance tests are uninformative and not worthy of reporting in these circumstances, it is common to see publications that describe all differences as statistically highly significant with p-values less than 0.0001.

Example from the Literature

Schag *et al.* (1992) evaluated the HIV Overview of Problems—Evaluation System (HOPES), comparing it with the MOS-HIV and other instruments, in patients with HIV infection. The patients were divided into the "known-groups" of: Asymptomatic, AIDS-related complex (ARC), AIDS, and AIDS with cancer (AIDS+C). The analysis of known-groups validity in Table 3.3 shows that high HOPES or low MOS-HIV scores indicate poor QoL and worse functioning.

For all scales, the asymptomatic group showed clear differences from the other three groups. The differences between ARC, AIDS and AIDS with cancer were much smaller. With one exception, the ANOVA returned highly significant p-values of less than 0.0001—mainly because of the extreme difference between the asymptomatic patients and the others.

Table 3.3 Known-groups validity of the HOPES and MOS-HIV instruments, in patients with HIV infection (Based on Schag *et al.*, 1992)

	Asymptomatic $n = 119$	ARC $n = 65$	AIDS $n = 78$	AIDS + C $n = 56$	ANOVA p-value
HOPES					
Global score	0.75	1.27	1.18	1.24	0.0001
Physical	0.44	1.03	1.09	1.08	0.0001
Psychosocial	1.02	1.49	1.24	1.42	0.0001
Medical interaction	0.30	0.70	0.62	0.55	0.0001
Sexual	1.29	1.54	1.67	1.98	0.0001
MOS-HIV					
Physical	81.78	53.07	40.98	46.72	0.0001
Mental health	70.25	59.61	66.54	64.20	0.01
Role function	82.62	44.62	30.77	39.29	0.0001
QoL	67.82	55.38	56.73	52.68	0.0001

CONVERGENT VALIDITY

Convergent validity is another important aspect of construct validity, and consists of showing that a postulated dimension of QoL correlates appreciably with all other dimensions that theory suggests should be related to it. That is, we may believe that some dimensions of QoL are related, and we therefore expect the observed measurements to be correlated. For example, one might anticipate that patients with severe pain are likely to be depressed, and that there should be a correlation between the pain scores and depression ratings.

Many of the dimensions of QoL are interrelated. Very ill patients tend to suffer from a variety of symptoms, and have high scores on a wide range of psychological dimensions. Many, and sometimes nearly all, dimensions of QoL are correlated with each other. Therefore assessment of convergent validity consists of predicting the strongest and weakest correlations, and confirming that subsequent observed values conform to the predictions. Analysis consists of calculating all pairwise correlation coefficients between scores for different QoL scales.

A very high correlation between two scales invites the question of whether both of the scales are measuring the same factor, and whether they could be combined into a single scale without any loss of information. The decision regarding the amalgamation of scales should take into account the composition of the separate scales, and whether there are clinical, psychological or other grounds for deciding that face validity could be compromised and that it is better to retain separate scales. Alternatively, a very high correlation might imply that one of the scales is redundant and can be deleted from the instrument. Convergent validity is usually considered together with discriminant validity.

DISCRIMINANT VALIDITY

Discriminant validity, or divergent validity, recognises that some dimensions of QoL are anticipated to be relatively unrelated, and that their correlations should be low. Convergent and discriminant validity represent the two extremes in a continuum of associations between the dimensions of QoL. One problem when assessing discriminant validity (and, to a lesser extent, convergent validity) is that two dimensions may correlate "spuriously" because of some third, possibly unrecognised, construct that links the two together. For example, if two dimensions are both affected by age, an apparent correlation can be introduced solely though the differing ages of the respondents. Another extraneous source of correlations could be "yea-saying", in which patients may report improving QoL on many dimensions simply to please staff or relatives. When specific independent variables are suspected of introducing spurious correlations, the statistical technique of "partial correlation" should be used; this is a method of estimating the correlation between two variables, or dimensions of QoL, whilst holding other "nuisance" variables constant. In practice, there are usually many extraneous variables each contributing a little to the spurious correlations.

Convergent validity and discriminant validity are commonly assessed across instruments rather than within an instrument, in which case those scales from each instrument that are intended to measure similar constructs should have higher correlations with each other than with scales that measure unrelated constructs.

Example from the literature

Schag *et al.* (1992) predicted the pattern of associations that they expected to observe between scales from the HOPES questionnaire and the MOS-HIV. Table 3.4 shows some of the corresponding observed correlations.

The authors commented that, as predicted, the MOS-HIV scales of cognitive function, mental health, health distress correlated most highly with the psychosocial summary scale of the HOPES. Similarly, other MOS-HIV subscales correlated most highly with the HOPES physical summary scale.

The high correlations supported the predictions of convergent validity, whilst the lower correlations between other subscales supported the discriminant validity.

Table 3.4 Correlations between HOPES physical and psychosocial scales and the MOS-HIV scales, in patients with HIV infection (Based on Schag *et al.*, 1992)

MOS-HIV	HOPES	
	Physical	Psychosocial
General health	0.74	0.41
Physical function	0.74	0.42
Role function	0.70	0.36
Social function	0.75	0.43
Cognitive function	0.55	0.55
Pain score	0.67	0.39
Mental health	0.55	0.70
Energy/fatigue	0.72	0.47
Health distress	0.65	0.67
QoL	0.52	0.44
Health transition	0.25	0.17

MULTITRAIT–MULTIMETHOD ANALYSIS

The *multitrait–multimethod* (MTMM) correlation matrix is a method for examining convergent and discriminant validity. The general principle of this technique is that two or more "methods", such as different instruments, are each used to assess the same "traits", for example QoL aspects, items or subscales. Then we can inspect and compare the correlations arising from the same subscale as estimated by the different methods. Various layouts are used for MTMM matrices, the most common being shown in Table 3.5.

In Table 3.5, the two instruments are methods, while the functioning scales are traits. Cells marked C show the correlations of the scores when different instruments are used to assess the same trait. *Convergent* validity is determined by the C cells. If the correlations in these cells are high, say above 0.7, this suggests that both instruments may be measuring the same thing. If the two instruments were developed independently of each other, this would support the inference that the traits are defined in a consistent and presumably meaningful manner.

Similarly, the D cells show the scale-to-scale correlations for each instrument, and these assess *discriminant* validity. Lower correlations are usually expected in these cells, since otherwise scales purporting to measure different aspects of QoL are in fact more strongly related than supposedly similar scales from different instruments.

The main diagonal cells, marked R, can be used to show *reliability* coefficients, as described later and in Chapter 4. These can be either Cronbach's α for internal reliability or, if repeated QoL assessments are available on patients whose condition is stable, test–retest correlations. Since repeated values of the same trait measured twice by the same method will usually be more similar than values of the same trait measured by different instruments, the R cells containing test–retest repeatability scores should usually contain the highest correlations.

One common variation on the theme of MTMM matrices is to carry out the patient assessments on two different occasions. The unshaded triangular area to the upper-right of Table 3.5 can be used to display the correlations at time 1, and the time 2 data can be shown in the shaded triangle that we have been describing above. The diagonal cells dividing the two triangles, marked R, should then show the test–retest repeatability correlations.

Table 3.5 Template for the multitrait–multimethod (MTMM) correlation matrix

		Emotional function		Social Function		Role function	
	Instrument	*1*	*2*	*1*	*2*	*1*	*2*
Emotional function	*1*	R					
	2	C	R				
Social function	*1*	D		R			
	2		D	C	R		
Role function	*1*	D		D		R	
	2		D		D	C	R

Example from the literature

Greenwald (1987) applied the SIP, POMS and MPQ to recently diagnosed cancer patients. The SIP and the POMS both measure physical dysfunction and emotional distress. The corresponding MTMM matrix is shown in Table 3.6. The diagonal was left blank, although reliability coefficients could have been shown there.

The shaded correlations were higher than the other correlations (convergent validity) and thus the authors concluded: "The MTMM matrix supports the hypothesis that subscales believed to measure similar disease impacts have the highest inter-correlations."

Table 3.6 Multitrait–multimethod correlation matrix of correlations for SIP and POMS physical dysfunction and emotional distress scores (Based on Greenwald HP (1987). The specificity of quality-of-life measures among the seriously ill. *Medical Care*, **25** (7), 642–651)

	Physical dysfunction		Emotional distress	
	SIP	POMS	SIP	POMS
Physical dysfunction				
SIP	–			
POMS	−0.44	–		
Emotional distress				
SIP	0.27	0.32	–	
POMS	0.24	−0.32	0.47	–

Example from the literature

The FLIC (Schipper *et al.*, 1984) and the EORTC QLQ-C30 are two instruments that ostensibly measure many of the same aspects of QoL. King, Dobson and Harnett (1996) used an MTMM matrix, summarised in Table 3.7, to compare these two instruments in patients with breast, ovarian or colon cancer. QoL scores do not have a Normal distribution, and so Spearman's rank correlation coefficient was used.

King *et al.* used a slightly different layout from Table 3.5 in that they subdivided the instruments into traits (QoL dimensions); also they do not show reliability coefficients. The correlation between the FLIC Role scale and the FLIC "Current QoL" scale is 0.64, while the correlation between the QLQ-C30 Global QoL and the FLIC Current QoL is 0.76. The negative correlation coefficients arise because high QLQ-C30 scores for symptom scales indicate high levels of symptomatology, whereas high scores for all FLIC scales and the QLQ function-scales indicate better functioning or fewer problems.

Convergent validity is determined by the shaded cells, which represent the correlation of two instruments when assessing the same traits. In this example, QLQ-C30 Global QoL, Role function, Nausea, Emotional function and Pain all correlate fairly strongly with the FLIC Current, Role and Nausea scales. However, QLQ-C30 Social function and FLIC Sociability have a low correlation of

Table 3.7 Multitrait–multimethod correlation matrix for FLIC scores and EORTC QLQ-C30 scores (Based on King *et al.*, 1996)

	FLIC scales						QLQ-C30 scales					
	Current QoL	Role	Sociability	Emotional	Pain	Nausea	Global QoL	Role function	Social function	Emotional function	Pain	Nausea
FLIC scales												
Current QoL	1											
Role	0.64	1										
Sociability	0.26	0.24	1									
Emotional	0.46	0.44	0.17	1								
Pain	0.58	0.56	0.12	0.28	1							
Nausea	0.37	0.35	0.32	0.17	0.34	1						
QLQ-C30 scales												
Global QoL	0.76	0.65	0.17	0.50	0.60	0.21	1					
Role function	0.50	0.74	0.23	0.26	0.55	0.28	0.52	1				
Social function	0.58	0.69	0.35	0.52	0.49	0.33	0.62	0.62	1			
Emotional function	0.48	0.45	0.25	0.67	0.28	0.18	0.50	0.39	0.66	1		
Pain	-0.53	-0.50	-0.07	-0.24	-0.65	-0.08	-0.67	-0.53	-0.46	-0.39	1	
Nausea	-0.41	-0.34	-0.18	-0.25	-0.39	-0.74	-0.36	-0.34	-0.39	-0.45	0.30	1

0.35, which suggests they are measuring different things. For both instruments, Pain and Global QoL showed correlations of approximately 0.6, which is a high value and represents relatively poor discriminant validity. However, a more obvious interpretation is that Pain is a causal item that has a strong impact upon QoL scores.

It is often useful to consider confidence intervals (*CIs*) of the correlation coefficients, as shown in Chapter 4. The *CIs* reflect the sample size of the study, and a small study will be associated with wide intervals. The intervals enable a critical inspection of whether differences between correlations may be due to chance, or whether there is reasonable confirmation of the expected correlation structure

3.5 RELIABILITY

Assessment of *reliability* consists of determining that a scale or measurement yields reproducible and consistent results. Confusingly, this same word is used for two very different levels of scale validation. Firstly, for scales containing multiple items, all the items should be consistent in the sense that they should all measure the same thing. This form of reliability, which is called "internal reliability", uses item correlations to assess the homogeneity of multi-item scales and is in many senses a form of validity. Secondly, reliability is also used as a term to describe aspects of repeatability and stability of measurements. Any measurement or summary score, whether based upon a single item or multiple items, should yield reproducible or similar values if it is used repeatedly on the same patient whilst the patient's condition has not changed materially. This second form of reliability is a desirable property of any quantitative measurement.

From a statistical point of view, both forms of reliability are assessed using related techniques. Thus *repeatability reliability* is based upon analysis of correlations between repeated measurements, where the measurements are either repeated over time (*test–retest reliability*), by different observers (*inter-rater reliability*) or by different variants of the instrument (*equivalent-forms reliability*). *Internal reliability*, which is also often called *internal consistency*, is based upon item-to-item correlations in multi-item scales, and is discussed in Chapter 4. Since these two concepts are mathematically related, estimates of the internal reliability of multi-item scales can often be used to predict the approximate value of their repeatability reliability.

A number of different measures have been proposed. Since reliability is the extent to which repeated measurements will give the same results when the true scale score remains constant, measurement concerns the level of agreement between two or more scores. We describe methods suitable for two assessments per patient.

BINARY DATA: PROPORTION OF AGREEMENT

Binary assessments include ratings such as yes/no, present/absent, positive/negative, or patients grouped into those greater/less than some threshold value. The simplest method of assessing repeatability is the *proportion of agreement* when the same instrument is applied on two occasions. When patients are assessed twice, the

Table 3.8 Notation for repeated binary data, with two assessments of the same N subjects

Second assessment	First assessment		Total
	Positive	Negative	
Positive	x_{11}	x_{12}	r_1
Negative	x_{21}	x_{22}	r_2
Total	c_1	c_2	N

resulting data can be tabulated as in Table 3.8. Here x_{11} is the number of patients whose QoL response is positive both times.

The number of agreements, that is the number of patients who respond in the same way in both assessments, is $x_{11} + x_{22}$, and so the proportion of agreements is

$$p_{Agree} = (x_{ii} + x_{22})/N. \tag{3.1}$$

BINARY DATA: κ

However, we would expect some agreement purely by chance, even if patients entered random responses on the questionnaire, and P_{Agree} does not reflect whether the agreement arises mainly from being positive twice, or negative twice. The kappa coefficient, κ, provides a better method by extending the above concept of proportion agreement to allow for some expected chance agreements. It can be shown that the expected number of chance agreements corresponding to cell x_{11} is $c_1 r_1/N$ and similarly for x_{22}, $c_2 r_2/N$. Thus the expected proportion of chance agreements is

$$p_{Chance} = \left(\frac{c_1 r_1}{N} + \frac{c_2 r_2}{N}\right)/N = (c_1 r_1 + c_2 r_2)/N^2. \tag{3.2}$$

The excess proportion of agreement above that expected is then $(p_{Agree} - p_{Chance})$. Furthermore, since the maximum proportion of agreements is 1 when $x_{11} + x_{22} = N$, the maximum value of is $(p_{Agree} - p_{Chance})$ is $(1 - p_{Chance})$. Hence we can scale the excess proportion of agreement so that it has a maximum value of 1. This leads to the κ index of agreement:

$$\kappa = (p_{Agree} - p_{Chance})/(1 - p_{Chance}). \tag{3.3}$$

The value of κ is equal to 1 if there is perfect agreement, and equals 0 if the agreement is no better than chance. Negative values indicate an agreement that is even less than what would be expected by chance. Interpretation of κ is subjective, but the guideline values in Table 3.9 are commonly used.

Although κ may seem intuitively appealing, it has been criticised. Misleading values are often obtained, mainly because κ is affected by the degree of asymmetry or imbalance in the table. The value of κ is also influenced by the total percentage of positives, and it is possible to obtain very different values of κ even when the proportion of agreement remains constant. Thus κ is no substitute for inspecting the

Table 3.9 Guideline values of κ to indicate the strength of agreement

κ	Agreement
<0.20	Poor
0.21–0.40	Slight
0.41–0.60	Moderate
0.61–0.80	Good
0.81–1.00	Very high

table of frequencies, and examining whether the table appears to be symmetrical or whether there is a tendency for patients to respond differently on the two occasions.

ORDERED CATEGORICAL DATA: WEIGHTED κ

QoL assessments frequently consist of ordered categorical response items that are scored according to the level of response. For example, items from some instruments are scored with $g = 4$ categories from 1 for "not at all" through to 4 for "very much".

If we construct the $g \times g$ two-way table of frequencies analogous to Table 3.8, we obtain

$$p_{Agree} = (\textstyle\sum x_{ii})/N \text{ and } p_{Chance} = (\textstyle\sum r_i c_i)/N^2, \qquad (3.4)$$

where the summation is from $i = 1$ to g. Equation (3.3) is then applied to give κ.

However, these equations give equal importance to any disagreement. Although it is possible to use this directly, it is generally more realistic to use a *weighted* form, κ_{Weight}. This takes into account the degree of disagreement, such that a difference between scores of 1 and 3 on the two occasions would be considered of greater importance than the difference between 1 and 2. In terms of the table of frequencies, values along the diagonal, corresponding to x_{11}, x_{22}, x_{33} etc., represent perfect agreement. Values that are off the diagonal in row i and column j are given scores or "weights" according to their distance from the diagonal, which corresponds to their degree of discrepancy. Two frequently used choices of weights are

$$w_{ij} = 1 - \frac{|i-j|}{g-1}, \text{ or } w_{ij} = 1 - \left(\frac{i-j}{g-1}\right)^2, \qquad (3.5)$$

where $|i-j|$ is the absolute difference of i and j, which ignores the sign of the difference. The first weighting in equation (3.5) is termed "linear", the second "quadratic".

Example

Suppose an item has $g = 4$ possible response categories, with 1 for "not at all", 2 for "a little", 3 for "quite a bit" and 4 for "very much". If the result of the first assessment on a patient is 1, then for second assessment values of 1, 2, 3 or 4 respectively, the corresponding linear weights would be 1, 0.67, 0.33 and 0, whilst the quadratic weights would be 1, 0.89, 0.56 and 0. For both weighting schemes 1 indicates perfect agreement and 0 the maximum disagreement. The quadratic weights place greater emphasis upon measurements that agree closely.

Quadratic weights are generally considered preferable, and lead to

$$p^w_{Agree} = \left(\sum_{i=1}^{g} \sum_{j=1}^{g} w_{ij} x_{ij} \right) / N, \; p^w_{Chance} = \left(\sum_{i=1}^{g} \sum_{j=1}^{g} w_{ij} r_i c_j \right) / N^2,$$

and hence

$$\kappa_{Weight} = (p^w_{Agree} - p^w_{Chance})/(1 - p^w_{Chance}). \tag{3.6}$$

Similar reservations apply to weighted κ_{Weight} as to simple κ. The value is highly affected by the symmetry of the table, and by the proportion of patients in each category. Also, the number of categories g affects κ_{Weight}. Thus, for example, κ_{Weight} will usually be greater if patients are evenly distributed over the range of values for QoL, and will be smaller if most patients have extreme values—for example, if most patients have very poor QoL.

Despite these reservations, when analysing proportions or items, which have only a few ordered categories, κ_{Weight} remains the appropriate measure for assessing the agreement between two items or between two repeats of an assessment. Quadratic-weighted κ_{Weight} is also analogous to the intraclass correlation coefficient described later.

Example from the literature

Frost *et al.* (1998) developed the VCM1, a questionnaire for measuring vision-related QoL. It contains ten items relating to physical, psychological and social issues, and is intended to be applicable to patients with a wide range of problems including cataract and corneal surgery, glaucoma, blind rehabilitation, and cytomegalovirus retinitis. Questions are scored from 0 (Not at all) to 4 (A lot).

Patients completed a test–retest study, with the median time between tests being 17 days. Table 3.10 shows that the effect of weighting κ is quite marked, and using κ_{Weight} with quadratic weights results in a substantial increase in the reported scores.

It can be difficult to know how to interpret or decide what are acceptable values of κ_{Weight} as it is greatly affected by the weights, making the guideline values of Table 3.9 inapplicable. One use of κ_{Weight} that does not depend upon guideline values is inference about the relative stability of different items: those items with largest κ are the most repeatable.

Table 3.10 Test–retest κ coefficients for the VCM1, measuring vision-related QoL (Based on Frost *et al.*, 1998)

Item	Absolute score difference				Number of observations	Unweighted κ	Quadratic-weighted κ_{Weight}
	0	1	2	3			
Embarrassment	20	5	2	0	27	0.43	0.79
Anger	15	9	2	1	27	0.39	0.75
Depression	20	5	2	0	27	0.36	0.75
Loneliness	24	3	0	0	27	0.57	0.69
Fear of deterioration in vision	16	10	1	0	27	0.44	0.86
Safety at home	20	7	1	0	28	0.35	0.65
Safety outside home	20	5	3	0	28	0.53	0.61
Coping with everyday life	21	6	1	0	28	0.49	0.67
Inability to do preferred activities	15	11	2	0	28	0.34	0.73
Life interference	14	10	1	1	26	0.33	0.66

PEARSON'S CORRELATION COEFFICIENT

The ordinary correlation coefficient, is also called *Pearson's correlation*, is described in Section 4.3 is often advocated as a measure of repeatability. This is to be deprecated, because correlation is a measure of association, and repeated measurements may be highly correlated yet systematically different. For example, if patients consistently score higher by exactly 10 points when a test is reapplied, there would be zero agreement between the first and second assessments. Despite this, the correlation coefficient would be 1, indicating perfect association. When one has continuous variables, a more appropriate approach to the assessment of reliability is the *intraclass correlation coefficient*.

INTRACLASS CORRELATION COEFFICIENT (*ICC*)

For continuous data, the *ICC* measures the strength of agreement between repeated measurements, by assessing the proportion of the total variance, σ^2 (the square of the *SD*), of an observation that is associated with the between-patient variability. Thus

$$ICC = \frac{\sigma^2_{Patient}}{\sigma^2_{Patient} + \sigma^2_{Error}} \tag{3.7}$$

If the *ICC* is large (close to 1), then the random error variability is low and a high proportion of the variance in the observations is attributable to variation between patients. The measurements are then described as having high reliability. Conversely, if the *ICC* is low (close to 0), then the random error variability dominates and the measurements have low reliability. If the error variability is regarded as "noise" and the true value of patients' scores as the "signal", the *ICC* measures the signal–noise ratio.

The *ICC* can be estimated from an analysis of variance (ANOVA), the rationale for which is described in greater detail in Chapter 8. In brief, ANOVA partitions the total variance into separate components, according to the source of the variability. A table for ANOVA in which p patients repeat the same QoL assessment on r occasions can be represented as in Table 3.11.

The "error" variability corresponding to equation (3.7) has been separated into two components, and is now equal to $\sigma^2_{Repeats} + \sigma^2_{Error}$. This leads to

$$ICC = \frac{\sigma^2_{Patient}}{\sigma^2_{Patient} + \sigma^2_{Repeats} + \sigma^2_{Error}}, \tag{3.8}$$

and solving the equations for $\sigma^2_{Patient}$, $\sigma^2_{Repeats}$ and σ^2_{Error} gives

$$ICC = \frac{p(V_{Patient} - V_{Error})}{pV_{Patient} + rV_{Repeats} + (p - r)V_{Error}} \tag{3.9}$$

which is the more general form of the *ICC* for repeated assessments.

Table 3.11 ANOVA table to estimate the intraclass–class correlation

Source	Sum of squares	Degrees of freedom	Mean squares	Variances
Between-patients	$S_{Patient}$	$p-1$	$V_{Patient} = \dfrac{S_{Patient}}{p-1}$	$= r\sigma^2_{Patient} + \sigma^2_{Error}$
Repeats (Within patients)	$S_{Repeats}$	$r-1$	$V_{Repeats} = \dfrac{S_{Repeats}}{r-1}$	$= p\sigma^2_{Repeats} + \sigma^2_{Error}$
Error	S_{Error}	$rp-r-p+1$	$V_{Error} = \dfrac{S_{Error}}{rp-r-p+1}$	$= \sigma^2_{Error}$
Total	S_{Total}	$rp-1$		

The *ICC* is the most commonly used method for assessing reliability with continuous data. It is also sometimes used for ordered categorical data that have more than four or five response categories. A reliability coefficient of at least 0.90 is often recommended if measurements are to be used for evaluating individual patients (Nunnally and Bernstein, 1994), although most QoL instruments fail to attain such a demanding level. For discriminating between groups of patients, as in a clinical trial, it is usually recommended that the reliability should exceed 0.70, although some authors suggest that values of 0.60 or even 0.50 are acceptable. The principal effect of using measurements with a low reliability in a clinical trial is that there will be a dilution of the between-treatments effect, and so the sample size will have to be increased accordingly to compensate.

Study size for reliability studies depends upon both the minimum acceptable reliability and the true reliability; for example, if it is desired to show that the reliability is above 0.7 and the anticipated reliability is 0.9, then two measurements on 18 patients would suffice; but if the anticipated reliability is only 0.8, then 118 patients are needed (Walter *et al.*, 1998).

TEST–RETEST RELIABILITY

If a patient is in a stable condition, an instrument should yield repeatable and reproducible results if it is used repeatedly on that patient. This is usually assessed using a test–retest study, with patients who are thought to have stable disease and who are not expected to experience changes due to treatment effects or toxicity. The patients are asked to complete the same QoL questionnaire on several occasions. The level of agreement between the occasions is a measure of the reliability of the instrument. It is important to select patients whose condition is stable, and to choose carefully a between-assessment time-gap that is neither too short nor too long. Too short a period might allow subjects to recall their earlier responses, and too long a period might allow a true change in the status of the subject. In diseases such as cancer, where one might anticipate that most treatments would cause QoL to vary over time in various ways, the requirement of stability often leads to patients being studied either pre- or post-treatment.

The range of acceptable values for test–retest reliability will depend upon the use to which the instrument will be put.

Example from the literature

Juniper *et al.* (1996) evaluated the Paediatric Asthma Quality of Life Questionnaire (PAQLQ) by examining reliability in children aged 7 to 17 who had stable asthma. The results are shown in Table 3.12, and it can be seen that all but one of the *ICC* values were above 0.80. These findings suggest that the PAQLQ has high test–retest reliability in stable patients.

Table 3.12   Test–retest reliability of the PAQLQ and its scales (Based on Juniper *et al.*, 1996)

	Within-subject SD	Between-subject SD	Intraclass correlation ICC
Overall QoL	0.17	0.73	0.95
Symptoms	0.22	0.84	0.93
Activities	0.42	0.96	0.84
Emotions	0.23	0.64	0.89

INTER-RATER RELIABILITY

Inter-rater reliability concerns the agreement between two raters. However, for QoL purposes we are principally interested in the patient's self-assessment. Many studies have shown that observers such as healthcare staff and patients' relatives make very different assessments from the patients themselves. Therefore, for validation of a QoL instrument, inter-rater reliability is usually of lesser concern than test–retest reliability.

Since the patients are usually regarded as the best assessor of themselves, there may be interest in determining whether observers are able to predict the patients' scores. This is particularly important when deciding whether to use proxies to assess QoL in patients who are unwilling, too ill, too young or unable to complete questionnaires. In this situation, absolute agreement between the two observers (patient and proxy) is not the issue of interest. Instead, one is usually more interested in prediction or estimation, using techniques such as regression analysis. However, if one does wish to assess agreement between two observers, the same methods may be used as for test–retest reliability.

Example from the literature

Many stroke survivors have cognitive and communication disorders, and may be unable to complete QoL questionnaires satisfactorily. Proxy ratings by "significant others" may be more informative than self-completed assessments. Sneeuw *et al.* (1997) studied a cohort of survivors from a larger study. Some were not able to communicate, but both self-reported and proxy ratings were obtained for those who could. The differences between proxy and patient SIP scores are shown in Table 3.13, together with the *ICC* values.

There were statistically significant differences between mean scores for the total SIP score and seven of the eleven subscales, with proxies generally rating patients as having more functional limitations than the patients claimed to have. However, Sneeuw *et al.* regarded the differences as small, and described the *ICC* values as ranging from "moderate for the eating scale (0.47) to excellent for ambulation (0.80) and body care and movement scales (0.82)".

Because of this good agreement between patient and proxy, it was concluded that non-communicative patients should be included in studies when proxies could be identified.

Table 3.13 Agreement between patient and proxy SIP scores in stroke survivors (Based on Sneeuw KCA, Aaronson NK, de Haan RJ and Limburg M (1997). Assessing quality of life after stroke: the value and limitations of proxy ratings. *Stroke*, **28**, 1541–1549)

	Difference (proxy – patient)			
	Mean	*SD*	Mean/*SD*	*ICC*
SIP subscales				
Sleep and rest	1.5	16.1	0.09	0.57
Emotional behaviour	2.7	15.4	0.18	0.59
Body care and movement	3.7	10.3	0.36	0.82
Household management	6.6	20.7	0.32	0.69
Mobility	5.1	16.5	0.31	0.66
Social interaction	6.2	13.9	0.45	0.52
Ambulation	0.1	12.2	0.01	0.80
Alertness behaviour	6.7	24.2	0.28	0.59
Communication	1.6	14.5	0.11	0.60
Recreation and pastimes	5.2	21.3	0.24	0.60
Eating	−0.4	9.4	−0.04	0.47
SIP dimension				
Physical	3.2	8.7	0.37	0.85
Psychosocial	4.5	11.6	0.39	0.61
Total SIP score	3.6	8.2	0.44	0.77

EQUIVALENT-FORMS RELIABILITY

Equivalent-forms reliability concerns the agreement between scores when using two or more instruments that are designed to measure the same attribute. For example, in principle a new QoL instrument could be compared against a well-established one or against a lengthier one. However, as with inter-rater reliability, agreement is often of lesser concern than is prediction; one of the instruments is usually regarded as the standard against which the other is being assessed, and linear regression analysis is more informative than a simple measure of agreement. It is less common to have two instruments that are believed to be equivalent to each other in QoL research than in areas such as education, where examination questionnaires often aim to use different, but equivalent, test items. When appropriate, the same methods as for test–retest reliability may be used. Ways of analysing method comparison studies are discussed by Bland and Altman (1986).

3.6 SENSITIVITY AND RESPONSIVENESS

Two closely related properties to repeatability are sensitivity and responsiveness. *Sensitivity* is the ability to detect differences between groups; for example between two treatment groups in a randomised clinical trial, or between groups of patients with mild disease and those with more severe disease. *Responsiveness* is the ability of a scale to detect changes. An instrument should not only be reliable, yielding reproducible results when a patient's condition is stable and unchanged, but in addition it should respond to relevant changes in a patient's condition. If disease progression causes deterioration in a patient's overall QoL, we would expect the measurements from a QoL instrument to respond accordingly. In addition, the measurement instrument should be sufficiently responsive to detect relevant changes when the condition of the patient is known to have altered. Similarly, if two groups of patients differ in their QoL, an instrument should be sufficiently sensitive to detect that change.

Both sensitivity and responsiveness are crucially important for any measurement, and a QoL instrument that lacks these properties will be less able to detect important changes in patients. Depending upon the intended application, sometimes one property is more important that the other. An *evaluative* QoL instrument intended for monitoring patients should be responsive to changes, and a *discriminative* one aimed at diagnosing individual patients will have to be more sensitive than a *discriminative* one that is intended for detection of group differences in clinical trials. However, if a QoL measurement can be shown to be sensitive to specific changes, then it is presumably also responsive to the condition causing those changes.

Sensitivity can be assessed by cross-sectional studies, but responsiveness is evaluated by longitudinal assessment of patients in whom a change is expected to occur. Disease-specific scales, being more focused and tailored towards problems of particular importance to the target group of patients, are generally more responsive than generic health status measures.

Two of the most widely used measures of sensitivity and responsiveness are the standardised response mean (*SRM*) and the effect size (*ES*), which are also used for indicating clinical significance (see Chapter 16). Briefly, the *SRM* is the ratio of the mean change to the *SD* of that change, and the *ES* is the ratio of the mean change to the *SD* of the initial measurement (Table 3.14). Thus *ES* ignores the variation in the change, whilst *SRM* is more similar to the paired *t*-test (except that the *t*-test uses the standard error, *SE*, rather than the *SD*). The *SRM* is more frequently used than *ES*.

Another approach is to argue that the most sensitive scale is the one most likely to result in statistically significant differences between groups of patients, and thus the scale with the largest *t*-statistic is the most sensitive. Therefore, when comparing two scales or items, the ratio of the two *t*-statistics would be a suitable measure. However, in practice, squared *t*-statistics are often used when calculating the ratios, giving the widely used measure that is called relative efficiency (*RE*) or relative validity (*RV*). When comparing more than two scales, it is customary to use the smallest of the *t*-statistics as the denominator when calculating the ratios, resulting in all coefficients being greater than 1, as illustrated in Table 3.15 (where *RE* is based on *F*-ratios). This amounts to defining the least sensitive scale as the baseline.

All of the above methods are based upon means and *SD*s, with an implicit assumption that the data follow a Normal distribution. Many QoL scales have a

Table 3.14   Summary of measures of sensitivity and responsiveness, for two measurements x_1 and x_2 with corresponding means $\bar{x}_1$, $\bar{x}_2$

Measure	Equation	Denominator
Effect size (*ES*)	$(\bar{x}_2 - \bar{x}_1)/SD(x_1)$	*SD* of baseline (x_1)
Standardised response mean (*SRM*)	$(\bar{x}_2 - \bar{x}_1)/SD(x_2 - x_1)$	*SD* of change
Paired *t*-statistic	$(\bar{x}_2 - \bar{x}_1)/SE(x_2 - x_1)$	*SE* of change
Responsiveness statistic (for stable patients)	$(\bar{x}_2 - \bar{x}_1)/SD^*(x_2 - x_1)$	*SD* of change
Relative efficiency, *RE* (Relative validity, *RV*) of two scales	Ratio of the squares of the *t*-statistics for the two scales	

non-Normal distribution, in which case medians and interquartile ranges may replace means and *SD*s. Unfortunately, little work has been carried out into this subject. It should also be noted that some scales are not only non-Normal, but may also suffer from "ceiling effects" in which a large number of patients place responses in the maximum category. This can compromise sensitivity and responsiveness.

Although Table 3.14 summarises the principal measures that may be encountered in the literature, there is controversy as to which is the best measure to use and a number of other alternatives have been proposed. As Wright and Young (1997) concluded when comparing five indices for their ability to rank responsiveness of different instruments: "Given that the indices provide different rank ordering, the preferred index is unclear."

When there are more than two groups or more than two measurements only the *RE* can be readily generalised. Just as the *t*-test is replaced by an *F*-test in ANOVA when comparing more than two means, so we can base the *RE* upon the ratio of two *F*-statistics when there are more than two groups. In the case of two groups, the *F*-statistic is identical to the squared *t*-statistic, and so these approaches are consistent with one another.

SENSITIVITY

Sensitivity is one of the most important attributes of an instrument. The usefulness of a measure is dependent upon its ability to detect clinically relevant differences. In clinical trials, therefore, sensitivity should be sufficient to detect differences of the order of magnitude that might occur between the treatment groups. The level of sensitivity that is adequate depends upon the intended application of the instrument. An instrument should be capable of distinguishing the differences of interest, using realistically-sized study groups. The more sensitive an instrument, the smaller the sample size that is necessary to detect relevant differences.

Usually, but by no means always, sensitive measurements will be reliable. This follows because reliability is usually a prerequisite for sensitivity. An unreliable measurement is one that has large background noise, and this will obscure the detection of any group differences that may be present. The converse need not apply; reliable measurements may lack sensitivity. For example, responses to the four-point single item "Do you have pain? (none, a little, quite a bit, very much)" may be highly reliable in the sense that repeated responses by stable patients are very consistent. However, such a question may be unable to detect small yet clinically important differences in pain levels unless there are large numbers of patients in each treatment group. To take an extreme situation, all patients in both groups could respond "quite a bit", with 100% reliability, and yet the patients in one group might have more pain than the other group. The pain scale would have zero sensitivity but perfect reliability. This example also serves to illustrate that "floor" and "ceiling" effects may be crucial. If most patients have very poor QoL and respond with the maximum, "ceiling" value, or with the minimum, "floor" value, the scale will not be sensitive and will not be capable of discriminating between different treatment groups.

Sensitivity is usually assessed by cross-sectional comparison of groups of patients in which there are expected to be QoL differences. Thus it is in practice closely related to known-groups validity. The main distinction is that with known-groups validity we are concerned with confirming that anticipated differences are present between groups of patients. Sensitivity analyses, on the other hand, aim to show that a reasonable-sized sample will suffice for the detection of differences of the magnitude that may exist between treatments (or other subdivisions of interest) and which are clinically relevant.

If the anticipated effects can be detected by a statistical significance test on the resulting data, this is often taken to be an indication of adequate sensitivity. However, it should be noted that statistical significance of group differences is also influenced by the selection of the patient sample. For example, a validation study might select a group of very ill patients to compare against patients who are disease-free. Then we know that there are undoubtedly group differences in QoL, and a significance test is of little practical interest. If the differences are large enough, a p-value of less than 0.0001 merely indicates that the sample size is also large enough to reject the possibility that the difference is zero. A sensitive instrument should be able to detect *small* differences, in *modest-sized* studies.

Example from the literature

When the HIV Overview of Problems Evaluation System (HOPES) was evaluated by Schag *et al.* (1992), the mean scores in various subgroups of patients were presented as "further evidence of the validity of the HOPES". Scores from the HOPES scales were compared against scales from other instruments including PACIS, MOS-HIV and POMS. Twelve out of the fifteen p-values were significant with $p < 0.0001$.

Rather than p-values, it would have been more informative to give the *RE* of the various scales.

On the one hand we want to be confident that the groups in the sensitivity study really do differ, but on the other hand we do not want to select groups that are known to have unusually large differences. For this reason, sensitivity studies that evaluate a new instrument should report a variety of comparisons, covering a range of situations that are typical of the areas of intended future application of the instrument.

It is perhaps easier to interpret the measures of sensitivity (and responsiveness) in terms of relative rather than absolute values. Different scales or instruments can then be compared, to determine which is the most sensitive. The *RE* provides a suitable comparative measure. Another advantage of the comparative approach is that it largely overcomes the criticism that measures of sensitivity are affected by the choice of patient sample and the actual group differences that are present. Thus the magnitude of the specific difference no longer matters; the most sensitive of the concurrently applied instruments is the one with the largest *RE*.

Example from the literature

Vickrey *et al.* (1997) compared the SF-36, a generic instrument, against the disease-specific QOLQ for multiple sclerosis (MS). They hypothesised that patients reporting least severe MS symptoms during the past year would report the best QoL

Table 3.15 shows the mean scores, *F*-ratios and *RE* for a subset of the scales. For all scales, the ordering of the mean scores tended to follow the hypothesised order. The SF-36 role limitation scale was defined as the reference group because it had the smallest *F*-ratio, and the *RE* values are calculated using this as the denominator. The physical function test of the SF-36 had the highest *RE*, but the SF-36 role limitations scales, pain scale, emotional well-being and energy scales all showed low *RE*.

The authors concluded: "Disease-targeted measures provide additional information about health-related quality of life beyond what is assessed by the SF-36." They also acknowledged that they did not evaluate responsiveness to change, and that "our findings may not generalise to all studies of MS, particularly longitudinal studies".

Table 3.15 Sensitivity of the SF-36 and the QOLQ in adults with multiple sclerosis: mean scores, ANOVA *F*-ratios, and *RE* (Based on Vickrey *et al.*, 1997)

Scale	Degree of MS symptom severity				*F*-ratio	*RE*
	None $n = 4$	Mild $n = 69$	Moderate $n = 73$	Extreme $n = 25$		
SF-36						
Physical function	71.3	55.0	25.6	8.5	25.7	23
Role limitations (physical)	75.0	45.3	26.1	13.0	7.2	7
Role limitation (emotional) [Reference group]	58.3	67.7	58.8	50.7	**1.1**	**1**
Pain	72.5	79.5	67.5	62.6	3.7	3
Emotional well-being	72.0	68.7	66.1	53.0	4.2	4
Energy	56.3	43.5	36.8	30.1	3.7	3
Social function	78.1	70.3	51.4	42.5	11.3	10
Current health	60.4	54.1	37.3	26.0	8.9	8
QOLQ for MS						
Self-selected physical problems	54.2	52.8	35.5	22.8	19.1	17
Mobility	68.3	69.2	48.3	34.4	17.2	16
Fatigue	65.6	60.7	48.5	35.3	8.5	8
Control	61.1	57.8	46.6	22.7	10.9	10
Emotional upset	63.1	60.6	57.1	41.8	4.7	4

Thus we can compare the different instruments or scales, and identify the ones with the highest sensitivity. The most sensitive ones will usually be the preferred scales for detecting differences between treatments, *provided* they are also thought to be clinically sensible and providing comprehensive coverage.

RESPONSIVENESS

Responsiveness is another important feature that is a requirement for any useful scale. It is closely related to sensitivity, but relates to changes *within* patients. In particular, if a patient's health status changes over time, can the instrument detect the changes? An instrument may be of limited applicability if it is not responsive to individual-patient changes over time. Responsiveness can also be regarded as providing additional evidence of validity of an instrument, since it confirms that the anticipated responses occur when the patient's status changes. A highly sensitive scale will usually also be highly responsive.

Example from the literature

Juniper *et al.* (1993) evaluated the properties of the Asthma Quality of Life Questionnaire (AQLQ). Patients were assessed at enrolment and after 4 and 8 weeks. At each of the two follow-up times, patients were shown their AQLQ scores from their previous visit. After each study period, the patients were classified into those with stable asthma and those whose asthma changed. This classification was based upon both clinical assessment including lung function tests, and the patients' global rating of change in overall QoL. For both groups of patients, the mean change in each AQLQ scale was calculated. The changes in AQLQ scores were scaled to be from −7 (a very great deal worse) through 0 (no change) to +7 (a very great deal better).

Table 3.16 shows the mean changes and *SD*s, and the results of a *t*-test comparing the difference between the two change scores. The authors described as "moderate" the mean QoL change of 1.06 in those whose asthma changed. Not only was this value statistically significantly different from the null hypothesis of no difference ($p < 0.001$), but the changes in the stable group were also significantly different from the changes in the other group (0.11 versus 1.06, $p < 0.001$). Similar patterns were seen for each of the scales, leading the authors to conclude that the AQLQ is responsive.

Table 3.16 Responsiveness of the Asthma Quality of Life Questionnaire (Based on Juniper *et al.*, 1993)

| | Change in AQLQ scores | | | | | |
| | Asthma stable | | Asthma changed | | | |
	Mean	*SD*	Mean	*SD*	Difference	*p*-value
Overall QoL	0.11	0.39	1.06	0.78	0.95	0.001
Activities	0.13	0.37	0.84	0.66	0.71	0.001
Symptoms	0.09	0.54	1.30	1.08	1.21	0.001
Emotions	0.09	0.46	1.18	1.01	1.09	0.001
Environment	0.07	0.45	0.66	0.72	0.59	0.007

Example from the literature

Beaton, Hogg-Johnson and Bombardier (1997) compared five generic instruments including the SF-36, NHP and SIP, in workers with musculoskeletal disorders. Table 3.17 shows the responsiveness analysis for some items from three instruments, for patients who reported no change between two repeated assessments (*ICC*) and for patients who reported a positive change (*ES* and *SRM*).

The authors concluded that the SF-36 was the most responsive of the instruments, and its reliability was adequate although it seemed to be less than for the other two instruments.

Table 3.17 Responsiveness analysis for selected scales of the SF-36, NHP and SIP (Based on Beaton *et al.*, 1997)

		Reliability (*ICC*)	Effect Size (*ES*)	Standardised response mean (*SRM*)
SF-36	Overall	0.85	0.67	1.09
	Pain	0.74	0.99	1.13
	Physical function	0.74	0.55	0.81
NHP	Overall	0.95	0.52	0.66
	Pain	0.87	0.57	0.70
	Physical function	0.76	0.48	0.64
SIP	Overall	0.93	0.42	0.66
	Physical function	0.94	0.39	0.51

3.7 CONCLUSIONS

This chapter has shown a variety of methods for examining the validity of measurement scores, to confirm that the scores appear to be consistent with their intended purpose. We also examined the assessment of the repeatability reliability, to ensure that the measurements appear to give consistent and repeatable results when applied to patients who are believed to be in a stable state. Finally, we showed ways of establishing that the scores are sufficiently sensitive or responsive to be able to detect differences between treatments or patients.

Sensitivity and responsiveness are amongst the most important attributes of a scale, because a non-sensitive scale is of little use for most practical applications. Furthermore, if a scale possesses face validity and is sensitive to the anticipated changes, it is likely to be measuring either the intended construct or something closely similar. However, a counter argument is that since many aspects of QoL are inter-correlated, sensitivity alone is not sufficient as confirmation of construct validity. If one dimension of QoL shows high sensitivity, it is likely that other scales correlated with this dimension will also show at least some degree of apparent sensitivity. Therefore, it is also important to consider other aspects of construct validity.

4 Multi-item Scales

Summary

In this chapter we consider methods that are specific to multi-item scales. We examine ways of exploring relationships amongst the constituent items of a multi-item scale, and between the individual items and the scale to which they are hypothesised to belong. Most of these methods rely upon examination of correlations. Do the items in a multi-item scale correlate strongly with each other? Do they correlate weakly with items from other scales? Do items correlate with the score of their own scale? Cronbach's α, multitrait-scaling analysis, and factor analysis are three of the most frequently used methods for exploring these correlations.

4.1 INTRODUCTION

Many QoL instruments contain one or more multi-item scales. For example, the HADS was designed with the intention that there would be anxiety and depression scales. Summary scores can be calculated for both scales. One of the reasons for using multiple items in a scale is that the reliability of the scale score should be higher than for a single item. For example, each of the seven items for anxiety in the HADS is assumed to reflect the same overall "true" anxiety score. Thus although individual measurements are imprecise and subject to random fluctuations, an average of several measurements should provide a more reliable estimate with smaller random variability. Therefore, each item in a multi-item scale should contribute to an increase in reliability; but does it? We describe methods of assessing *internal consistency* or *reliability for multi-item scales*. There is also the related assumption that the items in a scale reflect a single latent variable. We discuss how this *unidimensionality* can be examined.

Other aspects of *validation* can be explored when there are several multi-item scales in an instrument. The investigator should have a hypothetical model in mind when developing such instruments, and should be aware of the plausible relationships between the constructs and the items comprising them. Usually, items within any one scale should be highly correlated with each other but only weakly correlated with items from other scales—*construct validity*, including *convergent* and *discriminant validity* as discussed in Chapter 3, should apply also to items within a scale.

One important reason for constructing multi-item scales, as opposed to single-item measurements, is that the nature of the multiple items permits us to validate the consistency of the scales. For example, if all the items that belong to one multi-item scale are expected to be correlated and behave in a similar manner to each other, rogue items that do not reflect the investigator's intended construct can be detected. With single items, validation possibilities are far more restricted.

The methods of this chapter rely heavily upon the analysis of item-to-item correlations, and thus apply to Likert and other scales for which the theory of parallel tests applies. *Clinimetric* and other scales containing *causal variables* follow different rules. These scales are discussed at the end of this chapter.

4.2 SIGNIFICANCE TESTS

In statistical analyses we are frequently *estimating* values such as the mean value for a group of patients, the mean difference between two groups, or the degree of correlation (association) between two measurements. These estimates are invariably based upon patients in a study—that is, patients in a *sample*—and so the measurements observed and the estimated values calculated from them will vary from study to study. We might, for example, have carried out a randomised clinical trial to compare two treatments, and wish to determine whether the observed difference in response rates is large enough for us to conclude that there is definitely a treatment effect. The problem is, of course, that if another investigator replicates the study they are bound to obtain somewhat different values for the treatment response rates since they will be dealing with a different sample of patients. Consequently they may well obtain a very different value for the mean difference. Thus, if we have observed a fairly small difference in our study, there would not be very strong weight of evidence for claiming that we have definitely demonstrated that the treatments differ; it is quite possible that future trials could show that our findings were due to chance and not a treatment effect at all. The role of a statistical significance test is to quantify the weight of evidence, and we do so by calculating the probability that we could have observed at least as large a difference as that in our study, *purely by chance*.

One problem is that even if the two treatments have identical clinical effect, we may well observe an apparent difference in our particular sample of patients. Furthermore, it is impossible to prove statistically that two treatments do have identical effect; there is always a possibility that if measurements are taken more precisely, or if a larger number of patients is recruited, a difference (possibly very small) will eventually be detected. Hence it is convenient to start by assuming a *null hypothesis* of "no difference" between the treatments, and we assess the observed data to decide whether there is sufficient evidence to reject this null hypothesis. If there is not, we continue to *accept the null hypothesis* as still remaining plausible. This procedure is in fact very similar to international law: we assume innocence (null hypothesis) unless there is sufficient weight of evidence to ascribe guilt (rejection of the null hypothesis).

The formal method that we use to weigh the evidence is a *statistical significance test*, which calculates the probability, or *p-value*, that we could have observed such extreme results even if the null hypothesis is true. If the p-value is very small, we conclude that there is very little chance of having obtained such extreme results simply because of patient-to-patient variability, and thus we would *reject the null hypothesis* as being fairly implausible. In practice, most investigators take a *p*-value of 0.05 or less (that is, a chance of 5 in 100, or 5%) as implying that the results are unlikely to be due to chance, and therefore reject the null hypothesis. A p-value less than 0.01 (that is, 1 in 100, or 1%) indicates far more convincing evidence, and many would regard $p < 0.001$ as fairly conclusive evidence. However, it is important to recognise that out of all the many studies published each year where investigators claim "significant difference, $p < 0.05$", about 5% of publications will have reached this conclusion despite there being no treatment effect. This is because a p-value $<$ 0.05 simply means that roughly 5% of studies might have observed such extreme data purely by chance.

Chapter 8 shows how to calculate p-values for some commonly arising situations. Standard statistical books such as Altman (1991) provide more extensive details. Briefly, many tests take the form of equation (8.1), namely:

$$z = \frac{\text{Estimate}}{SE \text{ (Estimate)}}$$

where "Estimate" is, for example, the mean difference between treatments. SE is the *standard error*, or variability of the "estimate", that arises from the patient-to-patient variations. For many situations the calculated statistic, z, can be shown to be of one of the forms tabulated in the Appendix, Tables T1 to T5. The most common of these is the Normal distribution (Tables T1 and T2), and from T1 we see that a value of 1.96 corresponds to $p = 0.05$. Thus, if the value of z is greater than 1.96, we could "reject the null hypothesis with $p < 0.05$".

Chapter 14 discusses the impact of *sample size* upon significance tests, and the meaning of the *power* of a test.

4.3 CORRELATIONS

The methods described in this chapter make extensive use of correlations, both item-to-item and item-to-scale. For more extensive details about the use and misuse of correlations, readers are referred to Altman (1991).

Correlation coefficients are a measure of the degree of association between two continuous variables. The most common form of correlation is called Pearson's r, or the product-moment correlation coefficient. If there are n observations with two variables x_i and y_i (where i ranges from 1 to n),

$$r = \frac{\sum(x_i - \bar{x})(y_i - \bar{y})}{\sqrt{\sum(x_i - \bar{x})^2 \sum(y_i - \bar{y})^2}} \tag{4.1}$$

where $\bar{x}$ and $\bar{y}$ are the mean values of x and y. The equation is symmetric, and so it does not matter which variable is x and which y. Pearson's r measures the scatter of the observations around a straight line representing trend, and the greater the scatter the lower the correlation.

The values of r lie between -1 and $+1$. For uncorrelated points, $r = 0$, indicating no association between x and y. A value of $r = +1$ indicates perfect correlation, with all points lying on a straight line from bottom left to top right, that is, positive slope. Similarly, $r = -1$ for points on a straight line with negative slope.

RANGE OF VARIABLES

Many validation studies aim to include a heterogeneous group of patients with a variety of disease states and stages. However, correlations are greatly affected by the range of the variables. A homogenous group of patients will have similar symptomatology to each other, and the ranges of their scores for QoL items and scales may be less than those from a more heterogeneous group. Consequently, item-correlations for a homogenous group of patients will usually be much less than for a more heterogeneous group. Thus increasing sample heterogeneity is an easy way to "buy" higher correlations, but does not imply that the questions on the instrument are in any way more highly valid. Because of this, claims of high validity based upon correlations can be misleading, and may reflect merely sample heterogeneity; it is difficult to know what interpretation to place on the magnitude of the correlations. For instrument validation purposes, it is often easier to compare and contrast the *relative magnitude* of various correlations from within a single study than to interpret the absolute magnitude of correlations. Thus we emphasise such comparisons as whether an item correlates *more highly* with its own scale than with other scales. It remains appropriate to seek heterogeneous samples of patients for these comparisons.

SIGNIFICANCE TESTS

The null hypothesis of no association between x and y implies that there is truly zero correlation ($r = 0$) between them. The significance test compares the quantity

$$z = \frac{r}{\sqrt{(1 - r^2)/(n - 2)}} \tag{4.2}$$

against a t-distribution with $n - 2$ degrees of freedom.

In many contexts we know, *a priori*, that two variables are correlated. In such a situation it is of little practical interest to test a null hypothesis of $r = 0$, since that hypothesis is already known to be implausible. If a significance test is carried out and the result obtained happens to be "not significant", all we can say is that the sample size was too small. Conversely, if the sample size is adequate, the correlation coefficient will always differ significantly from zero. Thus a significance test for $r = 0$ should be carried out only when it is sensible to test whether r does indeed differ from zero.

CONFIDENCE INTERVALS

Instead of significance tests, it is usually far more informative to estimate the confidence interval (*CI*). Although r itself does not have a Normal distribution, there is a simple transformation that can convert r to a variable Z that does. This transformation is

$$Z = \frac{1}{2}\log_e\left(\frac{1 + r}{1 - r}\right) \tag{4.3}$$

Furthermore, it can be shown that, for a sample size of n, the standard error of Z is given by

$$SE(Z) = \frac{1}{\sqrt{n-3}} \qquad (4.4)$$

These equations assume that n is reasonably large—in practice, more than 50 observations.

A confidence interval for Z can then be calculated as for any data that follows a Normal distribution. For example, a 95% *CI* is

$$Z_{lower} = Z - 1.96 \times \frac{1}{\sqrt{n-3}} \text{ to } Z_{upper} = Z + 1.96 \times \frac{1}{\sqrt{n-3}} \qquad (4.5)$$

Finally, Z_{lower} and Z_{upper} can be converted back to obtain the *CI* for r itself, using

$$r_{lower} = (e^{2Z_{lower}} - 1)/(e^{2Z_{lower}} + 1), \qquad (4.6)$$

with a similar expression for r_{upper}.

Example

One correlation given by King, Dobson and Harnett (1996) and illustrated in Table 3.7 is $r = 0.58$ for the association between Current QoL and Pain using the FLIC. Her sample size was $n = 98$ and so

$$Z = \frac{1}{2}\log_e\left(\frac{1+0.58}{1-0.58}\right) = 0.6625 \text{ and } SE(Z) = \frac{1}{\sqrt{98-3}} = 0.1026.$$

The *CI* for Z is

$$Z_{lower} = 0.6625 - (1.96 \times 0.1026) = 0.4614 \text{ to}$$

$$Z_{upper} = 0.6625 + \frac{1.96}{\sqrt{98-3}} = 0.8636.$$

Therefore the 95% *CI* for r itself is

$$r_{lower} = (e^{2\times0.4614} - 1)/(e^{2\times0.4614} + 1) = 0.43 \text{ to}$$

$$r_{upper} = (e^{2\times0.8636} - 1)/(e^{2\times0.8636} + 1) = 0.70.$$

Hence we would expect that the true value of r is likely to lie between 0.43 and 0.70.

SIGNIFICANCE TEST TO COMPARE TWO CORRELATIONS

We can also use the Z-transformation and equations (4.3) and (4.4) for an approximate comparison of two correlation coefficients (r_1 and r_2) from samples of size n.

The correlations r_1 and r_2 are converted to Z_1 and Z_2, and the standard error of $Z_1 - Z_2$ is

$$SE(Z_1 - Z_2) = \sqrt{\frac{2}{n-3}} \qquad (4.7)$$

The difference $Z_1 - Z_2$ would be statistically significant (p-value < 0.05) if

$$z = \frac{Z_1 - Z_2}{SE(Z_1 - Z_2)} > 1.96. \qquad (4.8)$$

Example

In the FLIC scales example of Table 3.7, the correlation between Current QoL and Nausea scales is 0.37, and between Current QoL and Pain is 0.58. The Z-scores are

$$Z_1 = \frac{1}{2}\log_e\left(\frac{1+0.37}{1-0.37}\right) = 0.388, \ Z_2 = \frac{1}{2}\log_e\left(\frac{1+0.58}{1-0.58}\right) = 0.662.$$

Thus $Z_1 - Z_2 = 0.274$, and $SE(Z_1 - Z_2) = 0.415$. Thus $z = 0.274/0.145 = 1.89$. This is less than 1.96, and so is not statistically significant at the 5% level. Therefore we conclude that the observed difference between the correlations (0.58 and 0.37) could be due to chance.

However, equation (4.8) assumes that r_1 and r_2 come from independent samples. This is clearly not true for the above example, where r_1 and r_2 are correlations between items measured on one sample of patients. This will also usually be the case in examples from multitrait-scaling analysis. In this situation, any test based on equation (4.8) only provides a very rough guide as to statistical significance. For multitrait-scaling analysis, precise comparisons are unimportant and this approach provides an adequate, simple approximation.

RANK CORRELATION

The significance tests and CIs associated with Pearson's r require that at least one of the variables for the observations in the sample follow a Normal distribution. However, QoL items are frequently measured as categorical variables, often with a 4-point or 5-point scale, and these will not have a Normal distribution form. Depending upon the nature of the sample, there may also be many individuals with extreme scores. For example, patients with advanced disease may have uniformly high symptomatology, implying asymmetrically distributed ordered categories. In these circumstances Spearman's rank correlation, $r_{Spearman}$, is preferable.

To calculate $r_{Spearman}$ the values of the two variables are ranked in order, and then the calculation of equation (4.1) is performed using the values of the ranks in place of the original data. The distribution of $r_{Spearman}$ is similar to that of $r_{Pearson}$, and so the same methods can be utilised for confidence intervals and a test of whether two correlations differ significantly from one another.

CORRECTION FOR OVERLAP

When exploring the correlation structure of the QoL scales, we shall be interested in examining the relative magnitude of the correlations between the total scale score and each of the component items that form the scale. That will, for example, enable us to identify which items appear to be most consistent with the scale as a whole. However, when calculating the correlation between any one item, say x_1, and the total score of the scale in which the item is contained, a *correction for overlap* should be made. This is necessary because if the m items in a scale are $x_1, x_2, \ldots, x_m$, the correlation between, say, x_1 and the total $S = x_1+x_2+\ldots+x_m$ would be inflated since S also includes x_1 itself. Instead, x_1 should be correlated with the sum-score formed by omitting x_1 from the scale; that is, x_1 correlated with $S - x_1$.

Example

The cognitive functioning scale (CF) of the EORTC QLQ-C30 comprises the sum of two questions, difficulty in concentrating (q20) and difficulty remembering things (q25). Although it may make clinical sense to group these into a single scale, it is arguable that they represent two different dimensions. In a sample of 900 patients, the correlation between q20 and the CF scale score was 0.87, whilst that between q25 and CF it was 0.85. Both these correlations appear satisfactorily high. However, correcting for overlap, which amounts to correlating q20 with q25 because there are only two variables, the correlation is only 0.46.

In fact, it can be shown that if two completely independent (that is, uncorrelated), randomly distributed variables from a Normal distribution are combined into a single scale, the correlation between either variable and the sum score is approximately 0.71. However, this apparently high correlation is misleading. When the correction for overlap is applied, the "corrected" correlations will be approximately zero, confirming that neither of the two variables contributes to the scale as defined by the remaining (other) item.

4.4 CONSTRUCT VALIDITY

Multi-item scales open up a whole new range of techniques for construct validity beyond those described in Chapter 3. For the main part, we shall be making use of correlations: correlations between items in the same scale, correlations between an item and items in other scales, correlations between a scale score and its constituent items, and correlations between items and external scales or other external variables.

CONVERGENT AND DISCRIMINANT VALIDITY

Convergent and discriminant validity have been discussed in Chapter 3 in terms of relationships between different scales, or dimensions, of QoL. For multi-item scales, these concepts are extended to explore item-level relationships. In this setting, *convergent validity* states that items comprising any one scale should correlate with each other. This is closely related to internal consistency, and in effect declares that all items in a scale should be measuring the same thing. If theory leads us to expect two items to be similar, they should be strongly correlated; if they are not strongly correlated, that may imply that one or the other is not contributing to the scale score it was intended to measure. Convergence is often assessed by comparing the correlations between each item and the overall sum-score for the scale.

Equally important is *discriminant validity*, which states that if an instrument contains more than one scale, the items within any one scale should not correlate too highly with external items and other scales. Thus items that theory suggests are unrelated should not correlate strongly with each other. If an item correlates more strongly with those in another scale than its own, perhaps that item is more appropriately assigned to the other scale. If several items, or all the items, correlate highly with items in another scale, this may suggest there are insufficient grounds for declaring that two separate scales exist.

MULTITRAIT–MULTIMETHOD ANALYSIS

Multitrait–multimethod (MTMM) analysis, described in Chapter 3, can also be used to explore the relationships between items and scales. For this, the traits represent the items and the postulated scales become the methods. However, the number of item-to-item correlations can become quite large and unwieldy to present. Thus for the SF-36 there are 36 items, and each of these could be correlated with the other 35 items. An alternative approach is to restrict the focus upon item-to-scale correlations, which is termed *multitrait-scaling analysis*.

MULTITRAIT-SCALING ANALYSES

If an item *does not* correlate highly with the items from another scale, it may be expected to have a low correlation with the total score for that other scale. Similarly, if an item *does* correlate highly with other items in its own scale, it will also be correlated with the total sum-score for the scale. The principal objective of multitrait-scaling analysis is to examine these correlations, and thereby to confirm whether items are included in the scale with which they correlate most strongly, and whether the postulated scale structure therefore appears to be consistent with the data patterns. When calculating these correlations, the "correction for overlap" should be applied.

Widely used levels for acceptable correlation coefficients are the following. During initial scale development, *convergent validity* is supported if an item correlates moderately ($r = 0.3$ or greater) with the scale it is hypothesised to belong to, but when the instrument is undergoing final testing a more stringent criterion of at least 0.4 should be used. *Discriminant validity* is supported whenever a correlation between an item and its hypothesised scale is higher than its correlation with the other scales.

Example from the literature

McHorney *et al.* (1994) examined the convergent and discriminant validity of the SF-36, on 3445 patients with chronic medical and psychiatric conditions.

Table 4.1 shows examples of the correlations between individual items and the hypothesised scales, with correction for overlap as appropriate. The four items comprising RP (RP1, RP2, RP3 and RP4) had corrected correlations of 0.67, 0.70, 0.65 and 0.68 respectively with the RP scale (convergent validity). Each of these items had a significantly ($p < 0.05$) higher correlation with their own scale than with other scales (discriminant validity).

Table 4.1 Correlations between SF-36 items and hypothesised scales, for patients with chronic medical and psychiatric conditions (Based on McHorney *et al.*, 1994)

Item	PF	RP	BP	GH	VT	SF	RE	MH	TRAN
				Hypothesised scales					
RP1	0.58	0.67	0.55	0.42	0.43	0.41	0.28	0.20	0.12
RP2	0.51	0.70	0.51	0.42	0.47	0.46	0.40	0.27	0.17
RP3	0.44	0.65	0.46	0.39	0.51	0.39	0.41	0.28	0.12
RP4	0.49	0.68	0.56	0.41	0.50	0.45	0.39	0.32	0.14
BP1	0.53	0.54	0.70	0.44	0.46	0.43	0.27	0.29	0.21
BP2	0.53	0.61	0.70	0.44	0.48	0.51	0.33	0.33	0.19

PF = Physical functioning, RP = Role physical, BP = Bodily pain, GH = General health perceptions, VT = Vitality, SF = Social functioning, RE = Role emotional, MH = Mental health, TRAN = Reported change in health.

Unless there are clinical, other practical or theoretical grounds that outweigh the rules for convergent and discriminant validity, it is usually sensible to regard items that have poor convergent or discriminant properties as *scaling errors*. To allow for random variability and the sample size, the correlation coefficients may be compared using a statistical significance test. A *scaling success* is counted if the item to own-scale correlation is significantly higher than the correlations of the item to other scales. Similarly, if the item to own-scale correlation is significantly less than that of the item to another scale, a *definite scaling error* is assumed. If the correlations do not differ significantly a *possible scaling error* is counted. Usually, a *p*-value less than 0.05 is regarded as "significant" for this purpose.

Example from the literature

McHorney *et al.* (1994) examined correlations between all 36 items and the nine hypothesised scales of the SF-36. Table 4.2 summarises the convergent and discriminant scaling errors, and the scale homogeneity and internal consistency values. For example, in Table 4.1 the four RP items had correlations with their own scale of between 0.65 and 0.70, and the 32 correlations with other scales ranged from 0.12 (RP3 with TRAN) to 0.58 (RP1 with PF). Also, for each RP item, its own-scale correlation was compared against the correlations with the eight other scales, giving eight tests per item and a total 32 tests for the RP scale.

Tests confirmed that SF-36 items are more highly correlated with their own scales than with other scales. Thus in this sample the SF-36 items satisfy "scaling success" criteria.

Table 4.2 Item scaling tests: convergent and discriminant validity for SF-36 scales (Based on McHorney et al., 1994)

Scale	No. of items per scale	Convergent validity (range of correlations)	Discriminant validity (range of correlations)	Scaling Success[a]	Scaling success rate[b]	Homogeneity (average inter-item correlation)	Reliability (Cronbach's α)
PF	10	0.49–0.80	0.10–0.54	80/80	100	0.56	0.93
RP	4	0.65–0.70	0.12–0.58	32/32	100	0.57	0.84
BP	2	0.70	0.19–0.61	16/16	100	0.70	0.82
GH	5	0.38–0.72	0.09–0.58	40/40	100	0.42	0.78
VT	4	0.69–0.75	0.17–0.55	32/32	100	0.62	0.87
SF	2	0.74	0.20–0.62	16/16	100	0.74	0.85
RE	3	0.63–0.73	0.11–0.56	24/24	100	0.61	0.83
MH	5	0.65–0.81	0.11–0.59	40/40	100	0.64	0.90

[a] Number of convergent correlations significantly higher than discriminant correlations/The total number of correlations.
[b] Scaling success rate is the previous column as a percentage.

What sample size is necessary for multitrait-scaling analysis? If the sample size is too small, the correlations will be estimated imprecisely and this will be reflected by non-significant p-values for the significance tests comparing the correlation coefficients. Therefore, for scaling analyses, sample sizes of greater than 100 are recommended. In the above example, large sample size means that even small and unimportant differences in the level of correlations will be statistically significant, as shown in the column for scaling success.

The selection of an appropriate sample of patients is also important. A heterogeneous sample, with patients from a variety of disease states and with a range of disease severities, will result in a wide range of responses. This will tend to result in high correlations, especially for convergent validity. Thus most investigators aim to recruit a heterogeneous sample for their validation studies. To ensure that the instrument remains valid and sensitive for use with all types of patient, it is equally important to investigate performance in various subgroups.

Example

McHorney *et al.* (1994) checked convergent and discriminant validity of the SF-36 in 24 patient subgroups. They reported that convergent validity was excellent, and that scaling successes were high in nearly all subgroups. The worst groups were the small ones, namely psychiatric and complicated medical (87 patients), congestive heart failure (216), and recent myocardial infarction (107).

These results, together with other data they presented, led to the conclusion that scaling assumptions were well met across diverse medical and psychiatric groups.

Multitrait-scaling analysis is a simple yet effective method for checking that the pattern of the correlations corresponds to expectations, and that items have been assigned to the scale that they are most strongly correlated with. It also identifies items that are only weakly associated with the rest of their scale. However, statistical correlation can point only to areas in which there may be problems, and as we note in Section 4.6 it also assumes that the parallel tests model of Chapter 2 applies. Clinical sensibility should also be considered when interpreting seemingly inconsistent correlations.

Example from the literature

Bjordal *et al.* (1999) developed a 35-item questionnaire module for patients with head and neck cancer (Appendix E7), to be used together with the EORTC QLQ-C30. As one stage of the validation process, questionnaires were given to newly diagnosed head and neck cancer patients from Norway, Sweden and the Netherlands. Multitrait-scaling analysis was carried out for the combined sample, and separately by participating centre, disease groups (oral, pharynx, larynx), disease stage (early, advanced) and assessment times (before treatment, and up to five times during the subsequent year). Table 4.3 illustrates part of the pre-treatment multitrait-scaling analyses.

The authors noted that the last item of the *Pain scale* showed low correlations with its own scale (scaling errors) for most of the subanalyses, and somewhat higher correlations with the *Swallowing scale*, which makes clinical sense. Patients may have pain in the throat without having pain in the mouth, but if the patient reports pain in the throat, it is likely that swallowing problems are also present. However, it was felt important to retain this item in the *Pain scale*, in order to have a measure of pain in patients with hypopharyngeal and laryngeal cancer, and the scale was retained unchanged.

Thus multitrait-scaling analyses drew attention to potential problems, but upon further consideration it was decided that clinical sensibility indicated that these scaling errors could be safely ignored.

Example from the literature

Multitrait-scaling analysis of Table 4.3 indicated other potential problems. The *Nutrition scale* included seven items assessing various symptoms related to the oral cavity. Based upon clinical judgement, it was decided to join the two senses items into a separate *Senses scale*. The item assessing trouble eating had scaling errors in all subgroups. This item may assess the more social aspects of eating problems, and was moved to a *Social eating scale*.

Thus this time clinical considerations supported a modification of two scales and the creation of another.

Although the necessary calculations for multitrait-scaling analyses can be performed using standard statistical packages, care must be taken to ensure that correction for overlap is applied where appropriate. The MAP-R program (Ware *et al.*, 1998) is a computer package that has been designed specifically for multitrait-scaling and provides detailed item-scaling analyses.

FACTOR ANALYSIS AND DIMENSIONALITY

Factor analysis, which is a form of structural equation modelling (SEM), is one of the most important and powerful methods for establishing construct validity of psychometric tests. Whereas the methods of the previous sections rely to a large extent upon the scrutiny of inter-item and item-scale correlation matrices, factor analysis attempts to provide a formal method of exploring correlation structure. Although it provides a method for investigating the internal structure of an instrument, the results are difficult to interpret without a theoretical framework for the relationship between the items and scales. The simplicity of multitrait-scaling analysis, on the other hand, means that the results are easier to understand and more readily interpreted clinically.

In addition to its role in modelling complex latent structures, one particular aspect of factor analysis is important in the context of reliability assessment: it provides a means of examining and testing the dimensionality of scales. A scale is *unidimensional* if the items describe a single latent variable. Thus application of factor analysis should confirm that a single factor suffices to account for the item-variability in the scale. The term *homogeneity* is also often used as a synonym for

Table 4.3 Item-scale correlations for multitrait-scaling analysis of EORTC QLQ-H&N35, with data from head and neck cancer patients (Data from Bjordal et al., 1999)

Item	Pain	Swallowing	Nutrition	Speech	Social function	Body image and sexuality
			Hypothesised scales			
Pain scale						
Pain in mouth	0.75*	0.42	0.51	0.05	0.33	0.19
Pain in the jaw	0.61*	0.34	0.49	0.00	0.25	0.22
Soreness in the mouth	0.65*	0.40	0.45	0.01	0.28	0.20
Painful throat	0.37*	0.67	0.47	0.34	0.32	0.22
Swallowing scale						
Problems swallowing liquid	0.51	0.77*	0.43	0.27	0.28	0.11
Problems swallowing pureed food	0.51	0.83*	0.50	0.29	0.40	0.17
Problems swallowing solid food	0.58	0.71*	0.58	0.26	0.50	0.25
Choked when swallowing	0.23	0.37*	0.33	0.27	0.32	0.12
Nutrition scale						
Problems with teeth	0.31	0.14	0.25*	0.15	0.25	0.18
Problems opening mouth	0.48	0.37	0.41*	0.12	0.30	0.19
Dry mouth	0.29	0.23	0.34*	0.23	0.21	0.22
Sticky saliva	0.37	0.45	0.41*	0.33	0.28	0.15
Problems with sense of smell	0.13	0.09	0.28*	0.15	0.20	0.23
Problems with sense of taste	0.28	0.29	0.46*	0.19	0.33	0.21
Trouble eating	0.56	0.66	0.48*	0.24	0.61	0.25

Correlations marked * were corrected for overlap.

unidimensionality. However, confusingly, many authors regard homogeneity as meaning internal consistency as measured by Cronbach's α.

4.5 CRONBACH'S α AND INTERNAL CONSISTENCY

Internal consistency refers to the extent to which the items are interrelated. Cronbach's coefficient, $\alpha_{Cronbach}$, is one method of assessing internal consistency, and is the method used most widely for this purpose. It is also a form of reliability assessment, in that for parallel and certain related tests it is an estimate of reliability, and even for other tests it provides a lower bound for the true reliability. It is a function of both the average inter-item correlation and the number of items in a scale, and increases as either of these increases. Although internal consistency is often regarded as a distinct concept, it is closely related to convergent validity. Both methods make use of within-scale between-item correlations.

If a scale contains m items that describe a single latent variable θ, and the observed total score is S, then the reliability is defined as $R = \sigma_\theta^2/\sigma_S^2$, which is the ratio of the true score variance to the observed score variance. Now θ, being the latent variable, is unknown and so we do not have an estimate of its variance σ_θ^2. Hence the reliability cannot be determined but has to be estimated. For summated scales, Cronbach (1951) proposed the measure

$$\alpha_{Cronbach} = \frac{m}{m-1}\left(1 - \frac{\sum \text{Var}(x_i)}{\text{Var}(S)}\right). \tag{4.9}$$

Here, $\text{Var}(x_i)$ is the variance of the ith item in the scale, calculated from the sample of patients completing the QoL assessment, and $S = \Sigma x_i$.

The basis of Cronbach's α is that if the items were uncorrelated, $\text{Var}(S)$ would equal the sum of their individual variances, implying $\alpha_{Cronbach} = 0$. At the other extreme, if all the items are identical and have perfect correlation, all of the item variances would be equal and sum to the variance of the total score, making $\alpha_{Cronbach} = 1$. Cronbach's α can be shown to underestimate the true reliability, and is therefore a conservative measure. Coefficients above 0.7 are generally regarded as acceptable for psychometric scales, although it is often recommended that values should be above 0.8 (good) or even 0.9 (excellent). For individual patient assessment, it is recommended that values should be above 0.9.

Perhaps one of the most useful applications of Cronbach's α is in the development of scales and selection of items. If Cronbach's α changes little when an item is omitted, that item is a candidate for removal from the scale. Conversely, a new item may be worth including if it causes a substantial increase. However, in order to assess the benefit of adding an extra item we should first estimate the expected change in Cronbach's α due to lengthening the scale. This is expressed by the Spearman–Browne "prophecy formula" which relates the original Cronbach's α, written as α_0, and the relative increase in number of scale items to predict the resultant $\alpha_{Cronbach}$ for the longer scale:

$$\alpha_{Cronbach} = \frac{k\alpha_0}{1 + (k-1)\alpha_0}, \tag{4.10}$$

where k is the ratio of the number of items in the new scale over the number in the original scale. Thus merely having a longer scale automatically inflates Cronbach's α.

Example

> If, initially, the value of Cronbach's α is $\alpha_0 = 0.6$ for a scale, then (assuming all items have approximately similar inter-item correlations) doubling the length of the scale by including additional items would give a value of $k = 2$. This results in an increase of Cronbach's α to $\alpha_{Cronbach} = 2 \times 0.6/[1 + (2 - 1) \times 0.6] = 0.75$. In contrast, halving the number would result in $\alpha_{Cronbach} = 0.5 \times 0.6/[1 + (0.5 - 1) \times 0.6] = 0.43$.

Cronbach himself, in 1951, recognised the need to adjust for the number of items. He commented that a quart of homogenised milk is no more homogenised than a pint of milk, although $\alpha_{Cronbach}$, the measure of homogeneity, does increase according to the size (number of items) of a scale. Since Cronbach's α increases as the number of items in the scale is increased, high values can be obtained by lengthening the scale. Even the simple expedient of adding duplicate items with closely similar wording will suffice to increase it. This has led many to question whether it is sensible to specify criteria for acceptable levels of Cronbach's α without specifying the number of items in the scale.

Another consequence of the Spearman–Browne formula, equation (4.10), is that if the individual items in the scale are good estimators of the latent variable in the sense that they estimate it with little error, they will have high correlations and few items are needed in the scale. On the other hand, if the items have much error, many items will be needed.

The theory behind Cronbach's α assumes that the scale relates to a single latent variable, and is therefore unidimensional. Although it is often assumed that $\alpha_{Cronbach}$ is itself a check for dimensionality, and that a high result implies a unidimensional scale, this is incorrect. Results can be misleadingly high when calculated for multidimensional scales. Therefore dimensionality should always be checked by, for example, using factor analysis.

The consequences of multidimensionality can be readily seen: consider a scale consisting of the sum of bodyweight and height. Although this would have very high test–retest repeatability, since neither measurement varies very much in stable subjects, Cronbach's α—supposedly an indicator of reliability—would not be correspondingly high because these items are only moderately correlated.

It can be shown that Cronbach's α is a form of intra-class correlation (*ICC*, Chapter 3), and thus it can also be estimated using ANOVA. Therefore the issues regarding correlations will also apply. Thus a wide and heterogeneous range of patients will tend to result in higher values, whilst the values will be low if the patients are similar to each other. Since it is almost always obvious that Cronbach's α must be greater than zero, significance tests of the null hypothesis that $\alpha_{Cronbach} = 0$ are usually irrelevant although often reported. Provided the sample size is large enough, the p-value will invariably indicate statistical significance; a non-significant result indicates merely that the sample size is inadequate. More sensible, and far more informative, are confidence intervals. These are most conveniently estimated using the so-called "bootstrap" methods that are available in statistical packages such as STATA.

Example from the literature

> Table 4.2 showed Cronbach's α for the SF-36 obtained by McHorney *et al.*
> (1994). The smallest value is 0.78, and all other values are above 0.8, indicating
> that the scales show good internal reliability.

Example from the literature

> The EORTC QLQ-C30 (version 1.0) contained two items that assessed role
> functioning. These were "Are you limited in any way in doing either your work
> or doing household jobs?" and "Are you completely unable to work at a job or
> to do household jobs?" and took response options "No" and "Yes". Low
> values of Cronbach's α had been reported, ranging from 0.52 to 0.66. There
> were also concerns about the content validity because it was felt that role
> functioning ought to encompass hobbies and leisure-time activities. Two new
> questions were introduced, replacing the original questions. These were "Were
> you limited in doing either your work or other daily activities?" and "Were you
> limited in pursuing your hobbies or other leisure-time activities?" The binary
> response options were changed into four-category scales.
>
> Osoba *et al.* (1997) evaluated these modifications in patients who were assessed
> before, during and after chemotherapy or radiotherapy. With questions in the
> original format, Cronbach's α varied between 0.26 and 0.67. The revised items
> showed considerably higher internal reliability (0.78 to 0.88) and were accepted
> for the QLQ-C30 (version 2.0). Whilst the rewording may have contributed to
> these changes in reliability, a more likely explanation is that increasing the
> number of categories from two to four accounted for the differences.

4.6 IMPLICATIONS FOR CAUSAL ITEMS

Most methods generally assume that the items in a scale are parallel tests—that is,
that all the items in any one scale are selected so as to reflect the postulated latent
variable, and each item is presumed to be measuring much the same thing. On that
basis, the items should be correlated with each other. Sometimes this assumption is
either untrue or inappropriate. In particular, many QoL scales contain symptoms or
other causal variables. As we have seen in Chapter 2, the correlations between such
items can be misleading; these correlations do not indicate QoL constructs, but are
often merely consequences of symptom clusters arising from the disease or its
treatment. For example, in cancer patients, hair loss and nausea may both be
associated with chemotherapy and therefore highly correlated, even though in terms
of QoL concepts they may be unrelated to one another. The methods of this chapter
are usually inappropriate for clinimetric or other scales containing causal items.

Thus convergent and discriminant validity seem sensible criteria for instrument
validity when one is considering scales made from *indicator variables*. When *causal
variables* are present, neither criterion need apply. It may be clinically sensible to
retain certain causal items in a single QoL subscale even though they are only

---

Consequences for clinimetric and other scales containing causal items:

- Basic properties of measurement scales, such as content validity, sensitivity, responsiveness and test–retest reliability, are invariably important when devising any QoL instrument.

- Assessment of construct validity, including convergent and discriminant validity, is mainly based upon analysis of item-correlation structures, and is less relevant when causal items are involved.

- Cronbach's α is based upon item-to-item correlations, and is largely irrelevant for scales containing causal items.

Alternative criteria for clinimetric scales or scales with causal items:

- Clinical sensibility. This is equivalent to face validity.

- Comprehensive coverage of items.

- Emphasis upon items that patients rate as important.

- Emphasis upon items that patients experience frequently.

Figure 4.1   Clinimetric scales and scales with causal items

weakly correlated with each other and therefore have low convergent validity. Equally, it might make sound clinical sense to disregard high correlations and treat some causal items as comprising two or more distinct scales, irrespective of discriminant validity.

High internal consistency, as measured by Cronbach's α, is a fundamental requirement for instruments that are based upon indicator variables and designed upon the principles of parallel tests. When scales contain causal variables, there may be low convergent correlations and therefore low internal consistency. Similarly, definitions of reliability do not work well for items that have a causal relationship with the latent variable of interest.

The implications for causal items and clinimetric scales are summarised in Figure 4.1.

Example

An example of the problems presented by items that are not parallel tests was shown for the study of Bjordal *et al.* (1999) in Table 4.3. Painful throat had low convergent correlation with its own scale (0.37), and high correlation with both swallowing and nutrition scales.

Despite this, it was considered clinically sensible to have a single pain scale that contains questions about disease- or treatment-related pain in various parts of the body. A pain scale that did not include throat pain would have poor content validity from a clinical point of view. Low convergent and low discriminant validity are explained by these pain items being causal variables that arose as consequences of the cancer or its treatment.

In clinimetric scales the items are chosen primarily from the perspective of high content validity, and the internal reliability can be low. Properties such as sensitivity and responsiveness are also of paramount importance.

Example

> Apgar (1953) scores, mentioned in Chapter 2, are a well-known and useful index for the health of newborn babies. The items included (heart rate, respiratory rate, reflex responses, and the skin colour and muscle tone) were selected on the basis of being important yet distinct prognostic indicators. After many years of use, the Apgar score has been found to be an effective indicator of neonatal health. Despite this, the constituent items may have weak correlations and Cronbach's α is low.

It is also often inappropriate to use traditional psychometric methods when scales are designed on the basis of an item response model. In this case, items are deliberately chosen so as to be of varying difficulty, and the value of Cronbach's α, for example, may be misleading.

4.7 CONCLUSIONS

The methods described constitute a set of powerful tools for checking the validity of multi-item scales, to confirm that they appear to be consistent with the postulated structure of an instrument. However, confirming validity is never proof that the instrument, or the scales it contains, are really tapping into the intended constructs. Poor validity or reliability can suffice to indicate that an instrument is *not* performing as intended. Demonstration of good validity, on the other hand, is a never-ending process of collecting more and more information showing that there are no grounds to believe the instrument inadequate.

However, the techniques of this chapter rely upon analysis of inter-item correlations, and are suitable only for scales or subscales containing solely indicator variables. When QoL scales contain causal items, the intercorrelations between these items arise mainly because of disease or treatment effects, not because of association with the latent variable for QoL. This renders correlation-based methods inappropriate.

However, sometimes it is possible to use clinical judgement to select a group of symptoms that are expected to be interrelated, and correlation methods may be suitable within this restricted subset of items. For example, several symptoms related to digestive problems could be selected. Even though these are causal items for QoL changes, they might also represent a coherent set of items reflecting, say, a disease-related symptom cluster. They can then be regarded as indicator variables for disease state, and the methods of this chapter could be applied so as to produce a disease-based digestive function score. The validation methods for multi-item scales can therefore be used as a form of subscale validation, provided it is not claimed that this is evidence of a digestive construct indicating a QoL state.

For all instruments, clinical sensibility is crucial; this encompasses face and content validity, and comprehensive coverage of all important items. To be of practical value for clinical purposes or in randomised trials, sensitivity, responsiveness and test–retest repeatability are also extremely important. But the role of other aspects of validation is primarily to accrue evidence that the items behave in a sensible manner, and that the scales are consistent with the postulated constructs.

5   Factor Analysis

Summary

Factor analysis is a powerful technique for exploring the item correlations during scale validation. We illustrate factor analysis techniques with a detailed example of its application to the HADS, showing interpretation of the typical output that is obtained from most computer packages. We also discuss the reasons for using factor analysis in scale development and scale validation, and the limitations of this approach. Finally, we describe the more general approach of structural equation modelling.

5.1   INTRODUCTION

The methods of Chapter 4 were concerned primarily with examining item-to-item correlations in order to evaluate whether their patterns are consistent with the hypothesised scale structure. Factor analysis, on the other hand, can be used either as an automatic procedure to explore the patterns amongst the correlations (*Exploratory Factor Analysis*, or EFA), or as a *Confirmatory method* (CFA) for testing whether the correlations correspond to the anticipated scale structure. Thus factor analysis plays a major role in construct validation. Although CFA is the more flexible and powerful of the two, EFA is the form most commonly seen in QoL research because it does not require specification in advance of the details of the scale structures and the inter-item relationships. However, both EFA and CFA are concerned with detecting and analysing patterns in the inter-item correlation matrix.

5.2   CORRELATION PATTERNS

Since correlations provide the basic information for factor analysis, it is appropriate to start by considering a correlation matrix in which the correlations between all pairs of items are displayed. Since the correlation of x against y is the same as the correlation of y against x, we only need to show the "lower triangle" of correlations, as in Table 5.1.

The postulated structure of the HADS is relatively simple, with only two seven-item scales for anxiety and depression, and so it provides a convenient example for examining the techniques associated with factor analysis.

Example

The HADS questionnaire was completed by patients in many of the UK Medical Research Council (MRC) randomised clinical trials of cancer therapy. The results from six MRC trials have been pooled, yielding a dataset of 1952 patients with bladder, bronchus, colorectal, head and neck, and lung cancers of varying stages from early to advanced. Table 5.1 shows the (Pearson) correlation matrix for all pairs of items. Since half of the HADS items are deliberately worded positively and half negatively, the "negative" items have been recoded so that in all cases a response of 0 is the most favourable and 3 is least favourable. By making the scoring consistent, it becomes easier to interpret the correlations: the highly related items should have high (positive) correlation.

There are clearly many fairly highly correlated items, with correlations between 0.4 and 0.6. Although from prior information we know that the odd-numbered questions (Q_1, Q_3, Q_5, . . .) are the ones intended to reflect anxiety, it is difficult to see the pattern in this correlation matrix. However, rearranging the correlation matrix as in Table 5.2 makes the pattern very much clearer.

Items belonging to the two postulated scales are shown shaded in grey triangles, anxiety being the upper area and depression the lower. It is now clear that there are fairly high (greater than 0.4, say) correlations amongst most items within the anxiety scale except Q_{11} which is noticeably weaker, and similarly amongst the depression scale items. It is also reassuring to note that the unshaded rectangular area has lower correlations, which is consistent with the hypothesis that the anxiety items are only less strongly correlated with the depression items.

Tables 5.1 and 5.2 show the usual Pearson correlation coefficient, r. Since the HADS items take four-point responses, they are not strictly from a Normal

Table 5.1 Pearson correlations for the HADS questionnaire, from 1952 patients in MRC trials BA09, CR04, CH01, CH02, LU12 and LU16

	Q_1	Q_2	Q_3	Q_4	Q_5	Q_6	Q_7	Q_8	Q_9	Q_{10}	Q_{11}	Q_{12}	Q_{13}	Q_{14}
Q_1	1.0													
Q_2	0.31	1.0												
Q_3	0.54	0.26	1.0											
Q_4	0.34	0.47	0.36	1.0										
Q_5	0.56	0.27	0.60	0.36	1.0									
Q_6	0.41	0.50	0.37	0.58	0.41	1.0								
Q_7	0.50	0.41	0.41	0.43	0.43	0.47	1.0							
Q_8	0.28	0.52	0.23	0.33	0.27	0.37	0.33	1.0						
Q_9	0.49	0.20	0.58	0.28	0.52	0.32	0.38	0.17	1.0					
Q_{10}	0.30	0.40	0.27	0.38	0.27	0.41	0.34	0.36	0.23	1.0				
Q_{11}	0.34	0.15	0.32	0.18	0.32	0.19	0.34	0.16	0.30	0.17	1.0			
Q_{12}	0.33	0.59	0.32	0.54	0.31	0.52	0.44	0.44	0.26	0.45	0.17	1.0		
Q_{13}	0.54	0.26	0.60	0.33	0.56	0.37	0.43	0.23	0.57	0.33	0.38	0.30	1.0	
Q_{14}	0.30	0.42	0.27	0.44	0.30	0.47	0.40	0.31	0.30	0.36	0.19	0.42	0.31	1.0

Table 5.2 Correlations from Table 5.1 rearranged corresponding to the postulated subscales of anxiety (odd-numbered items) and depression (even-numbered)

	Anxiety							Depression						
	Q_1	Q_3	Q_5	Q_7	Q_9	Q_{11}	Q_{13}	Q_2	Q_4	Q_6	Q_8	Q_{10}	Q_{12}	Q_{14}
Q_1	1													
Q_3	0.54	1												
Q_5	0.56	0.60	1											
Q_7	0.50	0.41	0.43	1										
Q_8	0.49	0.58	0.52	0.38	1									
Q_{11}	0.34	0.32	0.32	0.34	0.30	1								
Q_{13}	0.54	0.60	0.56	0.43	0.57	0.38	1							
Q_2	0.31	0.26	0.27	0.41	0.20	0.15	0.26	1						
Q_4	0.34	0.36	0.36	0.43	0.28	0.18	0.33	0.47	1					
Q_6	0.41	0.37	0.41	0.47	0.32	0.19	0.37	0.50	0.58	1				
Q_8	0.28	0.23	0.27	0.33	0.17	0.16	0.23	0.52	0.33	0.37	1			
Q_{10}	0.30	0.27	0.27	0.34	0.23	0.17	0.33	0.40	0.38	0.41	0.36	1		
Q_{12}	0.33	0.32	0.31	0.44	0.26	0.17	0.30	0.59	0.54	0.52	0.44	0.45	1	
Q_{14}	0.30	0.27	0.30	0.40	0.30	0.19	0.31	0.42	0.44	0.47	0.31	0.36	0.42	1

distribution and other measures of correlation may be more suitable, as discussed in Section 5.8. Usually Pearson's r is adequate except in extreme situations, and similar results are in fact obtained when using the alternative methods with this HADS dataset.

A measure closely related to correlation is "covariance". Most people find correlations easier to interpret since, unlike covariances, they are scaled from -1 to $+1$. However, factor analysis programs often use the corresponding covariances instead, and the underlying theory of factor analysis is more closely based upon covariances. One may draw an analogy with standard deviation (SD) versus variance; there is a direct relationship (square-root) between SD and variance, but most people find SD is the easier measure to interpret even though variances are more convenient for generalisation and therefore used for ANOVA (analysis of variance). Hence we shall describe and illustrate the *correlation* structure of QoL data even though many factor analysis programs are in fact based upon analysis of covariances.

5.3 PATH DIAGRAMS

One way to represent the many interrelationships between the items is by means of a path diagram. Adopting standard conventions, we use circles to represent the latent variables or constructs, and boxes for the manifest variables or observable items. Lines link the items to their corresponding latent variable. Furthermore, if a construct is associated with particular items in the sense that a high value of the construct implies a high level for the item, we add directional arrows to the lines. Thus we regard the construct as implying a certain value of the item, or we might say the construct is "manifested" by the responses to the items. In extreme cases, the latent variable may be said to "cause" an outcome value for the item.

Example

> The path diagram corresponding to postulated structure of the HADS is shown in Figure 5.1. Thus if the anxiety has a high value, we would expect Q_1, Q_3, Q_5, Q_7, Q_9, Q_{11} and Q_{13} all to reflect this by manifesting high values. That is, we would expect reasonably strong correlations between these items and anxiety— although since anxiety is a latent variable, we do not know its value and cannot calculate this correlation directly. Furthermore, in any dataset consisting of patients with a range of levels of anxiety, we would expect all of the corresponding items Q_1, Q_3, ..., Q_{13} to reflect those levels, so that these items should show reasonably high correlations with each other. However, the lack of a direct link between, say, Q_1 and Q_3 indicates that if anxiety is constant (that is, if all patients have the same level of anxiety) then Q_1 and Q_3 would be uncorrelated; this is called "local independence". As we shall see in Chapter 6, local independence is crucial for item response theory, although factor analysis appears somewhat more robust against violation of this assumption.

When two latent variables are expected to be correlated with one another, a curved line with arrows at both ends is used to link them. This is illustrated in Figure 5.1, where anxiety and depression are linked in this manner. Thus these variables are assumed to be correlated, since persons with higher levels of anxiety are more likely also to have higher levels of depression, and vice versa. Without this correlation between anxiety and depression, there would have been no link between, say, Q_1 and Q_2, and then we would have expected those items to have zero correlation with one another. Instead, given the relationship between anxiety and depression, we would expect some degree of correlation between Q_1 and Q_2.

This example is a relatively simple one, with only seven items for each of two postulated constructs. If we were analysing a more general QoL questionnaire there might be far more items and also more constructs.

5.4 FACTOR ANALYSIS

Factor analysis is a statistical technique that examines a correlation matrix such as that in Table 5.2, and attempts to identify groups of variables such that there are strong correlations amongst all the variables within a group, but weak correlations between variables within the group and those outside the group. Thus since the model assumed in Figure 5.1 implies that each of the seven anxiety items are correlated with each other, factor analysis should identify these as constituting one "factor". If these items were indeed highly correlated, as we hope, the scale would be described as having "strong internal structure". Similarly, the seven depression items should form another factor. In principle one might be able to inspect a correlation matrix by eye, and verify whether this structure pertains. In practice this is usually difficult to do for all but the simplest of models, and so we often rely upon automatic techniques like factor analysis to explore the data for us.

Factor analysis as described here uses the correlation (or covariance) matrix as its staring point, and does not make use of any prior knowledge about the structure, or postulated structure, of the questionnaire. Therefore this is *exploratory factor analysis*.

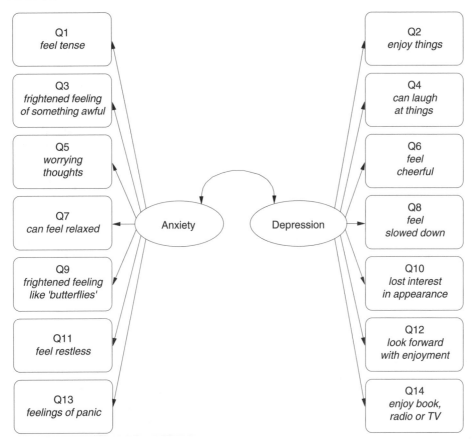

Figure 5.1   Postulated structure of the HADS questionnaire

5.5   FACTOR ANALYSIS OF THE HADS QUESTIONNAIRE

We explain how factor analysis works by using an illustrative example. The correlation matrix presented in Table 5.1 showed the interrelationships of the HADS items. Although pre-treatment data were used for this example, we would expect to find very similar results if during- or post-treatment assessments were considered. A standard statistical program, STATA (1999), is used to see how well the hypothesised factor structure is recovered. Very similar output would be obtained from most other packages. Most of the STATA default options are accepted. In general that might not be too wise; as will be discussed later, there are many choices to be made when carrying out factor analysis, and many of them can quite severely affect the analyses.

EIGENVALUES AND EXPLAINED VARIANCE

Most computer programs start by assuming there might be as many factors as there are variables (items). If each item proved to be completely independent of all other items, we would have to regard each item as a separate construct or latent variable.

In that case it would be inappropriate to construct any summary scale score, and the data would be summarised by factors that are the same as the original variables. This represents the "full model" with the maximal number of factors. Thus factor analysis programs commence by calculating the importance of each of the possible factors.

The *eigenvalues*, or *latent roots*, are obtained by matrix algebra; their precise mathematical meaning need not concern us, but a rough interpretation is that the eigenvalues are a measure of how much of the variation in the data is accounted for by each factor. Therefore the eigenvalues indicate the importance of each factor in explaining the variability and correlations in the observed sample of data. Usually these eigenvalues are scaled such that the total variability of the data is equal to the number of variables, and the sum of the eigenvalues will equal the number of items. The proportion of total variance explained by each factor is obtained by expressing the eigenvalues as percentages.

Most factor analysis programs will optionally use the eigenvalues to determine how many factors are present. A commonly used criterion is the so-called *eigenvalues greater than 1* rule. Applying this rule, the number of distinct factors is assumed to be equal to the number of eigenvalues that exceed 1.0.

Example

Table 5.3 shows the eigenvalues relating to the data in Table 5.1, with one row for each of the $n = 14$ potential factors. The eigenvalues sum to n. The proportion of variance explained is then obtained by dividing the eigenvalue by n; thus for the first factor, 5.84/14 = 0.42 or 42%. The first two factors account for 54% of the total variation. Using the "eigenvalues > 1.0" rule, there are assumed to be two factors. This conveniently confirms our prior expectation of two latent constructs.

Table 5.3 Factor analysis of Table 5.1: eigenvalues and proportion of variance explained

			Variance explained:	
Factor	Eigenvalue	Difference	Proportion	Cumulative
1	5.84	4.08	0.42	0.42
2	1.76	0.94	0.13	0.54
3	0.82	0.07	0.06	0.60
4	0.75	0.07	0.05	0.65
5	0.68	0.07	0.05	0.70
6	0.61	0.04	0.05	0.75
7	0.57	0.06	0.04	0.79
8	0.51	0.07	0.04	0.83
9	0.44	0.00	0.03	0.86
10	0.43	0.03	0.03	0.89
11	0.40	0.00	0.03	0.92
12	0.40	0.03	0.03	0.95
13	0.37	0.00	0.03	0.98
14	0.37	–	0.02	1.00

FACTOR LOADINGS

Having decided upon the number of factors in the model, the next stage is to obtain the factor pattern matrix, or factor loadings, corresponding to the factor solution. These numbers indicate the importance of the variables to each factor, and are broadly equivalent to regression coefficients. The loadings are also equal to the correlations between the factors and the items.

Example

The output continues with Table 5.4, which gives the factor pattern matrix corresponding to the two-factor solution. At first sight Table 5.4 does not look too promising: the first factor has broadly similar loadings for all variables, and is thus little more than an average of all 14 items. Factor 2 is difficult to interpret, although in this case it is noticeable that alternate items have positive and negative loadings.

Table 5.4 Factor loadings (unrotated) of two-factor solution for data in Table 5.1

Variable	Factor 1	Factor 2
Q_1	0.70	−0.31
Q_2	0.63	0.48
Q_3	0.69	−0.42
Q_4	0.67	0.29
Q_5	0.69	−0.36
Q_6	0.71	0.25
Q_7	0.70	−0.01
Q_8	0.54	0.38
Q_9	0.62	−0.46
Q_{10}	0.57	0.28
Q_{11}	0.44	−0.33
Q_{12}	0.67	0.42
Q_{13}	0.69	−0.41
Q_{14}	0.60	0.25

ROTATION

It can be shown mathematically that the initial solution is not the only one possible. Other two-factor solutions are equally good at explaining the same percentage of the variability, and in fact there are an infinite variety of alternative solutions. In general the initial factor solution will rarely show any interpretable patterns. Therefore it is usual to "rotate", or transform, the factors until a solution with a simpler structure is found. One of the most commonly used methods is "varimax", although many alternatives have been proposed. Briefly, varimax attempts to minimise the number of variables that have high loadings on each factor, thereby simplifying the overall structure. Thus we hope to obtain a new set of loadings for the factors, with fewer items having high values for each factor, but with the same amount of the total variance still explained by the factors.

Example

If we proceed to use varimax rotation in STATA, we obtain Table 5.5. To simplify the reading of Table 5.5, factor loadings above 0.4 have been shaded.

The anticipated relationships are apparent: the first factor relates to questions 2, 4, 6, (7), 8, 10, 12 and 14, whilst the second factor has questions 1, 3, 5, 7, 9, 11 and 13. Variable 11 in Factor 2 is weaker than most other items (loading of 0.55), which corresponds to the low correlations that were noted in Table 5.2. However, most noticeable is variable 7, which is included weakly in both factors. Inspecting Table 5.2 again, we see that Q_7 (fourth column in Table 5.2) has correlations above 0.4 with several depression items (Q_2, Q_4, Q_6, Q_{12} and Q_{14}), explaining its appearance in the depression factor. Apart from item Q_7, the fit may be regarded as extremely good and provides adequate confirmation of the postulated structure of the HADS. Others have found that Q_7, "I can sit at ease and feel relaxed", is anomalous and does not appear to perform very well; it must be a candidate for revision in any future version of HADS.

Table 5.5 Rotated matrix of factor loadings from Table 5.4: varimax rotation

Variable	Factor 1	Factor 2
Q_1	0.27	0.71
Q_2	0.79	0.11
Q_3	0.19	0.78
Q_4	0.68	0.26
Q_5	0.23	0.75
Q_6	0.68	0.32
Q_7	0.49	0.50
Q_8	0.65	0.11
Q_9	0.11	0.76
Q_{10}	0.60	0.20
Q_{11}	0.07	0.54
Q_{12}	0.77	0.18
Q_{13}	0.19	0.78
Q_{14}	0.60	0.24

When there are only two factors, the pairs of factor loadings can be displayed in a scatter plot. This aids interpretation by displaying graphically the factor space and the interrelationships of the items. Items that do not fit well into any factor can be easily identified, as can items that appear to relate to more than one factor. Multiple plots can be drawn when there are more than two factors, one for each pair of factors.

Example

Figure 5.2 shows the two varimax-rotated factors diagrammatically. The pairs of factor loadings of the 14 items in Factor 1 and Factor 2 have been plotted

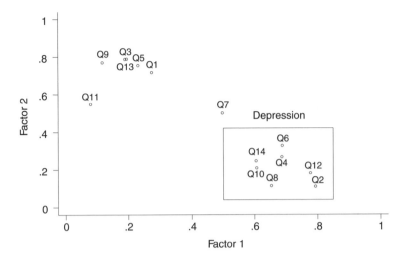

Figure 5.2 Plot of Factor 2 against Factor 1, using the rotated factors from Table 5.5

against one another. The even-numbered items cluster together, demonstrating that the depression scale is coherent and contains consistent items. Most items of the anxiety scale are also clustered together, with the exception of Q_7 which is closer to depression, and Q_{11} which is an outlier from the otherwise closely knit anxiety items.

5.6 USES OF FACTOR ANALYSIS

HISTORICAL PERSPECTIVE

A useful insight into the role of factor analysis may be obtained by considering its origins; this also provides a useful background when discussing its limitations for validation of QoL scales.

Factor analysis was developed initially by Spearman around 1904, building upon earlier work by Karl Pearson. Spearman was interested in modelling intelligence, with a view to testing whether intelligence could be separated into two components: a general ability, which was thought to be innate, and a specific ability which could vary according to subject (such as verbal skills, or mathematics) and which could be influenced by education. Thus Spearman wished to show that the results from a battery of intelligence tests covering different school subjects would reveal one general factor, and that the remaining variability in the data could be explained by specific factors associated with each test. Although Spearman is commonly regarded as the father of factor analysis, over the years there has been much criticism of the way in which he used it. In particular, there has been recognition that unrotated factors almost invariably result in a model similar to that which Spearman was seeking, with the first factor being a general factor; this is an artefact of factor analysis as a statistical method, and does not serve to verify the model. Furthermore, there is now awareness that, although rotation of factors is necessary, it is also ill-defined in that multiple solutions are possible. Therefore the current view of conventional factor analysis is that it is an exploratory technique, suitable for generating hypotheses about the structure of the data, and this is recognised by calling it *exploratory factor analysis* or EFA. The newer technique of *confirmatory factor analysis* is better for testing whether a postulated model fits the data.

Another characteristic of the conceptual model underlying EFA is that intelligence tests, like most psychological tests, should follow the basic pattern shown in Figure 5.1. Hence, if the person being assessed has a high intelligence (anxiety or depression in our example) we would expect this to be reflected in corresponding high scores for each of the individual items comprising the test. Any item in the test that does *not* satisfy this requirement would, under psychometric theory of tests, be regarded as a poor test-item and would be a candidate for removal from the questionnaire. Psychological, psychometric and educational tests are all typically constructed with the intention of measuring a few, possibly as few as one or two, subscales and contain a number of items that are expected to be homogeneous within each subscale. The HADS instrument is thus fully representative of such a test. This is rather different from many QoL instruments, which may contain a few items for each of many subscales. For example, the EORTC QLQ-C30 contains five functional scales, three symptom scales, and a number of single items; furthermore, only three of the scales comprise more than two items.

SCALE VALIDATION

The main objective of applying factor analysis to QoL scales is for construct validation, and two situations can be recognised. Firstly, if there are strong preconceptions concerning the structure of the scale, factor analysis may:

- confirm that the postulated number of factors are present (two in the example of the HADS)
- confirm the grouping of the items.

Secondly, when there is less certainty about the underlying model, an investigator may want to know:

- how many factors (or scales or constructs) are present
- how the individual items relate to the factors
- having identified the items that load on to each of the factors, whether this leads to definition of the substantive content or a meaning for the factors.

SCALE DEVELOPMENT

Another role for factor analysis lies in the checking of new scales. An illustration of this can be seen in the example of the HADS. The intention was that seven questions related to anxiety, and seven to depression. However, as we have seen, Q_7 is associated with both scales and so perhaps the wording should be modified or a different and better-targeted item substituted. The factor analysis implies that Q_7 is as strongly associated with depression as with anxiety, and that either factor could influence the value of Q_7.

Factor analysis can also draw attention to items that appear to contribute little to their intended scale. That, too, can be seen in the HADS example. Item 11 loads relatively weakly upon the anxiety scale. This suggests that Q_{11}, "I feel restless as if I have to be on the move", does not reflect anxiety as strongly as the other anxiety items, and that a better question should be devised.

Thus factor analysis can draw attention to items that load on to more than one scale, and also to items that do not load convincingly on to any scale. It also facilitates the checking for excessively strong correlations between two or more items: if very high correlations are observed between two of the items included in one factor, it would be sensible to drop one item since all information is already contained in the other.

SCALE SCORING

When a scale or subscale is composed of several items, a scale score or summary statistic will be required; for example, individual patient scale scores for anxiety and depression are the natural summary from the HADS questionnaire. As we have seen, quite often a simple summated score is used, with the assumption of equal weighting being given to each item, which is perhaps a naïve way to combine items. Accordingly, various methods have been proposed for determining differential weights, and factor analysis is commonly advocated. Indeed, since factor analysis and related methods are commonly used to assess construct validity, a natural extension is to consider using the same techniques to ascribe weights to the items, based upon factor loadings. Applying the resultant weights to the observed item values results in *factor scores* for each patient, with scale scores corresponding to each factor.

Psychometricians, however, rarely use factor scores as a method of deriving outcome scores; more commonly, factor analysis is used only to identify those items that should be included in a particular factor or construct, and then either equal weights or weights derived from other investigations are used for scoring. The reason for exercising caution against using factor scores is that the scores are often neither very precise nor uniquely defined. Also, any data-derived scores based upon one study may be inappropriate in the context of a different study drawn from another patient population. Thus, in general, we would advise against using factor analysis as anything other than a numerical process for reducing dimensionality for subsequent analyses.

5.7 APPLYING FACTOR ANALYSIS: CHOICES AND DECISIONS

Factor analyses are rarely as simple and straightforward as the HADS example, in which:

- there were few variables (14) and, more importantly, few factors (2)
- the postulated model was well-defined and the HADS scale had been developed with each item carefully chosen to load on to one of the two factors

- the sample size was fairly large (1952 patients)
- the patients were likely to have a wide range of levels of anxiety and depression, making it easier to discern the relationships.

Thus it was a relatively easy task to obtain a convincing confirmation of the HADS scale using these data. However, the rest of this chapter explores the use of factor analysis in more detail, and discusses the range of decisions that must be made when carrying out analyses. Some of the choices can be quite crucial for obtaining a satisfactory solution.

SAMPLE SIZE

Sample size is important for all studies, as discussed in Chapter 14, but it has particular impact upon factor analysis. In factor analysis, where the factor structure is being explored, a small sample size will lead to large standard errors for the estimated parameters. Even more importantly, it may result in incorrect estimation of both the number of factors and the structure of the factors. With a small sample size there will often be insufficient information to enable determination and extraction of more than one or two factors. On the other hand, with a very large sample size even trivial factors would become statistically highly significant, and so then there can be a tendency to extract too many factors. Therefore caution must be exercised in interpreting the results from large studies as well as small studies.

There is no general agreement about methods of estimating the suitable sample size. Sample size requirements will depend crucially upon the values in the between-item covariance matrix, and this is generally unknown before the study is carried out. Similarly, it will depend upon the distribution of responses to the questions, and this is likely to vary according to the population being studied and is rarely known in advance. Furthermore, many QoL items may be non-Normally distributed and strongly asymmetric, with high frequencies of subjects either reporting "no difficulty" or "very great difficulty" for individual items, thereby making simple approximations based upon Normal distributions of little practical relevance.

When the distribution of the variables and their correlation matrix is known or can be hypothesised, it is possible to carry out computer-based simulation studies to evaluate the effect of different sample sizes. Although some such studies have been reported, these have generally been for models with three or fewer factors, Normally distributed variables and simple correlation structures.

Many authors have provided conflicting recommendations and rules-of-thumb. Recommendations for the minimum number of subjects have ranged from 100 to 400 or more. Others have suggested five or ten times the number of observed variables. Various functions of the number of factors and observed variables have also been proposed. There is little theoretical basis for most of these rules. In addition, if the variables have low reliabilities or the interrelationships are weak, then many more individuals will be needed.

Although these problems may make sample size estimation appear impractical, inadequate sample size has clearly been a problem in many studies even though this is often appreciated only with hindsight, either upon completion of the study or when other investigators report conflicting factor analysis results. Thus sample size calculations cannot be simply dismissed. The best advice is to be conservative and aim for large sized studies. QoL scales are often expected to have five or more factors, and perhaps contain 30 or more items with few items per factor. The items are often discrete and form highly skewed scales with floor or ceiling effects. Then it seems likely that a minimum of a few hundred patients is required, and ideally there should be many hundreds.

NUMBER OF FACTORS

The first step in factor analysis is to determine the number of factors that are to be extracted. This is one of the more important decisions to be made since a totally different and erroneous factor structure may be estimated if an incorrect number of factors is used. If too many, or too few, factors are mistakenly entered into the model, the analyses can yield solutions that are extremely difficult to interpret. On the other hand, it is frequently possible to ascribe plausible meanings to many combinations of variables, and it can be very difficult to identify whether factors are meaningful and which models are likely to be correct. Therefore much research has been carried out into methods for deciding the number of factors that are present.

One of the oldest and most widely used approaches is the Kaiser (1960) rule *eigenvalues greater than 1*, as used in our example. Probably one (not very sound) reason for its near-universal application in computer packages is the simplicity of the method. Various foundations have been proposed for this rule, such as noting that the average eigenvalue is 1.0 and so the rule excludes all eigenvalues below the average. On the other hand, if there are 10 variables this rule will include factors that explain at least 10% of the variance, but if there were 50 variables then factors explaining as little as 2% would be retained. In general, this rule tends to include too many factors.

Another widely used method is the *scree plot*, which is simply a plot of successive eigenvalues. The scree plot is fairly good at separating the important factors from the later "factors" that are really little more than random noise; the scree is the random rubble of stones at the foot of the cliff face. Although interpretation of scree plots is subjective, frequently, as in Figure 5.3, a change in slope is fairly evident.

Example

Figure 5.3 shows the scree plot for the HADS dataset, corresponding to the eigenvalues of Table 5.3. There is a clear elbow in the plot, with the first two factors lying above the sloping line formed by the eigenvalues for factors 3 to 14. This implies that a two-factor solution is appropriate. This conclusion is also in agreement with the "eigenvalues greater than 1" rule, as indicated by the horizontal straight line.

A third widely used method for estimating the number of factors is based upon *maximum-likelihood estimation* (ML), although it has also been shown that for this purpose ML factor analysis is quite sensitive to the variability in the data ("residual" variability) and requires large sample sizes to yield reliable estimates. In our example, ML estimation successfully identified the two-factor solution.

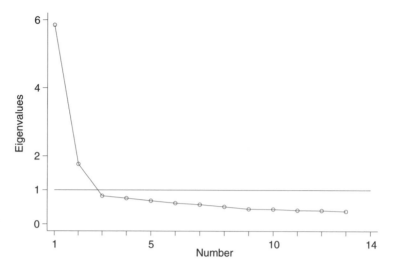

Figure 5.3 Scree plot of the eigenvalues in Table 5.3

Despite reservations, in practice both the "eigenvalues greater than 1" rule and the scree plot seem to have reasonable characteristics. When the same number of factors is suggested by all three methods, as in this example, the solution is quite convincing.

METHOD OF ESTIMATION

A variety of methods are available for estimating the factors, all leading to different solutions. Most statistical packages offer at least five or six methods for factor extraction. The only thing in common with all estimation procedures is that they define some arbitrary measure of fit which is then maximised (or, if a measure of deviation from fit is used, minimised). Methods commonly used include ML, which produces estimates that are most likely to have yielded the observed correlation matrix under assumptions of Normal distributions. Unweighted least squares minimises the sum of the squared differences between the observed and model-predicted correlation matrices. Alpha factoring maximises the Cronbach's alpha reliability of the factors, so that (for example) the first factor has the maximum reliability or internal consistency. Principal-axes factoring maximises the accounted-for variance. Minimum-residual factoring minimises the off-diagonal residuals of the total variance–covariance matrix. Many further methods also exist, each with their proponents.

When the data possess a strongly defined factor structure, theoretical and empiri-cal studies suggest that most methods of extraction will yield similar results. How-ever, in other situations there may be considerable divergence in the factor solutions, especially when there are small sample sizes, few explanatory variables, and a weak factor structure.

Statisticians generally prefer ML, because it is based upon sound mathematical theory that is widely applicable to many situations. ML estimation also provides foundations for hypothesis testing, including tests for the number of factors. Furthermore, unlike other methods, ML yields the same results whether a correlation matrix or a covariance matrix is factored. Although it is commonly thought to be a disadvantage that ML estimation explicitly assumes that the sample is from a multivariate Normal distribution, ML estimation of factor structure is fairly robust against departures from Normality. However, under non-Normality the significance tests will be invalid; violation of the distributional assumptions can reduce ML to being no better than other techniques. Overall, we recommend ML estimation as the preferred method.

The role of the factor estimation step is to find an initial solution, which can then be rotated to provide a simpler structure. Although the initial factor estimates may appear to vary considerably according to the method used, it is often found that similar results are obtained after rotation, no matter which method of factor estimation was used.

ORTHOGONAL ROTATION

Since there is no unique solution for the factor decomposition of a dataset, it is conventional to adopt an arbitrary procedure for rotation such that as many as possible of the items contribute to single factors. In other words, the aim of rotation is to simplify the initial factorisation, obtaining a solution that keeps as many variables and factors distinct from one another as possible. Thus rotation is an essential part of the factor analysis method, as the initial factor solution is frequently uninterpretable. The simplest rotations are "orthogonal", which assumes that the underlying factors are not correlated with each other, and of these "varimax" is the most widely used and generally appears to yield sensible solutions. In mathematical terms, varimax aims to maximise the variance of the squared loadings of variables in each factor; and thus minimises the number of high loadings associated with each factor. In practical terms, varimax results in a "simple" factor decomposition, because each factor will include the smallest possible number of explanatory variables. If there are preconceived ideas about the factor structure, it may be more appropriate to use goodness-of-fit tests to examine specific hypotheses, but for exploratory analysis the apparent simplicity and the sensible results following varimax have led to its near universal implementation in all computer packages.

However, many other methods do exist, most notably quartimax, which attempts to simplify the factor loadings associated with each variable (instead of the variable loadings associated with each factor). Orthomax and equamax are yet two other methods, and combine properties of both quartimax and varimax. If you are not satisfied with the arbitrary choice of varimax, there are plenty of alternatives.

OBLIQUE AXES

One assumption built into the model so far is that the factors are orthogonal and uncorrelated with each other. In many cases that is an unrealistic assumption. For example, there is a tendency for seriously ill patients to suffer from both anxiety and depression, and these two factors will be correlated. In statistical terms, we should allow "oblique axes" instead of insisting upon orthogonality. This leads to a whole set of other rotation methods, and Gorsuch (1983) lists a total of 19 orthogonal and oblique methods out of the many that are available. Most statistics packages offer a variety of these methods. Unfortunately, different procedures can result in appreciably different solutions unless the underlying structure of the data happens to be particularly clear and simple.

Promax, which is derived from varimax, is the most frequently recommended oblique rotation method. Starting from the varimax solution, promax attempts to make the low variable loadings even lower by relaxing the assumption that factors should be uncorrelated with each other; therefore it results in an even simpler structure in terms of variable loadings on to factors. Promax is therefore simple in concept, and results in simple factor structures. Not surprisingly, given its nature, promax usually results in similar—but simpler—factors to those derived by varimax. The most widely used alternative to promax is oblimin, which is a generalisation of earlier procedures called quartimin, covarimin and biquartimin; these attempt to minimise various covariance functions.

As with so much of exploratory factor analysis, it is difficult—and controversial—to make recommendations regarding the choice of method. One procedure of desperation is to apply several rotational procedures to each of two random halves of the total pool of individuals; it is reassuring if different rotational procedures result in the same factors, and if these same factors appear in both random halves. In other words, rotation is a necessary part of the exploratory factor analysis procedure, but one should be cautious and circumspect whenever using rotation.

Example

Table 5.5 showed the effect of a varimax rotation, which revealed the two factors postulated to underlie the HADS questionnaire. However, as shown in Figure 5.1, it has been suggested that the anxiety and depression factors would be correlated. Therefore an oblique rotation is may be more appropriate. Table 5.6 shows the effect of oblique rotation, using promax.

In this example, the strong factor structure of the HADS prevailed, and the oblique rotation yielded similar solutions to the varimax rotation. The negative signs attached to Factor 1 of the promax solution are immaterial, and reflect the arbitrary viewpoint from which the factors may be observed in geometrical space; the important features are the magnitudes of the loadings and the relative signs of the loadings within each factor. Perhaps the most noticeable difference from the varimax results in Table 5.5 is that the loadings of variable 7 have been diminished, yet again emphasising that this variable does not perform satisfactorily.

5.8   ASSUMPTIONS FOR FACTOR ANALYSIS

As with any statistical modelling technique, various assumptions are built into the factor analysis model and the associated estimation procedures. In many fields of research these assumptions may well be valid, but in the context of QoL scales there can be a number of problems arising from the frequently gross violation of the inherent assumptions.

Table 5.6 Oblique (promax) rotation of the factor loadings from Table 5.4

Variable	Factor 1	Factor 2
Q_1	−0.10	0.70
Q_2	−0.85	−0.11
Q_3	0.00	0.81
Q_4	−0.68	0.08
Q_5	−0.05	0.76
Q_6	−0.67	0.15
Q_7	−0.41	0.40
Q_8	−0.69	−0.07
Q_9	0.07	0.81
Q_{10}	−0.61	0.04
Q_{11}	0.06	0.58
Q_{12}	−0.81	−0.03
Q_{13}	−0.00	0.81
Q_{14}	−0.60	0.09

DISTRIBUTIONAL ASSUMPTIONS

The standard factor analysis model makes no special assumptions about data being continuous and Normally distributed. Since the commonly used estimation procedures are based upon either ML or "least squares", they assume continuous data from a Normal distribution. Furthermore, most methods of estimation of factors are based upon the Pearson product-moment correlation matrix (or, equivalently, the covariance matrix) with "Normally distributed error structure". If these distributional assumptions are violated, any test for goodness-of-fit may be compromised. However, goodness-of-fit measures are central to ML factor analysis in order to determine the number of factors to be retained, and as noted above this number is crucial to the subsequent extraction of the factor loadings.

In reporting studies it is important to specify the software that was used, as well as the model and methods of fitting and rotation of factors. Although some published reports of QoL studies do indicate the software or model used, few discuss distributional properties of their data such as whether it is continuous and Normally distributed. Presumably, the authors are unaware of the importance of these assumptions.

The two main types of departure from assumptions are that data may be discrete, possibly with only a few categories, or may be continuous but non-Normally distributed (for example, highly asymmetrical or "skewed"). Many forms of QoL data are both categorical and highly asymmetrical at the same time.

CATEGORICAL DATA

Although a few QoL instruments use linear analogue scales, by far the majority contain questions taking discrete ordinal responses, commonly with as few as four or five categories. Mathematical theory for factor analysis of categorical data has been developed by, for example, Lee, Poon and Bentler (1995) and Bartholemew (1987), and software is beginning to become more widely available. However, this is largely an untested and unexplored area and it remains unclear as to how effectively these techniques will be able to estimate the underlying latent structure, and what sample sizes will be required in order to obtain stable and consistent estimation of factors.

Since many investigators use standard factor analysis even when they have four- or five-point scales, one should at least consider the effect of this violation of the assumptions. How robust is factor analysis? A few reports, based upon experience or computer simulations, have claimed that scales with as few as five points yield stable factors. However, it remains unclear whether factor analysis using Pearson's correlation coefficient is adequate provided the five-point scale can be regarded as arising from an underlying Normal distribution with cut-points. Furthermore, the situation regarding four-point scales remains even more dubious. At one extreme, it has been suggested that correlations are fairly robust and that even ordinal scales with at least three points can be included, but this has not been supported by others who generally recommend a minimum of five response categories. It also seems likely that sample size should be increased so as to compensate for the loss of information in shorter scales.

Since the numerical solution of factor analysis uses the correlation (or sometimes the covariance) matrix, it is natural to consider techniques intended for estimating correlations based upon discrete ordinal data. "Polychoric correlations" are formed by assuming that the discrete categorical observed values are a manifestation of data with an underlying (Normal) continuous distribution. The mathematical theory leads to relatively complex estimation procedures, but computer algorithms for their estimation are available. Few studies have made use of such methods, and again there are fears about the effect upon sample size. It is best to be very cautious about applying them to samples of less than 500–1000 observations.

NORMALITY

We have commented on the effect of non-Normality upon ML estimation, but it can also prejudice other aspects of factor analysis. However, there are two reasons for anticipating highly non-Normal data in QoL research. Firstly, there is no reason to assume that categories labelled "Not at all", "A little", "Quite a bit", and "Very much" will yield equal-interval scales for patients' responses to any or all of the questions. Secondly, some of the items are likely to take extreme values depending upon the disease or the effects of its treatment. For example, cancer patients receiving certain forms of chemotherapy will almost invariably experience considerable nausea. Hence, for these patients, items such as nausea will have a highly asymmetric distribution with a "ceiling effect" of many responses towards "very much". Thus QoL items frequently possess highly skewed non-Normal distributions. Unfortunately, little work has been done on the impact of this.

Example

Figure 5.4 shows the HADS data from cancer trials of the MRC, where many items are markedly skewed and no items appear to have Normal distributions. Several items also suffer from "floor effects" and tend to take minimum values

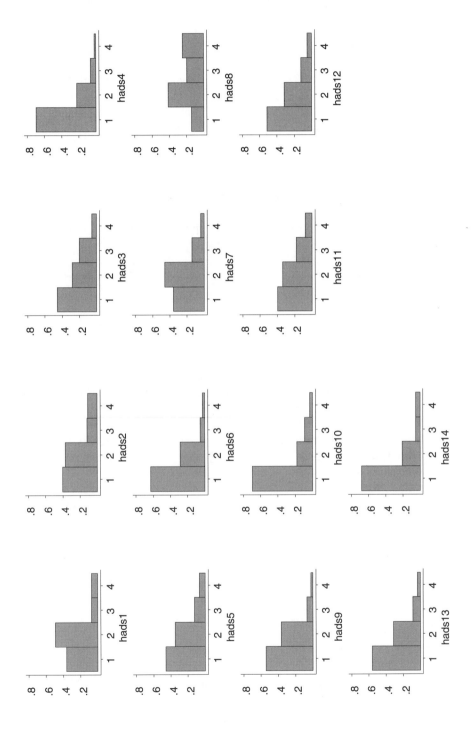

Figure 5.4 Histograms of the 14 HADS items, using the dataset from Table 5.1

for most patients, notably items Q_4, Q_6, Q_{10} and Q_{14}, and all items except Q_8 have very few patients with high responses.

Many other QoL scales may be expected similarly to contain items that deviate markedly regarding Normality.

There have been attempts to develop so-called "asymptotically distribution-free" (ADF) factor analysis that makes no assumptions about the distribution of the data (for example, Bartholomew, 1987). However, results suggest that huge sample sizes may be necessary for acceptable performance—for example, ADF on 15 variables with three "strong" factors may require samples of between 2500 and 5000 observations.

Example from the literature

When Muthén and Kaplan (1992) simulated five-point variables of various degrees of skewness for four models (2–4 factors, 6–15 variables), with 500 and 1000 observations they found "Chi-squared tests and standard errors . . . are not as robust to non-Normality as previously believed. ADF does not appear to work well."

DOES THE VIOLATION OF ASSUMPTIONS MATTER?

Since most models for factor analysis assume continuous data with Normally distributed error terms, whilst QoL data depart substantially from this by being both categorical and non-Normal, what is the overall impact? The effect of these violations of assumptions is largely unknown, although empirical results and simulation studies suggest that the techniques may be relatively robust to reasonable degrees of departures. However, it seems likely that sample size, which in QoL studies is sometimes small by any standards, should be increased so as to compensate for this. As already noted for ML estimation, it is commonly found in practice that departures from Normality may have a marked effect upon testing goodness-of-fit and the estimation of the number of factors, but has rather less impact upon the factor extraction.

Unfortunately there is no simple rule of thumb to decide when ML estimation may be applied. Any sign of appreciable deviation from Normality will be criticised as making analysis invalid, yet will be dismissed by the authors as of little consequence.

5.9 FACTOR ANALYSIS IN QoL RESEARCH

Given all the attendant problems and difficulties it is perhaps surprising that factor analysis of QoL instruments so often results in apparently sensible factors! However, this may be simply a reflection of the strong and obvious correlation structure that underlies many "constructs"; often the results, not surprisingly, confirm the expected QoL dimensions. Thus, provided there is adequate sample size, many

studies do report finding factors that represent groupings of variables that could
have been anticipated *a priori* to be correlated. However, many authors do also
report major discrepancies in the factor structure when they repeat analyses with
different datasets.

Example

Fayers and Hand (1997a) reviewed publications about seven studies reporting
factor analysis of the RSCL. All publications agreed that the first factor
represents general psychological distress and contains a broad average of the
psychological items, and that other factors were combinations of various
physical symptoms and side-effects. However, there was considerable
divergence about the details of the physical factors, with studies claiming to
find two, four, five, seven or even nine factors. Several authors acknowledged
that the extracted factors were curious and not easy to interpret. For example,
one study combined dizziness, shivering, sore mouth and abdominal aches as a
factor.

Instability of factors, especially after the first one or two factors have been
extracted, is evidently a problem. Contributory reasons include the following:

1. Some variables have weak intercorrelations. This may occur because the
    underlying relationship really is weak, or because in a particular dataset the
    observed correlations are weak.
2. Some studies may be under-sized. This will tend to result in unreliable estima-
    tion of the number of factors, and in poor estimation of the factor structure.
3. Some studies may be so large that, if care is not exercised, too many factors will
    be identified because with very large numbers of measurements even weak
    intercorrelations will suffice to pull a few variables together into a less mean-
    ingful factor.
4. Different sets of data may yield different factor structures. For example, in a
    cancer clinical trial the chemotherapy patients may experience both nausea and
    hair loss, with these items appearing strongly correlated. In contrast, in a
    hormone therapy trial, the same items could be relatively uncorrelated. Thus
    they would form a single factor in the first study, but would appear unrelated in
    the second. Factors for symptoms and side-effects can vary in different subsets
    of patients and, for example in oncology, can depend upon site of cancer,
    disease stage, treatment modality, patients' gender and age.
5. Heterogeneous samples may yield strange factors. In a clinical trial comparing
    different treatment modalities, for example, factor analyses may produce factors
    that are essentially group differences (see the example in Section 5.10). These
    factors are not-obvious, difficult to interpret, and not consistent with the
    expectations of the latent structure. If it is known that there are separate
    subgroups, one possibility is to use pooled within-group correlation matrices.
6. Some symptoms may be uncorrelated, yet contribute to the same scale. For
    example, it might be thought clinically logical to regard eating problems as part
    of a single scale, even though some patients (for example, with head and neck

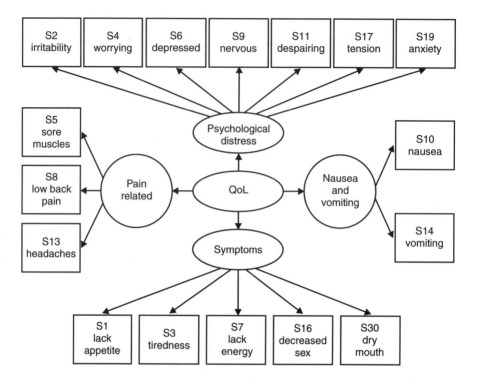

Figure 5.5 Conventional EFA model for the RSCL, with one psychological distress factor and factors relating to pain, nausea and vomiting, and symptoms / side effects. Only 17 out of the 30 items on the main RSCL are shown

cancer) may be unable to eat because of an oral problem, whilst others (with oesophageal cancer) may be unable to swallow because of throat obstruction. A serious limitation with respect to either item can have a major impact upon the patients' eating, social functioning and QoL. Thus although the correlation between these two items might be low, for many QoL purposes it could be appropriate to combine them into a single scale.

5.10 CAUSAL MODELS

The models described so far have all been based upon the assumption that QoL scales can be represented as in Figure 5.1, with observed variables that reflect the value of the latent variable. For example, in the HADS, presence of anxiety is expected to be manifested by high levels of Q_1, Q_3, Q_5, Q_7, Q_9, Q_{11} and Q_{13}. However, many QoL instruments include a large number of items covering diverse aspects of QoL. For example, the RSCL includes 30 items relating to general QoL, symptoms and side-effects; it also incorporates an activity scale and a global question about overall QoL. For simplicity, we restrict consideration to 17 items. Adopting a conventional EFA model, a path diagram such as that of Figure 5.5 might be considered.

This model assumes that a poor QoL is likely to be manifested by psychological distress, and that "psychological distress" is a latent variable that tends to result in anxiety, depression, despair, irritability and similar signs of distress. This much does seem a plausible model. However, a patient with poor QoL need not necessarily have high levels of all treatment-related symptoms. For example, a patient receiving chemotherapy may well suffer from hair loss, nausea, vomiting, and other treatment-related side-effects that cause deterioration in QoL. However, other cancer patients receiving non-chemotherapy treatments could be suffering from a completely different set of symptoms and side-effects that cause poor QoL for other reasons.

Thus a poor QoL does not necessarily imply that, say, a patient is probably experiencing nausea; this is in contrast to the psychological distress indicators, all of which may well be affected if the patient experiences distress because of their condition. On the other hand, if a patient *does* have severe nausea, that is likely to result in—or cause—a diminished QoL. Hence a more realistic model is as in Figure 5.6, where symptoms and side-effects are shown as *causal indicators* with the directional arrows pointing from the observed variables towards the "symptoms and side-effects" factor, which in turn causes changes in QoL. The observed items reflecting psychological distress are called *effect indicators*, to distinguish them from the causal indicators. Thus effect indicators can provide a measure of the QoL experienced by patients, whilst the causal indicators affect or influence patients' QoL.

Example from the literature

Fayers and Hand (1997a) analysed RSCL data from an MRC trial of chemotherapy with or without interferon for patients with advanced colorectal cancer. There appeared to be four factors, representing psychological distress, symptoms, nausea and vomiting, and pains and aches. At first sight the second factor, labelled "symptoms", contained a strange combination of items: lack of appetite, decreased sexual interest, dry mouth, tiredness and lack of energy. However, these five symptoms were precisely the items that the study team had reported as the main treatment differences in the randomised trial. In other words, the second factor is an interferon-related cluster of symptoms, and the item correlations arise from treatment differences and not through any sense of this necessarily being a single meaningful QoL construct.

Exploratory factor analysis is ill-equipped to deal with causal variables. Instead, a more general approach has to be considered, with models that can represent structures such as those of Figure 5.6 and can estimate the coefficients and parameters describing the various paths. This approach is known as *structural equation modelling* (SEM). At present, SEM requires the use of specialised software, and is not included as a standard part of most statistical packages. Programs for SEM models include AMOS (Arbuckle, 1997), EQS (Bentler, 1995) or LISREL (Jöreskog and Sörbom, 1996).

One major difference between EFA and SEM is the emphasis that the latter places upon prior specification of the postulated structure. Thus one form of SEM is also known as *confirmatory factor analysis*, since a factor-analytic structure is

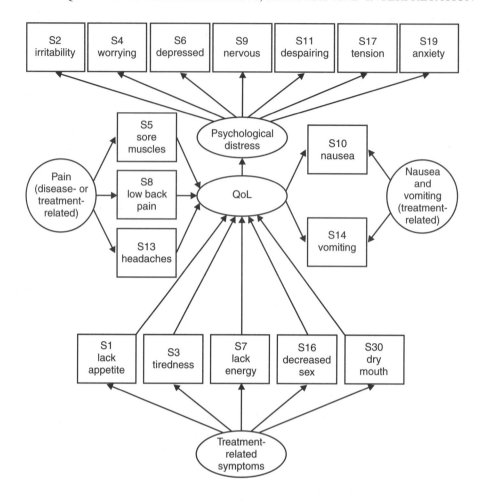

Figure 5.6 Postulated causal structure for 17 items on the RSCL. Treatment- or disease-related symptoms and side effects may be causal rather than effect indicators

pre-specified and one major purpose of the modelling is to test—or confirm—how well the data fit this hypothesised structure. Thus the testing takes the form of "goodness-of-fit" tests, with the model being accepted as adequate provided there is no strong counter-evidence against it. Although such techniques have been widely used in areas such as educational and personality testing, they are as yet little practised in the field of QoL. However, given the many disadvantages associated with EFA, it should be apparent that SEM is likely to be a far more appropriate approach. Despite this, it should still be emphasised that many of the problems remain unresolved for SEM just as much as for EFA. In particular, categorical data are hard to handle, non-Normality of data remains a major issue since Normality underpins most of the goodness-of-fit measures, and sample size is difficult to estimate in advance of carrying out the study.

Although SEM is suitable for fitting causal models, it often cannot distinguish between causal and non-causal models; both may be found to provide seemingly adequate fit to the dataset. This is because the underlying models that are appropriate for representing QoL constructs are rarely of sufficiently clear forms that enable SEM to reject the non-causal version whilst conclusively accepting the causal model as preferable. Thus SEM can rarely be used for inferring causality of individual QoL items.

One of the largest hurdles for SEM in QoL research is that many models will inevitably be complex. For example, "feedback" mechanisms may be present, with many variables being a mixture of causal and effect indicators: difficulty sleeping may cause reduced QoL which may in turn cause anxiety which causes further sleeping problems and yet further affects QoL. Diagrams such as Figures 5.5 and 5.6 are a simplification of reality. In addition, it may be impossible with data from ordinary QoL studies to distinguish between alternative models: when variables can be both effect and causal simultaneously, there are estimation problems and sometimes the solutions cannot be determined uniquely. Many alternative models may all fit the observed data equally well. In fact, one of the most important features of CFA is that it simply tests whether the pre-specified model is adequate to fit the observed data; this does not indicate that a model is correct, but merely that there is insufficient evidence against it. Thus a small study will almost inevitably be unable to provide evidence of a poor fit unless the model is totally inappropriate. On the other hand, unless the model is perfect—and, by definition, a model is only a model and is never perfect—a study that is large enough will almost always find evidence of statistically significant departures from perfect fit. Therefore, statistical significance is only of minor relevance in CFA; small-sized studies rarely have "significant" goodness-of-fit indices, whilst very large studies almost always do. Instead, conclusions should be based largely upon the magnitude of the goodness-of-fit indices. Unfortunately many goodness-of-fit indices have been proposed, each with varying properties, and it is difficult to make a specific recommendation.

5.11 CONCLUSIONS

Causal models, SEM and CFA hold great potential for QoL research, but at present they have been little used in QoL research, and there remain many controversial issues to be resolved before they can be recommended for routine usage. On the other hand, EFA has many disadvantages, not the least of which is that it will frequently be an inappropriate model for QoL instruments because of the occurrence of causal indicators. Perhaps the main advantage of EFA is its relative ease of application. EFA is available through many of the commonly used statistical packages, and analyses using EFA can readily be carried out. SEM, on the other hand, requires specialised software. Also, SEM models are considerably more difficult to specify, even though most SEM packages are moving towards model specification using graphical path diagrams. The results of analyses as displayed by SEM packages are also more difficult to interpret.

One overall conclusion should be that EFA, CFA and SEM are not "black box" procedures that can be applied blindly. Before embarking on any such analysis, the investigator must consider the possible path structures for the relationships between the explanatory variables and the latent structures. Usually there will be a number of alternative models that are thought plausible. The role of the approaches we have described is to examine whether any of these models appears reasonable, and if it does the investigator may feel satisfied. But this neither "proves" that the model is correct, nor that the scale has been truly "validated"; it confirms only that there is no evidence of bad fit.

5.12   FURTHER READING

The book by Gorsuch (1983) is recommended for a detailed description of factor analysis and related techniques. Unlike many books on this topic, it avoids detailed mathematics whilst covering factor analysis in depth; for example, Gorsuch has a whole chapter about selecting the number of factors, and two chapters about rotation methods. Nunnally and Bernstein (1994) contains extensive chapters about EFA and CFA, and has the advantage of greater emphasis on psychometric scales. Structural equation and latent variable models are fully described by Bollen (1989).

6 Item Response Theory and Differential Item Functioning

Summary

In contrast to the traditional psychometrics, item response theory introduces a different underlying model for the responses to questions. It is now assumed that patients with a particular level of QoL or functioning will have a certain probability of responding positively to each question. This probability will depend upon the "difficulty" of the item in question. For example, many patients with cancer might respond "yes" to "easy" questions such as "Do you have any pain?", but only patients with a high level of pain are likely to reply "yes" to the more "difficult" question "Have you got very much pain?" This chapter explains the role of item response models, and how to fit them. Use of these models to examine the psychometric properties of QoL scales, and in particular differential item functioning, is also described.

6.1 INTRODUCTION

As we have seen, under the traditional psychometric model of parallel test items with summated scales, it is assumed that each item is a representation of the same single latent variable. This is therefore a simple form of unidimensional scaling, in which it is frequently assumed that the items are of equal importance for measuring the latent variable, and that summated scales with equal weights can be used. It is also implicit to this model that the intervals between the levels (responses) for each category are equal, so that (for example, on a typical four-category QoL scale) a change from 1 to 2 is of equal importance as a change from 2 to 3. Since it is assumed that each item is an equally strong estimator of the latent variable, the purpose of increasing the number of items is to increase the reliability of the scale and hence improve the precision of the scale score as an estimate of the latent construct.

In contrast, *item response theory* (IRT) offers an alternative scaling procedure. IRT was developed largely in fields such as education, and initially focused upon the simple situation of binary items such as those that are frequently found in educational tests and which are scored "correct" or "wrong". There are four particular reasons explaining the importance of IRT in education. Firstly, traditional psychometric theory of parallel tests tends to result in items of equal difficulty. In educational tests this is not appropriate, as it tends to polarise students into those who find all questions easy and those who do not have the ability to answer any question. IRT methods lead to examinations that include questions of varying difficulty, enabling students to be classified into levels of ability. Secondly, educational tests should not discriminate unfairly between students of equal ability but of different sex, race, culture, religious background or other factors deemed irrelevant. IRT provides sensitive methods for detecting differential item functioning (item bias) in different subgroups. Thirdly, in annual examinations the questions will have to change in each successive year, to prevent students learning of the correct solutions. IRT provides methods for standardisation, to ensure that each year the examinations contain questions of similar difficulty and result in comparable overall scores. Fourthly, when students are faced by questions that are beyond their capability, if the valid responses are "yes" and "no" it is likely that a proportion of the correct responses were simply lucky guesses. IRT models support adjustment for guessing.

Many of these aspects of IRT are of obvious relevance to QoL assessment. Most QoL items, however, permit responses at more than two levels and multi-category IRT theory is less highly developed. Also, as with all models, IRT makes particular assumptions about the structure of the data, but some of these assumptions may be questionable when applied to QoL scales. IRT is mainly of relevance when considering scales that aim to classify patients into levels of "ability", for example activities of daily living (ADL) or other physical performance scales. These scales usually contain questions describing tasks of increasing difficulty, such as "Can you walk short distances?", "Can you walk long distances?", and "Can you do vigorous activities?" with Yes or No response items. As a consequence the earliest examples of IRT in relation to QoL research have been in the area of ADL assessment. Pain scoring is another potential field of application, since level of pain may be regarded as analogous to level of ability.

Many of the concepts, and many of the standard terms, such as "test difficulty" and "item bias", are most easily explained with reference to educational examinations.

Considering extreme cases can highlight the differences between the traditional parallel test and IRT approaches. A simple traditional test might consist of a single item, scored with multiple categories ranging from very poor (lowest category) to excellent (highest category). Then ability is assessed by the level of the response category. To increase precision and reliability, using traditional theory, additional parallel tests would be introduced and the average (or sum score) used as the measure. In contrast, under the IRT model, each test may take a simple binary "able" or "unable" response, and the tests are chosen to be of varying difficulty. To increase precision and reliability, any additional tests that are introduced are chosen so as to have difficulties evenly distributed over the range of the continuum that is of greatest interest. Although originally IRT-based tests were nearly always dichotomous, there has been a trend towards multi-category tests that can take three or four response levels.

6.2   ITEM CHARACTERISTIC CURVES

The principal concept in IRT is the *item characteristic curve*, usually abbreviated as ICC. The ICC relates the probability of a positive response to the level of the latent variable. If we consider a questionnaire that is intended to measure physical functioning, the ICC for a single item is constructed as follows.

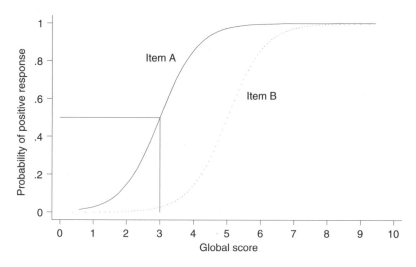

Figure 6.1 Item characteristic curves (ICC) for two items of differing difficulty

First, we require an estimate of the latent variable, overall physical functioning, for each patient. Ideally there would be an independent estimate of the "true" value of their physical functioning, but in practice that is unknown. Possible choices include use of (a) a global question such as "Overall, how would you rate your physical condition"; (b) an internally derived estimate based upon a number of items on the questionnaire; or (c) another, possibly lengthier, questionnaire that has already been validated. For each level of the latent variable it is possible to calculate the percentage or probability of patients who respond positively to the item. When items have multiple response categories, it is customary to collapse them into two levels for estimating the probability of, for example having "no difficulty or limitations" versus "some difficulty". Usually the ICC obtained will look similar to those in Figure 6.1. The "global score" is assumed to be an estimate of the true value of a latent variable, θ, such as physical functioning. Thus patients with a global score of 3 will on average give a positive response to item A approximately half of the time, but have only a very small probability (less than 0.2) of responding positively on item B.

ITEM DIFFICULTY

In educational examinations there is the concept of *difficulty* when comparing items. The more intelligent or more successful pupils are able to answer even difficult questions successfully. In Figure 6.1 the two items shown vary in their "difficulty". If the global score described educational attainment, item B would represent a more difficult question since for any particular global score the probability of answering B correctly is less than that for A. Although difficulty is also a suitable word for describing ability to perform physical functions, it may be intuitively less obvious for describing some other aspects of QoL assessment. It simply means that for a given value of the latent variable fewer patients will answer positively to a question related to a more advanced symptom or a more demanding task.

One of the most useful features of IRT is that it provides a solid theoretical framework for estimating this item difficulty. Thus IRT facilitates the design of questionnaires containing items with a spread of levels of difficulty, and enables formal procedures to be used for selecting these items. It also leads to the development of scaling and scoring procedures for the aggregation of items into summary measures of ability. It provides methods for comparing different questionnaires, and enables measures of patients' ability scores to be standardised across instruments.

Another important aspect of IRT is that it is "sample free", because the *relative* item difficulties should remain the same irrespective of the particular sample of subjects. Thus, the most difficult item remains the most difficult item irrespective of the sample and the mix of patient ability levels. It is this feature that enables IRT to be used for providing standardised tests.

ITEM DISCRIMINATION

In Figure 6.1, a patient who responds positively to item A is most likely to have a global score of 3 or more; however, even about 10% of patients with a global score of 2 are expected to respond positively. Thus a positive response to A does not provide a clear indication of the global score. An ideal test item is one with an ICC nearly vertical, since the central sloping region of the S-shaped curve represents the region of uncertainty in which we cannot be certain whether patients with a specified value of the global score will respond positively or negatively to the item. Conversely, an extremely poor item would be one with an ICC close to horizontal ICC at 0.5, for which all patients, irrespective of their global score, would answer positively half the time; this item would contain no information about the patients' ability.

The ability of a test to separate subjects into high and low levels of ability is known as its *discrimination*. Thus discrimination corresponds to steepness of the curve, and the steeper the better. In Figure 6.2, item A discriminates between patients better than item B. Thus, for item A, patients whose global score is less than 2 will answer positively with low probability, and patients with score greater than 4 will do so with high probability. Only those patients whose score is between 2 to 4 may or may not respond positively—a range of uncertainty of 4–2. In contrast, item B has a wider range of uncertainty of approximately 7–3.

Difficulty and discrimination are the two fundamental properties of binary items in questionnaires. If an item has poor discrimination, it may help to include several other items of similar difficulty so as to improve the reliability of the test. If an item has good discrimination it is less necessary to have additional items with closely similar difficulty. An ideal test would consist of evenly spaced, near vertical, ICCs that cover the range of abilities that are of interest.

6.3 LOGISTIC MODELS

Although IRT is a generic term for a variety of models, the most common form is the logistic item response model. It has been found that logistic curves provide a good fit to many psychological, educational and other measurements. If a patient, h, has an ability which is represented by the latent variable θ_h, then for a single item in a test the basic equation for the logistic model takes the form

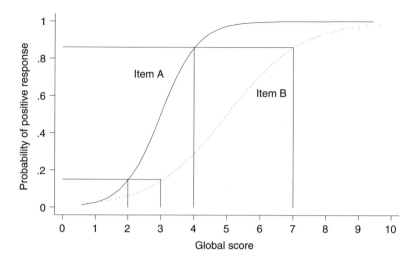

Figure 6.2 Item characteristic curves for two items of differing discrimination and difficulty

$$P(\theta_h) = \frac{\exp\{\theta_h - b\}}{1 + \exp\{\theta_h - b\}},$$ (6.1)

where $P(\theta_h)$ is the probability of a positive response by patient h, exp is the expo-nential function, and b is the item difficulty that we wish to estimate. Alternatively, this equation can be rearranged and written in the so-called "logit" form

$$\log\left(\frac{P(\theta_h)}{1 - P(\theta_h)}\right) = (\theta_h - b),$$ (6.2)

and thus b is the value of θ_h that has a probability of 0.5 for being positive. In Figure 6.1, $b = 3$ for item A, and $b = 5$ for item B.

Since Equation (6.1) requires only a single parameter b to be estimated, it is commonly described as the "one-parameter logistic model". It is also often called the *Rasch model* in honour of the Danish mathematician who promoted its usage in this area (Rasch, 1960). This equation can be generalised by adding a second parameter, a. It then becomes:

$$P(\theta_h) = \frac{\exp\{a(\theta_h - b)\}}{1 + \exp\{a(\theta_h - b)\}}.$$ (6.3)

The parameter a in equation (6.3) measures the slope of the ICC curve and is called the *discrimination* of the test. This is known as the *two-parameter logistic model*. Figure 6.2 shows ICCs with the same values of b as in Figure 6.1, but with a taking the values 1.75 for item A and 1.0 for item B. When there are n items on the questionnaire it is possible to fit a generalised form of equation (6.3), with different values of a and b for each item.

The "three-parameter model" introduces a third parameter, c, which allows the baseline intercept to vary. Representative curves are shown in Figure 6.3,

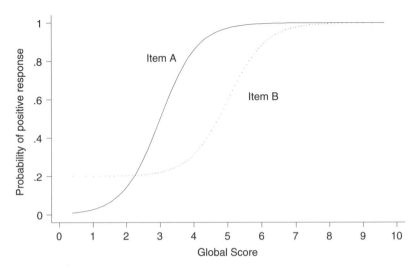

Figure 6.3 Item characteristic curves for two items with differing intercepts and difficulty

where item B from Figure 6.1 has been redrawn with $c = 0.2$. The corresponding equation is

$$P(\theta_h) = c + \frac{(1-c)\exp\{a(\theta_h - b)\}}{1 + \exp\{a(\theta_h - b)\}}. \tag{6.4}$$

In educational testing, c allows for pupils who guess at the answer. An equivalent situation in QoL measurement might arise if some patients tend to respond "yes" to items measuring symptoms even when they do not have the symptom or when their QoL is unaffected by the presence of the symptom.

One of the important properties of the logistic item response model is that it proves unnecessary to have estimates of the latent variable θ, provided one is interested only in the relative difficulties and discrimination of the items. The reason for this is that one can identify the relative positions of the curves without knowing the true values of the latent variable. These relative positions, corresponding to the relative sizes of the b parameters, are usually expressed in terms of log-odds ratios (logits). A logit difficulty is the mean of the log-odds that a patient of average ability will be able to move from one category to the next higher one. Typically the logits will range from –4 to +4, with +4 being the most difficult test.

LOGISTIC REGRESSION

Although Rasch and other item response models are logistic models, there are crucial distinctions between estimation for IRT and standard statistical logistic regression. In logistic regression θ is known and is the dependent or "y-value"; in the Rasch model it is unknown. In the Rasch model θ_h takes different values for each patient, h, leading to as many unknown parameters as there are subjects. Hence IRT is related to the so-called "conditional logistic regression". For each item, i, one or more of the corresponding item parameters a_i, b_i and c_i have to be estimated according to whether the one-, two- or three-parameter model is used.

ASSUMPTIONS FOR LOGISTIC IRT MODELS

Under the logistic IRT model, each ICC must be smoothly increasing. That is, the probability of a positive response should always increase as the ability increases, and thus the ICC curves should increase as the latent variable increases; this is called *monotonically increasing*.

In addition, as with traditional psychometric scales, the latent variable should be *unidimensional*. This means that a single latent trait underlies all the items in the model, and is sufficient to explain all but the random variability that was observed in the data. Related to this is the concept of *local independence*, which states that for patients with equal levels of ability there should be no correlation between any pair of items within the scale. That is, although we would expect to observe a (possibly strong) correlation between any two items in a scale if we calculate the correlation for a group of patients, this correlation should arise solely because both items reflect the same latent trait. Therefore, if we take account of the value of the latent trait, all remaining variability should be attributable to random fluctuations and the correlation should be zero after the latent trait is "held constant". Unidimensionality implies local independence, since both assumptions simply state that ability, and ability alone, is the only factor that affects the patients' responses. In terms of QoL, when two items in a QoL scale appear to be correlated, that correlation should arise solely because both items are measuring the same single dimension within the QoL construct.

Local independence is a crucial assumption for fitting and estimating the parameters of the logistic IRT model. Without that assumption there are too many unknown parameters to estimate and it becomes impossible to obtain a solution to the IRT equations.

When causal variables are involved, the IRT model becomes inappropriate. Firstly, local independence is usually strongly violated because causal variables are correlated by virtue of having been themselves caused by disease or treatment; they are not independent for given levels of the latent variable. Symptom clusters are, by definition, groups of highly intercorrelated symptoms and, for example, QoL scales may contain many symptom clusters. Secondly, "difficulty" is a central concept to the whole IRT approach. However, the frequency of occurrence of a symptom does not relate to its difficulty. Pain, for example, might occur with the same frequency as another (minor) symptom, yet for those patients with pain its affect upon QoL can be extreme. Also, if we consider patients with a given level of ability (QoL), the frequency of different symptoms does not reflect their "item difficulty" or their importance as determinants of QoL.

Any scale consisting of heterogeneous symptoms associated with disease or treatments, and which may therefore contain causal variables of QoL, should be carefully checked. The most suitable scales for logistic IRT modelling are those in which there is a clear underlying construct and where the items are expected to reflect levels of difficulty. Hence we have used physical functioning as our prime example: in most disease areas, items such as walking short distances, walking long distances, climbing flights of stairs, and carrying heavy loads are likely to reflect the overall level of physical functioning. Thus although these items may be causal variables with respect to levels of QoL, they are also indicators of the level of physical functioning.

FITTING THE MODEL

Fitting IRT models and estimation of difficulties and abilities is complex and usually requires iterative calculations. Most standard statistical packages do not have specific facilities for IRT modelling, although as noted above conditional logistic regression can be used. However, specialised software incorporates better estimation facilities and display of results, and has the added advantage that IRT diagnostics such as goodness-of-fit indices are usually provided. Large numbers of patients are required for the estimation procedure. Although it is difficult to be specific, sample sizes of at least 400 are recommended for the one-parameter model, 1000 are often found necessary for the more complex two-parameter model, and the numerically less stable three-parameter model may require many thousands of patients.

Software for logistic IRT analysis usually displays estimates of the logit values and their accompanying standard errors. The estimated logits can be compared with each other, and their differences tested for significance using t-tests.

Goodness-of-fit indexes enable the adequacy of the model to be assessed, and a poor fit implies that one or more of the assumptions has been violated. Thus, a poor fit for a one-parameter model could imply that the two- or three-parameter version is more appropriate, or that local independence is violated, or that the logistic model is inappropriate. Usually goodness-of-fit statistics will be produced for the overall model and "misfit indices" may be given for individual items (item-misfit index) and for patients (person-misfit index). Although the precise statistics used can vary, in general a large value for the misfit statistics indicates that an item is frequently scored wrongly (item-misfit) or that a patient has given inconsistent responses (person-misfit). For example, the item-misfit index would be large for an item that is expected to be easy (low difficulty) if it cannot be accomplished by a number of patients with high overall levels of ability. Similarly, the value will be high if those with low overall ability are able to answer "difficult" items. Most goodness-of-fit statistics follow an approximate χ^2 distribution (Table T4), and thus a significant p-value is evidence that the model does not provide a perfect fit.

It is important, however, to remember that most models are nothing more than an approximation to reality. If the dataset is sufficiently large, even well-fitting and potentially useful models may fail to provide perfect fit to the observed dataset, and the p-value may be significant. On the other hand, if the dataset is small there will be insufficient information to detect poor fit even when the model is inappropriate. Statistical tests of goodness-of-fit should be used with caution.

Example from the literature

Haley, McHorney and Ware (1994) used IRT to examine the relative difficulty and the reproducibility of item positions of the 10-item physical functioning scale of the MOS SF-36, in a sample of 3445 patients with chronic medical or psychiatric conditions. The Rasch one-parameter logistic model was used, with each item first dichotomised into "limitations" or "no limitations".

The item difficulty values of Table 6.1 were estimated in terms of Rasch logit values, and largely confirmed the authors" prior expectations. "Bathing or dressing" was the easiest task (with a value −3.44), and "vigorous activities" the most difficult (+3.67). The standard errors (*SE*s) of the *b*-values show the observed differences to be highly significant (greater than 2 × *SE*).

Item difficulties are clustered in the central region of the scale, with four items between −0.5 and +0.5. There is weaker coverage of the two extremes of the scale. The goodness-of-fit statistics, however, indicate that the Rasch model does not fit very well, with three items scoring item-misfit indices greater than +2, and another 5 items scoring less than −2.

Table 6.1 Rasch analysis of the PF-10 subscale in the SF-36 (Based on Haley *et al.*, 1994)

PF-10 items	*b* Item difficulty	*SE*	Goodness- of-fit
Vigorous activities	3.67	0.04	2.3
Climbing several flights of stairs	1.44	0.04	−3.4
Walking more than one mile	1.27	0.04	−0.2
Bending, kneeling, stooping	0.36	0.04	6.2
Moderate activities	0.18	0.04	−2.7
Walking several blocks	−0.11	0.04	−3.1
Lifting, carrying groceries	−0.36	0.04	0.0
Climbing one flight of stairs	−1.07	0.05	−5.1
Walking one block	−1.93	0.06	−3.2
Bathing or dressing	−3.44	0.07	8.9

Example from the literature

Stucki *et al.* (1996) also applied Rasch analysis to the PF-10 subscale, but divided the items into "limited a lot" versus "limited a little" or "not limited at all". Therefore it is difficult to make direct comparison of these results with those of Hayley *et al.* (1994), and this might also explain the apparent substantial differences between the two sets of results. For example, Stucki *et al.* reported that the items with worst fit to the model were "vigorous activities", "walking more than one mile", and "moderate activities"; while "bathing or dressing", and "bending, kneeling, stooping" all fitted the model very well— almost the opposite of the findings of Hayley *et al.* The estimates of item difficulty also varied, as did their rank order.

Stucki *et al.* also estimated item difficulty for the SF-36 in two other ways. They calculated the proportion of patients who had difficulty with each item, and also calculated the mean scores for each item across patients. They showed that all three methods gave broadly similar results, and that the Rasch estimates of item difficulty corresponded in rank order to the other simpler measures of difficulty. However, the Rasch method has the advantage of enabling the spacing of the item difficulties to be examined.

6.4 FITTING IRT MODELS: TIPS

IRT models place heavy demands upon datasets. The parameter estimates may be imprecise and associated with large standard errors; models may be unstable, and computer programs may fail to converge to a solution. The following tips are analogous to those that can be applied to other forms of modelling, including linear regression, but they assume special importance for estimating IRT models.

1. Use large datasets!
2. Use purpose-built computer software with output that is tailored for IRT modelling and provides IRT-specific diagnostic information such as goodness-of-fit and misfit indexes.
3. Studies should be designed so that the observations cover the full range of item values. If there are few patients with extreme values, it can become infeasible to obtain reliable estimates of the item difficulties. For example, when evaluating physical function in a group of elderly patients, the majority of patients may have poor overall physical function and respond "NO" to difficult questions such as those about carrying heavy loads, walking long distances and going up stairs. It may then be impossible to estimate these item difficulties
4. "Person-misfit indexes" identify individuals who fail to fit the model well. The stability of the model estimation can be greatly improved by excluding these patients from analyses. For example, some patients might state that they are unable to take a short walk, yet inconsistently also indicate that they can take long walks. Such conflicting responses cause problems when fitting IRT models.
5. Item-misfit indexes can identify items that should be excluded before re-running the IRT analyses. For example, the question "Do you have any trouble going up stairs?" might have a high level of misfit since some patients who cannot go up stairs will reorganise their lifestyle accordingly. If they believe that the questionnaire concerns the degree to which they are inconvenienced or troubled, they might truthfully respond "no problems, because I no longer have any need to go upstairs".
6. Item parameter estimates should be invariant if some of the other items are dropped.
7. Person scores should be relatively invariant even if some items are dropped.

6.5 TEST DESIGN

One of the most important aspects of IRT is that it can help towards the design of optimal scales. IRT can identify items that are not providing much information, either because they have low discrimination or because they are of similar difficulty to other items and provide little extra information. If it is important to evaluate all levels of the latent variable, items should be spaced fairly uniformly in terms of their difficulty and should cover the full range of the latent variable. If, on the other hand, one were only interested in subjects with high levels of ability, it would be sensible to concentrate most items in that region of difficulty. Also, if items have poor discrimination level it may be necessary to have several parallel items of approximately equal difficulty so as to increase the overall reliability or discrimination of the scale. Alternatively, it may be possible to explore why certain items on the questionnaire have poor discrimination (for example, by interviewing patients with extreme high or low ability and for whom the item response differs from that expected), and to consider substituting other questions instead. When IRT is used for test design purposes it can be useful to start with a large pool of potential or candidate items, and estimate the difficulty and discrimination of each item. The questionnaire can then be developed by selecting a set of items that appear to provide adequate coverage of the scale and which have reasonable discrimination.

Information functions can summarise the overall value of including individual items. Items that contribute little information are natural candidates for either removal or modification. Information functions can also expose areas in the test that are inadequately covered, and which would benefit by the addition of extra test items. The reading material listed at the end of this chapter describes how to estimate and use information functions.

6.6 IRT VERSUS TRADITIONAL AND GUTTMAN SCALES

Each item in a traditional psychometric scale will often be either multi-category or continuous, and the level of the item provides an estimate of the latent variable. A single item would be prone to errors such as subjects incorrectly scoring responses, and would lack precision. Thus the main purpose of having multiple parallel items, in which all items have equal difficulty, is to reduce the error variability. This error variability is measured by reliability coefficients, which is why Cronbach's α is regarded as of fundamental importance in psychometric scale development and is commonly used in order to decide which items to retain in the final scale.

Scales based upon IRT models, in contrast, frequently use binary items. Estimation of the latent variable now depends upon having many items of *different* levels of difficulty. In this context Cronbach's α is largely irrelevant to the selection of test items, since a high α can arise when items have *equal* difficulty—which is of course the opposite of what is required.

IRT can also be useful for testing the assumption of parallel items. Logistic models can be fitted, confirming that the items are indeed of equal difficulty and have equal discrimination. To do this, the item categories can be grouped to reduce multi-category items into dichotomous ones. IRT then provides a sensitive statistical test for validation of traditional scales, confirming that the scales perform as intended.

Guttman scales are multi-item scales that require each successive item to be more difficult than its predecessor, and are thus conceptually closely related to IRT models. For example, the item "Can you take short walks?" is easier than and therefore comes before "Can you take long walks?", which in turn would be followed by even more difficult tasks. Although Guttman scales are seemingly similar to IRT models, they make a strong assumption that the items are strictly hierarchical. Thus if a patient indicates inability to accomplish the easiest item then they *must* respond similarly for the more difficult items. Conversely if a patient answers "Yes" to a difficult question then all prior, easier questions must be "Yes", too. Hence in a perfect Guttman scale the response pattern is fully determined by the subject's level of ability. Under this model the ICCs are assumed to have almost vertical lines, leading to nearly perfect item discrimination. Such extreme assumptions may occasionally be realistic, as for example in childhood physical development (crawling, walking, and running), but is likely to be rarely appropriate for QoL scales. IRT, based upon non-perfect discrimination and logistic probability models, seems far more appropriate.

6.7   OTHER LATENT TRAIT MODELS

Although various other IRT models have been proposed for particular applications, such as psychomotor assessment, we have focused upon those IRT models that are most commonly encountered in QoL research. However, an extension that is of particular interest in QoL is the generalisation of the Rasch model for multiple categories, avoiding the need to reduce items to two categories by combining multiple categories as in the example of Hayley *et al.* (1994). One approach that has been proposed for this ordered categorical data involves dichotomising the data repeatedly at different levels, so that each g-category item is effectively decomposed into $g - 1$ binary questions. Thus an item that has three levels (such as Not limited, Limited a little, Limited a lot) can be regarded as equivalent to two binary questions: "Were you limited a little in doing vigorous activities?" (Yes or No), and "Were you limited a lot in doing vigorous activities?" (Yes or No). In this way the PF-10, for example, is equivalent to 20 binary questions that can be analysed by a Rasch analysis.

6.8   DIFFERENTIAL ITEM FUNCTIONING

Differential item functioning (DIF) arises when one or more items in a scale perform differently in various subgroups of patients. Suppose a physical functioning scale contains a number of questions, one of which is "Do you have trouble going to work?" Such a question might be a good indicator of physical problems for many patients, but could be expected to be less useful for patients who have reached retirement age. They would not experience trouble going to work if they were no longer in employment. As a consequence a summated scale which includes this question could yield misleading results. If retirement age is 65, say, there might appear to be an improvement in the average scale score at the age of 66 when compared with 64, simply because fewer 66-year-olds report trouble going to work. The item "trouble going to work" could therefore result in a biased score being obtained for older patients.

One example of a QoL instrument that contains exactly this question is RSCL, although the RSCL prudently contains qualifying patient instructions that say: "A number of activities is listed below. We do not want to know whether you actually do these, but only whether you are able to perform them presently." Those instructions make it clear that the authors of the RSCL were aware of potential item bias, and that they sought to eliminate the problem by using carefully worded instructions.

Example from the literature

> It is difficult to be certain that all patients will read the instructions thoroughly
> and act upon them. The UK Medical Research Council (MRC) colorectal trial
> CR04 used the RSCL, and found that 88% of patients over the age of 65
> reported trouble going to work, as opposed to 57% under that age. This is
> consistent with the suggestion of age-related DIF. It was also noted that 25% of
> patients left that item blank on the form, with most of these missing responses
> being amongst older patients. This further supports the idea of DIF since it
> implies that those patients had difficulty answering that item or regarded it as
> non-applicable; by contrast, fewer than 6% of patients left any of the other
> physical activity items blank.

Although the term *item bias* is widely used as a synonym for DIF, most authors
prefer the latter as a less emotive term. DIF simply assesses whether items behave
differently within different subgroups of patients, while ascribing the term "bias" to
an item constitutes a judgement as to the role and impact of the DIF.

A more general definition is that biased items result in systematically different
results for members of a particular subgroup. Rankings within the subgroup may be
relatively accurate, but comparisons between members of different subgroups would
be confounded by bias in the test item. In the colorectal trial example, subjects over
the age of 65 were not directly comparable with those under 65 because those retired
tended to interpret differently the question about trouble working.

DIF can be an issue whenever one group of patients responds differently from
another group, but is most commonly associated with gender, age, social class,
socioeconomic status and employment differences. It has rarely been explored in
relation to QoL measurements, and the extent of DIF problems is largely unknown.
Fortunately the problems may be less severe in treatment comparisons made within
a randomised clinical trial, since randomisation should ensure that roughly similar
proportions of patients from each relevant subgroup will be allocated to each
treatment arm. DIF may, however, distort estimates of the absolute levels of QoL-
related problems for the two treatment arms.

Several methods have been developed for DIF analysis, and comprehensive
details are given in Osterlind (1983) and Camilli and Shepard (1994). Many of the
methods involve fitting an appropriate IRT model, but we describe an alternative
method that is simpler to apply.

Example from the literature

> Groenvold *et al.* (1995) tested the EORTC QLQ-C30 for item bias, using data
> from 1189 surgically treated breast cancer patients with primary histologically
> proven breast cancer. They examined each of the 30 items, using age and treat-
> ment (whether they received adjuvant chemotherapy or not) as the two external
> variables for forming patient subgroups.
>
> The QLQ-C30 contains five items relating to physical activities. For the DIF
> analysis, each item was scored 0 (no problem doing activity) or 1 (unable to
> do, or only with some trouble), so that the summated scores of the physical

functioning ranged from 0 to 5. When a patient scored 0 for physical functioning, all five of the items must have been zero. Similarly, those scoring 5 must have responded with 1 for each item. These patients provide no information about DIF and were excluded, leaving 564 patients to be examined for evidence of DIF.

Table 6.2 shows that the item "Do you have to stay in a bed or chair for most of the day" behaves differently from the other items in the same scale. At each level of the physical functioning scale, this particular item behaves differently in relation to age. Younger patients are more likely to reply "Yes" to this question. A significance test confirmed that this was unlikely to be a chance finding ($p < 0.006$). This item was also biased in relation to treatment.

Groenvold *et al.* note that the bias seen here may reflect an effect of chemotherapy (mainly given to patients below 50 years of age): some patients may have been in bed owing to nausea, not to a bad overall physical function. Groenvold *et al.* also found that the pain item "Did pain interfere with your daily activities?" and the cognitive function item "Have you had difficulty remembering things?" were biased in relation to treatment.

Table 6.2   DIF analysis of the EORTC QLQ-C30 physical functioning scale (Based on Groenvold *et al.*, 1995)

Physical functioning score (PF)	Age	Have to stay in bed or a chair		No. of patients
		0 (no)	1 (yes)	
1	25–50	97.3	2.7	113
	51–60	99.0	1.0	104
	61–75	100	0	92
2	25–50	92.3	7.7	52
	51–60	96.7	3.3	61
	61–75	100	0	85
3/4	25–50	28.6	71.4	21
	51–60	46.7	53.3	15
	61–75	47.6	52.4	21

IRT AND DIF

IRT provides a natural method for examining DIF. In principle, the ICC should be the same for all subgroups of patients but DIF occurs if, for example, males of a given ability find a test more difficult than females of the same ability. The null hypothesis is that there is no DIF, so that the ICCs are equal. Thus, for the three-parameter logistic model this implies:

$$b_{male} = b_{female}, \quad a_{male} = a_{female}, \quad c_{male} = c_{female}.$$

The use of IRT for testing DIF has, however, been criticised (by, for example, Hambleton, Swaminathan and Rogers, 1991). It should be used only when there is evidence that IRT models provide a good fit to the items and that all the assumptions for IRT are valid. We describe alternative methods, based upon stratified analysis of patient scale-scores, which are computationally simpler and more robust against violation of the assumptions.

In the example of Table 6.2, age defined the subgroups in each two-way table and Groenvold *et al.* used a test statistic called "partial-gamma". An alternative method is the Mantel–Haenszel approach for testing significance in multiple contingency tables, using a χ^2 test. This is easier to calculate by hand, and is widely available in statistical packages. Whereas the partial-gamma test can analyse multiple levels of age, we now have to reduce the data to a series of 2×2 tables by creating age subgroups of 25–50 years and 51–75 years.

To apply this method, the data are recast in the form of a contingency table with $2 \times 2 \times S$ cells, where S represents the levels of the test score (physical functioning scores 1, 2, and 3+4). Thus at each of the S levels there is a 2×2 table of item score against the two age subgroups that are being examined for DIF.

Suppose each of the S 2×2 tables is of the form:

	Item score		
Subgroup	1	2	Totals
I	a	b	r
II	c	d	s
Totals	m	n	N

Then we can calculate the expected value of a, under the assumption of null hypothesis of no DIF. This is given by

$$E(a) = \frac{rm}{N}. \tag{6.5}$$

The corresponding variance and odds ratio are

$$Var(a) = \frac{mnrs}{N^2(N-1)}, \quad OR = \frac{ad}{bc}. \tag{6.6}$$

The Mantel–Haenszel statistic examines the differences between the observed a and its expected value, $E(a)$, at each of the S levels of the test score, giving in large-study situations:

$$\chi^2_{MH} = \frac{\left\{ \sum_{j=1}^{S} [a_j - E(a_j)] \right\}}{\sum_{j=1}^{S} Var(a_j)}, \tag{6.7}$$

where $j = 1, 2, \ldots S$. This is tested using a χ^2 test with one degree of freedom (*df*).

Furthermore, an estimate of the amount of DIF is given by the average *OR* across the S tables, which is

$$ OR_{MH} = \frac{\sum\limits_{j=1}^{S} a_j d_j / N_j}{\sum\limits_{j=1}^{S} b_j c_j / N_j}. \tag{6.8}$$

A value of $OR_{MH} = 1$ means no DIF, and other values indicate DIF favouring subgroup I ($OR_{MH} > 1$) or subgroup II ($OR_{MH} < 1$).

Example

The data of Groenvold *et al.* (1995), summarised in Table 6.2, can be collapsed into 2×2 tables, as in Table 6.3.

Using equations (6.5) and (6.6) we calculate the expected value and variance of a, and the OR for each table, giving Table 6.4.

The three odds ratios are less than 1, reflecting that at all levels of PF there were fewer patients in the older age group who were limited to having to stay in a bed or chair. From Equation (6.8), $OR_{MH} = 0.306$. Applying equation (6.7), the Mantel–Haenszel statistic is 6.65. Table T3 for χ^2, with df $= 1$, shows this to be statistically significant ($p = 0.0099$). Groenvold *et al.* report a slightly smaller p-value when using partial-gamma, but the Mantel–Haenszel test is regarded as sensitive and the difference between the two results is small.

Table 6.3 DIF analysis of the number of patients having to stay in bed or a chair (Data corresponding to Table 6.2)

Physical functioning score (PF)	Age	Have to stay in bed or a chair		No. of patients
		0 (no)	1 (yes)	
1	25–50	110	3	113
	51–75	195	1	196
2	25–50	48	4	52
	51–75	144	2	146
3/4	25–50	6	15	21
	51–75	17	19	36

Table 6.4 Results for the Mantel–Haenszel test used for detecting DIF

PF score	a	$E(a)$	$Var(a)$	Odds ratio
1	110	111.54	0.919	0.188
2	48	50.42	1.132	0.167
3/4	6	8.47	3.249	0.447

6.9 ADAPTIVE TESTING

One potential use for IRT in QoL research is the development of "tailored" or adaptive tests. If a group of patients are known to be severely limited in their physical ability, it may be felt unnecessary to ask them many questions relating to difficult or strenuous tasks. Conversely, other patients may be fit and healthy, and it is less relevant to ask them detailed questions about easy tasks. Therefore specific variants of a questionnaire may be used for different subgroups of patients. Logistic IRT modelling provides the means by which these variants can be standardised, so that they all relate to different segments within one ability scale.

One extension of this approach that has been adopted in some fields of research is to adapt the questions dynamically in the light of respondents' previous replies. Nunnally and Bernstein (1994) describe the use of computer-assisted questionnaires, in which questions of appropriate difficulty are selected on the basis of earlier responses. This can result in more precise grading of ability, whilst at the same time reducing the number of questions each person needs to answer.

Example from the literature

Fisher (1993) illustrated an Assessment of Motor and Process Skills (AMPS) instrument with more than 50 tasks. This assesses the ability of persons to perform activities of daily living. Rasch models were used to calibrate the tasks in terms of their relative difficulty with respect to the motor and process skills.

This enabled future assessments to be made using only a few tasks. The person being evaluated is provided with the opportunity to choose and perform two or three familiar tasks, out of the total set of more than 50. They are then rated on 15 motor skills and 20 process skills. Since the task difficulties are known, the person-ability measures could be adjusted to account for the differing challenges of the tasks.

Another application for tailored tests relates to DIF. In some scales it may be difficult to avoid item bias, and the investigators may even decide deliberately to include DIF items. As a rather contrived example, suppose an instrument is required for use in a clinical trial that will be entering patients aged from 10 to 70. It might be desired to obtain a single indicator of physical function even though it can be argued that "good physical functioning" will take on a different meaning for children as opposed to adults. In such a situation the investigator might have one question for adults about going to work, a different question for children about going to school, and possibly other questions aimed at other subgroups of patients such as the retired. Then each question would be relevant only for its own target subgroup, and would function differently for other patients. The results might be analysed by converting the individually targeted questions into the equivalent of the single compound question. Of course in such a simple example one could in principle have a compound question instead; for example: "Do you have trouble going to school/to work/doing housework/performing retirement activities?" However, this could become confusing and easily misunderstood.

We are not aware of examples from QoL literature where instruments target several subgroups of patients using questions that are specific to individual subgroups. However, paediatric assessment is one area in which this would be relevant, with different sets of questions applicable to different age groups and a standardised score providing a measure of QoL irrespective of age.

6.10 CONCLUSIONS

IRT has rarely been applied to QoL data. In part this may be a consequence of the mathematical complexity of many of the models, the need for large sample sizes, the problems of including multi-category items, and the need for specialised computer software. Unfortunately IRT makes strong assumptions about the response patterns of the items, and is sensitive to departures from the model. Much QoL data are not as tidy and homogenous as the items in educational examination. The examples that we considered by Haley *et al.* (1994) and Stucki *et al.* (1996) found that a Rasch model did not fit items in the physical functioning scale of the SF-36 very well. Perhaps this is not surprising: the assumption of local independence is a very demanding requirement, yet it is crucial to the estimation procedures used for IRT. Scales that include causal variables influencing QoL, such as treatment- or disease-related symptoms, will usually violate this assumption because the external variable (treatment or disease) introduces correlations that cannot be fully explained by the latent variable (QoL). Although scales such as physical functioning may appear to be homogenous and contain items that are more closely hierarchical (increasing difficulty), the requirements for IRT are still highly demanding. For example, tasks such as bending and stooping may generally be related to physical functioning, but some patients who can walk long distances may have trouble bending and others may be able to bend but cannot even manage short walks. Thus the seemingly hierarchical nature of the items may be violated, with some patients providing apparently anomalous responses.

One important feature of IRT is that the mathematical nature of the model enables the inherent assumptions to be tested, and goodness-of-fit should always be examined. The logistic models can help identify items that give problems, but when items do not fit the model it becomes difficult to include them in subsequent IRT analyses. Estimates of relative difficulty of items appear to be reasonably robust, but caution should be used when extending the model to other analyses. Tests of DIF are probably most easily applied using non-IRT approaches such as the Mantel–Haenszel χ^2 test.

Perhaps IRT is not suitable for regular use in QoL scale development. The necessary assumptions are too frequently violated. It is, however, a very useful supplement to the toolbox and can provide insights which traditional techniques cannot offer. It is particularly useful in screening items for inclusion in new questionnaires, and for checking the validity of assumptions even in traditional tests. For these purposes alone, it certainly deserves wider usage than it has received in the past. The most exciting roles for IRT in QoL research, however, lie firstly in the standardisation of different instruments so that QoL as assessed by disease- and treatment-specific instruments can be compared across different groups of patients, and secondly in the development of computer-administered adaptive testing. Both of these objectives require extremely large databases for the exploration of IRT models.

IRT is a complex subject, and a good starting point for further reading is the book *Fundamentals of Item Response Theory*, by Hambleton, Swaminathan and Rogers (1991). In the same series, *Methods for Identifying Biased Test Items* by Camilli and Shepard (1994) discusses item bias and DIF. Item bias is also the subject of the book by Osterlind (1983). The Rasch model is described in detail by Andrich, in *Rasch Models for Measurement* (1988).

7 Questionnaire Development and Scoring

Summary

Previous chapters have reviewed the aims, principles and psychometric techniques of questionnaire design, validation and testing. We now consider the practical aspects, and show how the methods of the earlier chapters relate to the development of new instruments.

7.1 INTRODUCTION

The development of a new QoL instrument requires a considerable amount of painstakingly detailed work, demanding patience, time and resources. Some evidence of this can be seen from the series of publications that are associated with such QoL instruments as the SF-36, the FACT and the EORTC QLQ-C30. These and similar instruments have initial publications detailing aspects of their general design issues, followed by reports of numerous validation and field-testing studies.

Many aspects of psychometric validation depend upon collecting and analysing data from samples of patients or others. However, the statistical and psychometric techniques can only confirm that the scale is valid in so far as it performs in the manner that is expected. These quantitative techniques rely upon the assumption that the scale has been carefully and sensibly designed in the first place. To that end, the scale development process should follow a specific sequence of stages, and details of the methods and the results of each stage should be documented thoroughly. Reference to this documentation will, in due course, provide much of the justification for content validity. It will also provide the foundation for the hypothetical models concerning the relationships between the items on the questionnaire and the postulated domains of QoL, which are then explored as construct validity.

7.2 GENERAL ISSUES

Before embarking on developing a questionnaire for QoL assessment, the research questions should have been formulated clearly. This will include specification of the objectives in measuring QoL, a working definition of what is meant by "quality of life," identification of the intended groups of respondents, and proposals as to the aspects or main dimensions of QoL that are to be assessed. Examples of *objectives* are whether the instrument is intended for comparison of treatment groups in clinical trials (a discriminative instrument), or for individual patient evaluation and management. Possible *definitions* of QoL might place greater or lesser importance upon symptoms, psychological, spiritual or other aspects. According to the specific definition of the target respondents, there may be particular emphasis upon disease- and treatment-related issues. All these considerations will affect decisions about the *dimensions* of QoL to be assessed, the number of questions, feasible length of the questionnaire and the scope and content of the questions.

When an instrument is intended for use in clinical trials, there is a choice between aiming at a general assessment of health-related QoL that is applicable to a wide range of patients, or a detailed evaluation of treatment- or disease-specific problems. The former has the advantage of providing results that can be contrasted across patients from trials in completely different disease-groups. This can be important when determining healthcare priorities and allocation of funding. The SF-36 is an example of such an instrument. However, disease-specific instruments can provide information that focuses upon the issues considered to be of particular importance to the patient-groups under investigation. Treatment-specific instruments will clearly be the most sensitive ones for detecting differences between the treatment groups.

7.3 DEFINING THE TARGET POPULATION

Before considering the issues to be addressed by the instrument, it is essential to establish the specification of the target population. What is the range of diseases to be investigated, and are the symptomatology and QoL issues the same for all disease subgroups? What is the range of treatments for which the questionnaire should be applicable? For example, in cancer there can be a wide range of completely different treatment modalities, from hormonal treatment to surgery. Even within a class of treatments, there may be considerable variability; the drugs used in cancer chemo-therapy include many with completely different characteristics and toxic side-effects. A QoL instrument that will be used for more than the immediate study should ensure that it is appropriate for the full range of intended treatments. Similarly, patient characteristics should be considered. For example, what is the age range of the patients, and might it include young children who have very different priorities and may also require help in completing the questionnaire? Will the target group include very ill patients, who may have high levels of symptomatology and who may find it difficult or even distressing to answer some questions? Might a high proportion of patients be relatively healthy, with few symptoms? If so, will the questions be sufficiently sensitive to discriminate between patients who report "no problems" in response to most items?

The detailed specification of the intended patient population and their target disease states is second in importance only to the specification of the scientific question and the definition of QoL or of the aspects of QoL that are to be investigated. All of these aspects should be specified and recorded carefully.

7.4 ITEM GENERATION

The first phase of developing a QoL instrument is to generate an exhaustive list of all QoL issues that are relevant to the domains of interest, using literature searches, interviews with healthcare workers, and discussions with patients. It is essential to have exhaustive coverage of all symptoms that patients rate as being severe or important. After identifying all of the relevant issues, items can be generated to reflect these issues. Some issues, such as anxiety, are often assessed using several items in order to increase the reliability of the measurement. The two principal approaches for selecting items for this purpose are Likert summated scales using parallel tests, or item response theory (IRT) models. On the other hand, symptoms or other causal variables are more commonly assessed using single items.

LITERATURE SEARCH

The initial stage in item generation usually involves literature searches of relevant journals and bibliographic databases, to ensure that all issues previously though to be relevant are included. Any existing instruments that address the same or related areas of QoL assessment should be identified and reviewed. From these sources, a list of potential QoL issues for inclusion in the questionnaire can be identified.

Example from the literature

Bjordal *et al.* (1994a) describe the development of a head and neck (H&N) cancer-specific questionnaire, designed as a supplementary module to the EORTC QLQ-C30. Literature searches were made for relevant QoL issues, using the medical bibliographic databases of MEDLINE and CANCERLIT. Textbooks on medical oncology and radiotherapy were also used. Forty-six relevant references were found, from which 57 issues were identified for possible inclusion in the QoL module. These issues were divided into five areas: pain-related issues, nutritional problems, dental status, other symptoms, and functional aspects.

SPECIALIST INTERVIEWS

The list generated by the initial search should be reviewed by a number of healthcare workers who are experienced in treating or managing patients from the disease area in question. This will usually include physicians and nurses, but may well also involve psychiatrists and social workers. They should address issues of content validity: Are the issues that are currently proposed relevant, or should some be deleted? If they are recommended for deletion, why? Some possible reasons for deletion of an issue may be: (a) it overlaps closely with other issues that are included, possibly by being too broad in scope; (b) it is irrelevant to the target group of patients; (c) it lacks importance to QoL evaluation; and (d) it concerns extremely rare conditions and affects only a small minority of patients. Care should be taken to ensure that issues are not deleted at this stage simply because of fixed opinions of the development team.

Of equal importance is that the questionnaire should be comprehensive. What other issues should be added to the list? If new issues are proposed, details of the reasons should be recorded for subsequent justification in reports or publications.

Following this stage, a revised list of issues will have been generated.

Example from the Literature

> Bjordal *et al.* (1994a) interviewed 21 specialist nurses, oncologists and surgeons. Seventeen of the 57 issues identified in the literature search were regarded as being irrelevant, too rare, or too broad in scope. Although five specialists felt that questions about body image and sexuality were irrelevant, these items were retained because previous statements by patients had indicated that they might be important. Fifty-nine new issues were also proposed, and eleven of these were added, resulting in a provisional list of 43 issues.

PATIENT INTERVIEWS

The revised list of issues should be reviewed by a group of patients who are representative of those in the intended target population. For example, the group should contain patients of different ages and with a range of disease severities. Their brief will be similar to that of the healthcare specialists: to recommend candidate items for deletion, and identify omissions.

Example from the literature

> Bjordal *et al.* (1994a) interviewed 40 patients with H&N cancer and, as a result, six of the issues that were felt by them to be of low relevance or unimportant were deleted. In contrast, 21 new symptoms or problem issues and five new function issues were identified. However, none of these was proposed by more than one or two patients, and they were hence not regarded as of general interest. The revised list covered 37 issues.

7.5 FORMING SCALES

A decision must be made regarding the format of the questions. Most of the individual questions to be found on QoL questionnaires either take responses in binary format, such as yes/no, or are ordinal in nature. *Ordinal scales* are those in which the patients rank themselves between low and high, not at all and very much, or some similar range of grading. Usually the responses to such questions are assigned arbitrary scores of successive integers starting from 0 or 1, although a few instruments assign nonlinear scores. Thus the modified Barthel Index assigns scores 0, 2, 5, 8, 10 to successive categories of the feeding item. The example instruments in the Appendix illustrate a variety of formats for ordinal scales. Chapter 8 describes analysis of ordinal data.

ORDERED CATEGORICAL OR LIKERT SCALES

The most common ordinal scale is the *labelled categorical scale*. For example, the EORTC QLQ-C30 items have four-point labelled categories of "Not at all", "A little", "Quite a bit" and "Very much". These labels have been chosen by defining the two extremes, and then devising two intermediate labels with the intention of obtaining a very roughly even spread. However, there is little evidence that the difference between, say, categories "Not at all" and "A little" is emotionally, psychophysically or in any other sense equal to the difference between "A little" and "Quite a bit" or between "Quite a bit" and "Very much". Thus there are no grounds for claiming that these *ordinal scales* have the property of being *interval scales*.

Labelled categorical scales usually have four or five categories, although six or even seven are sometimes used. Fewer than four categories is usually regarded as too few, whilst studies have shown that many respondents cannot reliably and repeatedly discriminate between categories if there are more than six or seven. There are divided opinions about the advantages or disadvantages of having an odd number of categories for a symmetrical scale. For example, question 11 of the SF-36 ranges from "Definitely true" to "Definitely false", leading to a middle category of "Don't know". Some investigators argue that it is better to have an even number of categories instead, so that there is no central "Don't know" and respondents must make a choice.

Scales with more than five categories are also often presented with only the two end-points labelled. For example, question 30 on the EORTC QLQ-C30, "How would you rate your overall quality of life during the past week?", takes responses 1 to 7, with only the two ends labelled: "Very poor" to "Excellent". Although it may seem more likely that this could be an interval scale, there is little scientific evidence to support the intervals between successive score-points as being equal.

Ordered categorical scales, when scored in steps of one, are commonly called *Likert scales*. Despite the ongoing arguments about the lack of equal-interval properties, these scales have consistently shown themselves to provide useful summaries that appear to be meaningful even when averaged across groups of patients.

VISUAL ANALOGUE SCALES

Visual analogue scales (VAS) consist of lines, usually horizontal and 10 cm long, the ends of which are marked with the extreme states of the item being measured. Patients are asked to mark the line at a point that represents their position between these two extremes. The responses are coded by measuring their distance from the left-hand end of the line. These scales have been used in QoL assessment for many years. Although some patients may take some time to get used to them, most find them easy to complete.

VAS are generally thought to have equal-interval properties, although this is not necessarily true. In particular, McCormack, Horne and Sheather (1988) have reviewed the distribution of responses to VAS questions and have suggested that many respondents cluster their answers as high, middle or low. For analyses or the readings, some investigators use the reading in millimetres of the distance along the scale, resulting in readings between 0 and 100. Others regard the mark as being the manifestation of a yes/no binary response and so, by analogy with logistic regression and IRT models, use a logit transformation of the VAS score; that is, $\text{logit(VAS)} = \log[\text{VAS}/(\text{VAS} - 100)]$.

VAS scales can take many forms. An example of an instrument with a scale that is similar to a VAS is the EQ-5D (Appendix E4), which contains a "thermometer" scale. It is vertical, and graduated with 100 tick-marks and labelled at every tenth.

PLEASE SCORE HOW YOU FEEL EACH OF THESE ASPECTS OF YOUR
LIFE WAS AFFECTED BY THE STATE OF YOUR HEALTH DURING TODAY (24H)

Nausea
extremely severe _____ no nausea
nausea

Physical activity
completely unable_____ normal physical
to move my body   activity for me

Depression
extremely   _____ not depressed
depressed   at all

Figure 7.1   The Linear Analogue Self Assessment scale (LASA) is an example of a visual analogue scale (Based on Selby PJ, Chapman JA, Etazadi-Amoli J, Dalley D and Boyd NF (1984). The development of a method for assessing the quality of life in cancer patients. *British Journal of Cancer*, **50**, 13–22, by permission of the publisher Churchill Livingstone)

It has been claimed that the VAS is more sensitive and easier for patients to complete than ordered categorical scales, although this has been disputed in some reviews (McCormack *et al.*, 1988). However, VAS is used less frequently in QoL instruments than ordered categorical scales, possibly because they take greater space on the page and demand more resources for measuring the responses. It will be interesting to see whether VAS become more widely used now that interactive computer data-capture methods are available.

Example from the literature

Selby *et al.* (1984) describe an instrument containing VAS, for assessing QoL in cancer patients. They called the scales "linear analogue self-assessment" (LASA) scales. These included a "Uniscale" assessing overall QoL, and 30 scales for individual items. Each scale was 10 cm long. Three items are shown in Figure 7.1.

GUTTMAN SCALES

A Guttman scale consists of several items of varying difficulty. An example is found in many activities-of-daily-living (ADL) scales. These usually consist of a number of items that represent common functions or tasks, sequenced in order of increasing difficulty. Guttman scales are also sometimes called "hierarchical" scales, since the questions can be ranked as a hierarchy in terms of their difficulty or challenge to the respondents.

In a strict sense, a Guttman scale is a rigidly hierarchical scale. If a patient can accomplish a difficult task at the upper end of the scale, they *must* be able to accomplish all of the easier tasks. For the EORTC QLQ-C30, and for most other ADL and physical functioning scales, this is clearly untrue. Although climbing stairs, for example, might be regarded as more difficult than taking a short walk, a few patients might be able to climb stairs yet be unable to take a walk. Thus this

		No	Yes
1.	Do you have any trouble doing strenuous activities, like carrying a heavy shopping bag or a suitcase?	1	2
2.	Do you have any trouble taking a long walk?	1	2
3.	Do you have any trouble taking a short walk outside of the house?	1	2
4.	Do you need to stay in bed or a chair during the day?	1	2
5.	Do you need help with eating, dressing, washing yourself or using the toilet?	1	2

Figure 7.2   Physical functioning scale of the EORTC QLQ-C30 versions 1.0 and 2.0

scale is not a true Guttman scale, because the ordering of item difficulty is not fixed and constant for all patients. IRT provides a more appropriate model. It assumes that items are of varying difficulty with a probability of positive response that varies according to each patient's ability. That is, IRT incorporates a probabilistic element for responses, whereas a Guttman scale is strictly deterministic and depends solely upon the patient's ability. Hence, Guttman scales are rarely used nowadays.

Example

The physical functioning scale of the EORTC QLQ-C30 contains five items of varying difficulty, shown in Figure 7.2. In versions 1.0 to 2.0, each item was scored "Yes" or "No". The scale is hierarchical in concept, with items ranging from easy (eating, dressing, washing) to difficult (carrying heavy loads).

7.6   SCORING MULTI-ITEM SCALES

There are three main reasons for combining and scoring multiple items as one scale. Some scales are specifically designed to be multi-item, to increase reliability or precision. Sometimes items are grouped simply as a convenient way of combining related items; often this will follow the application of methods such as factor analysis, which may suggest that several items are measuring one construct and can be grouped together. Also, a multi-item scale may arise as a clinimetric index, in which the judgement of a number of clinicians and patients is used as the basis for combining heterogeneous items into a single index.

The simplest and most widely practised method of combining or *aggregating* items is the method of *summated ratings*, also known as *Likert summated scales*. If each item has been scored on a k-point ordered categorical scale, with scores either from 1 to k or 0 to $k-1$, the total sum-score is obtained by adding together the scores from the individual items. For a scale containing m items, each scored from 0 to $k-1$, the sum-score will range from 0 to $m \times (k-1)$. Since different scales may have different numbers of items or categories per item, it is common practice to "standardise" the sum-scores to range from 0 to 100. This may be done by multiplying the sum-score by $100/(m \times (k-1))$. It should be noted that if some questions use positive wording and others negative, it may be necessary to reverse the scoring of some items so that they are all scored in a consistent manner with a high item score indicating, for example, a high level of problems.

Example

The emotional functioning scale of the EORTC QLQ-C30 (Appendix E6) consists of questions 21–24. These four items are scored from 1 to 4. A patient responding 2, 2, 3 and 4 for these items has a sum-score of 11. The range of possible scores is from 4 to 16. Thus we can standardise these scores to lie between 0 and 100 by first subtracting 4, giving a new range of 0 to 12, and then multiplying by 100/12. Hence the standardised score is $(11 - 4)\times100/12 = 58.3$. However, the *Scoring Manual* for the EORTC QLQ-C30 (Fayers *et al.*, 1999) specifies that high scores for functioning scales should indicate high levels of functioning, whereas high responses for the individual items indicate poor functioning. To achieve this the scale score is subtracted from 100, giving a patient score of 41.7.

Likert summated scales are optimal for parallel tests, because for these each item is an equally good indicator of the same underlying construct (see Chapter 2). Perhaps surprisingly, they have in practice also been found to be remarkably robust in a wide range of other situations. The main requirement is that the items should be *indicator variables*. Each item should also have the same possible range of score values.

The items of the physical functioning scale of the EORTC QLQ-C30 are clearly not parallel items. However, a summated scale has the property that higher scores correspond to greater numbers of problems. Thus although Likert scales are intended for parallel tests, the same procedure is sensible for use with many other types of scale. In particular, this is the approach recommended by the EORTC Quality of Life Study Group for scoring the physical functioning scale (Fayers *et al.*, 1999).

It is sometimes suggested that *weights* should be applied to those items that are regarded as most important. Thus, for example, an important item could be given double its normal score, or a *weight* of 2, so that it would have values 0 to $2 \times (k-1)$. If there are three items in a scale, and one is given double weight, that is equivalent to saying that this item is just as important as the other two combined. If the ith item has a score x_i, we can assign weights w_i to the items and the sum-score becomes $\sum w_i x_i$. However, empirical investigations of weighting schemes have generally found them to have little advantage over simple summated scales.

Other methods for aggregating items into scores have been proposed, including Guttman scalogram analysis, the method of equal-appearing intervals, and multi-dimensional scaling. These methods are rarely used for QoL scales nowadays. In the past, factor weights derived from exploratory factor analysis have occasionally been used when aggregating items; in Chapter 5 we showed that this is unsound. For indicator variables, the principal alternative to summated scales is IRT (see Chapter 6).

For scales containing *causal variables* there are other considerations. Although summated scores are frequently used, causal variables should be included in Likert scales only with caution. Fayers *et al.* (1997a) show that if a scale contains several causal items that are, say, symptoms, it is surely inconceivable that each symptom must be equally important in its effect upon patients' QoL. Whilst some symptoms, even when scored "very much", may have a relatively minor impact, others may have a devastating effect upon patients. Instead of a simple summated scale, giving equal weight (importance) to each item, symptom scores should be weighted, and the weights should be derived from patients' ratings of the importance and severity of different symptoms.

As noted in Chapter 2, if the causal variables are also *sufficient causes*, linear models such as Likert summated scales and weighted sum-scores will not be satisfactory predictors of QoL. Nonlinear functions may be more appropriate. A high score on any one of the sufficient-cause symptoms would suffice to reduce QoL, even if no other symptoms are present. A maximum of the symptom scores could be a better predictor of QoL than the average symptom level. Utility functions are another possibility (see, for example, Torrance *et al.*, 1996), and these lead to estimation of QoL by functions of the form $\sum w_i \log(1 - x_i)$.

7.7 WORDING OF QUESTIONS

Having identified the issues considered relevant and having made some decisions regarding the format of the questions, the next stage is to convert the items into questions. It should go without saying that questions should be brief, clearly worded, easily understood, unambiguous, and easy to respond to. However, the experience of many investigators is that seemingly simple, lucid questions may present unanticipated problems to patients, and that all questions should be extensively tested on patients before being used in a large study or a clinical trial.

The book by Sudman and Bradburn (1982) focuses on wording and designing questionnaires. The following suggestions are merely a sample of the many points to consider.

1. Make questions and instructions brief and simple. Ill patients and the elderly, especially, may be confused by long, complicated sentences.
2. Avoid small, unclear typefaces. Elderly patients may not have good eyesight.
3. Questions that are not applicable to some patients may result in missing or ambiguous answers. For example, "Do you experience difficulty going up stairs?" is not applicable to someone who is confined to bed. Some patients may leave it blank because it is not applicable, some might mark it "Yes" because they would have difficulty if they tried, and others might mark it "No" because they never need to try and therefore experience no difficulty. The responses cannot be interpreted.
4. If potentially embarrassing or offending questions are necessary, consider putting them at the end of the instrument or making them optional. For example, the FACT-G has a question about satisfaction with sex life, but precedes this with "*If you prefer not to answer it, please check this box and go to the next section.*"

5. Avoid double negatives. For example, a question such as "I don't feel less interest in sex (Yes/No)" is ill-advised.
6. If two or more questions are similar in their wording, use underlining, bold or italics to draw patients' attention to the differences. For example, questions 4 and 5 of the SF-36 are very similar apart from the underlined phrases "<u>as a result of your physical health</u>" and "<u>as a result of any emotional problems</u>".
7. Use underlining and similar methods also to draw attention to key words or phrases. For example, many of the instruments underline the time frame of the questions, such as "<u>during the past 7 days</u>".
8. Consider including items that are positively phrased as well as negatively phrased items. For example, the HADS includes equal numbers of positive and negative items, such as "I feel tense or 'wound up'" and "I can sit at ease and feel relaxed."

7.8 PRE-TESTING THE QUESTIONNAIRE

It is essential that new QoL questionnaires be extensively tested on groups of patients before being released for general use. This testing is best carried out in two stages. First, before the main "field-test", a pilot or "pre-test" study should be conducted. The purpose of this initial study is to identify and solve potential problems. These might include ambiguity or difficult phrasing of the questions and responses, or might relate to the layout and flow of the questions.

For the pre-test, patients should first be asked to complete the provisional questionnaire, and then debriefed using a pre-structured interview. Sprangers *et al.* (1998) suggest that they could be asked about individual items; for example: "Was this question difficult to respond to?", "Was it annoying, confusing or upsetting?", "How would you have asked this question?" and "Is this experience related to your disease or treatment?"

If resources do not permit an item-by-item scrutiny, the whole instrument could be reviewed instead; for example: "Were there any questions that you found irrelevant?", "Were there questions that you found confusing or difficult to answer?", "Were any questions upsetting or annoying?"

Whichever approach is used, there should be some general questions about the whole instrument: "Can you think of other important issues that should be covered?" and "Do you have other comments about this questionnaire?" There should also be questions about how long the questionnaire took to complete, and whether assistance was obtained from anyone.

The results of the pre-testing should identify any potentially serious problems with the questionnaire. Before carrying out the field study, wording of items may need to be changed, items deleted, or additional items introduced.

REPRESENTATIVE SAMPLE

The pre-testing will usually involve between 10 and 30 patients, selected as representing the range of patients in the target population. These should not be the same patients as those who were used when identifying the issues to be addressed. If a questionnaire is intended to be applicable to various subgroups of patients for whom the QoL issues might vary, it is important to ensure that there is adequate representation of all these types of patients and the sample size may have to be increased accordingly. Thus if a QoL questionnaire is intended to address issues associated with different modalities of treatment, it should be tested separately with patients receiving each of these forms of therapy. For example, an instrument for cancer patients could be tested in those receiving surgery, chemotherapy or radiotherapy. It is crucial to ensure that patients with each of these cancers are able to complete the questionnaire without difficulty, distress or embarrassment, and that all patients feel the relevant issues have been covered.

Example from the literature

The module of Bjordal *et al.* (1994a) is intended to cover problems over the whole range of H&N cancers. This is a heterogeneous group of patients, since the disease affects different anatomical sites, and they receive different treatment modalities. The symptomatology and the QoL issues that concern these patients vary considerably. For example, patients receiving radiotherapy for early laryngeal cancer may report problems with speech, social function and role function, whereas patients receiving surgery or radiotherapy for cancer of the oral cavity are more likely to experience pain, problems with their teeth, trouble eating, body image concerns and sexuality problems.

As a consequence, Bjordal *et al.* (1994a) recruited representative groups of patients with cancer of the oral cavity, larynx, pharynx, sinus and salivary glands. A total of 60 patients from five countries were included, compared with the usual 10–30 patients in such studies.

WORDING OF QUESTIONS

An important aspect of the pre-testing phase is the identification of items that have ambiguous, difficult or poorly worded questions. These items should be rephrased before the main field study is carried out.

Example from the literature

Bjordal *et al.* (1994a) reported that some patients found it confusing to answer certain positively worded functional items. For example, the patients were asked "Have you been able to talk on the telephone? (never, sometimes, often, very often)", but this was reworded to "Have you had any trouble talking on the telephone? (not at all, a little, quite a bit, very much)".

A different wording problem was detected when asking about swallowing problems, which are common for H&N cancer patients. Patients with extreme swallowing difficulty may have a tube inserted, and some of them left this question blank as being "not applicable". Others reported "no problems swallowing" because they no longer needed to swallow, and yet others responded that they had "a lot of problems" because they could not swallow. The question was ambiguous to patients with a feeding tube.

MISSING DATA

Interpretation of results is difficult when there is much missing data, and it is best to take precautions to minimise the problems. For example, questions about sexual interest, ability or activity may cause problems. In some clinical trials these questions might be regarded as of little relevance, and it may be reasonable to anticipate similar low levels of sexual problems in both treatment arms. This raises the question of whether it is advisable to exclude these potentially embarrassing items so as to avoid compromising patient compliance over questionnaire completion.

Example from the literature

Fayers *et al.* (1997b) reported that in a wide range of UK MRC cancer trials, approximately 19% of patients left blank a question about "(have you been bothered by) decreased sexual interest". Females were twice as likely as males to leave this item blank. Possible interpretations are that some patients found the question embarrassing, or that they did not have an active sexual interest before their illness and therefore regarded the question as not applicable. Perhaps wording should be adapted so that lack of sexual activity before the illness (not applicable) can be distinguished from other reasons for missing data.

7.9 STRATEGIES FOR VALIDATION

Both the pre-testing and field-testing phases aim to provide quantitative data for validation purposes, and in order to decide the appropriate sample sizes and the composition of the patient to be sampled it is necessary to consider the validation strategy. It was emphasised that the methods of Chapter 3 are important for all measurement scales, and that content validity is invariably important since it involves clinical sensibility. The need for emphasis on construct validation is more controversial, and as discussed there are problems when applying the methods of Chapter 4 to scales containing causal items. In particular, although there is always a need to evaluate individual new items, in some circumstances it might be reasonable to assume that the overall latent structure of the constructs is already well understood. Thus it is important to use methods such as multitrait scaling analysis for checking whether each of the chosen items really does belong to the scale it has been assigned to, and whether each item performs satisfactorily; but how crucial are other aspects of construct validity?

When developing an instrument for assessing general QoL in a new disease area, it may be possible to adopt the design constructs of existing instruments. Thus, for example, many instruments use a model that assumes distinct dimensions for physical, emotional, social and role functioning. Under these circumstances there are reasonable *a priori* grounds for believing that these constructs will satisfy the broader terms of construct validity—methods such as factor analysis are unlikely to reveal unexpected structures.

In addition, when adapting instruments to cover a new disease area, or when developing a disease-specific module to supplement an existing instrument, it is likely that many of the new items that are introduced will target disease-related problems such as symptoms or treatment issues. These are usually causal items, and so the reservations of Chapter 4 will hold.

However, very different considerations may apply when developing an instrument or scale to measure a particular aspect of QoL, such as fatigue, depression or pain. In this situation there may be far less prior knowledge about the constructs that it is aimed to measure, and there may even be research questions concerning the dimensionality and factor structure. Construct validity now assumes a far more important role. Furthermore, when assessing these dimensions, it is likely that many or all of the items may be indicator variables, and therefore all the methods of Chapter 4 can be pertinent.

Example

> The MFI-20 in Appendix E14 is intended to assess fatigue. The MFI-20 was developed using a five-dimensional model for fatigue, although this model remains controversial and other instruments have assumed a different structure for fatigue. Assessment of construct validity is therefore crucial, and methods such as factor analysis provide valuable insight into this instrument.

7.10   TRANSLATION

Since a field study will normally be conducted in a number of different countries, the QoL questionnaire will need to be translated into other languages. The translation process should be carried out just as rigorously as the instrument development process, to avoid introducing either errors into the questionnaire or shifts in nuances that might affect the way patients respond to items. The aims of the translation process should be to ensure that all versions of the questionnaire are equally clear, precise and equivalent in all ways to the original.

As a minimum, translation should involve a two-stage process. A native speaker of the target language who is also fluent in the original language should first make a forward translation. Then another translator who is a native speaker of the original language should take the translated version and make a back-translation into the original language. This second translator must be "blind" to the original questionnaire. Next, an independent person should formally compare each item from this forward–backward translation against the original, and must prepare a written report of all differences. The whole process may need to be iterated until it is agreed that the forward–backward version corresponds precisely in content and meaning to the original.

Following each translation, a patient-based study has to be carried out. This will be similar in concept to the pre-testing study that we described, and will examine whether patients find the translated version of any item confusing, difficult to understand, ambiguous, irritating or annoying.

7.11   FIELD-TESTING

The final stage in the development of a new questionnaire is the field-testing. The objective of field-testing is to determine and confirm the acceptability, validity, sensitivity, responsiveness, reliability and general applicability of the instrument to cultural groups or other subgroups.

The field study should involve a large heterogeneous group of patients, and this should include patients who are representative of the full range of intended responders. We have already emphasised the need to include a wide range of patients when determining the issues to be assessed and developing the wording of the questions. At the field-testing stage, it becomes even more crucial to ensure that the sample includes patients who are representative of the full range of the target population, and that sample sizes are adequate to test the applicability of the instrument to all types of patient. For example, it may be relevant to include males and females, elderly and young, sick and healthy, highly educated and less educated. Societies often include individuals from diverse cultures and ethnic origins, and even an instrument intended for use within a single country should be tested for applicability within the relevant cultural, ethnic or linguistic groups. Questions that are perceived as relevant and unambiguous by one group may be misunderstood, misinterpreted and answered in ways that are unexpected by the investigator. In some cases, questions that are acceptable to the majority of people may prove embarrassing or cause distress to minority groups.

A debriefing questionnaire should be used. This will be similar in style to the questionnaire administered during the pre-test stage: How long did the questionnaire take to complete? Did anyone help complete the questionnaire, and what was the nature of that help? Were any questions difficult to answer, confusing, upsetting? Were all questions relevant, and were any important issues missed? Any other comments?

The analyses of the field study should make use of the techniques described in Chapters 3 and 4 to examine validity, reliability, sensitivity and responsiveness. In addition, the following basic issues should be considered.

MISSING ITEMS

The extent of missing data should be determined and reported. This includes not only missing responses in which the answers are left blank, but also invalid or uninterpretable responses that will have to be scored "missing" for analyses of the data. For example, a patient might mark two answers to a categorical question that permits only a single response. If a question is unclear or ambiguous, there can be a high proportion of invalid responses of this form. If the reason for missing data is known, this too should be reported. For example, patients might indicate on the debriefing form that a question is difficult to complete or upsetting.

In general, it is to be expected that for any one item there will always be a few (1% or 2%) patients with missing data. This figure will obviously be reduced if there are resources for trained staff to check each questionnaire immediately upon completion, asking patients to fill in the omitted or unclear responses. Whenever items have missing values for more than 3–4% of patients, the questions should be re-examined. Possible reasons for missing values include:

- *Problems with the wording of response options to a question.* Patients may feel that none of the categories describes their condition. Alternatively, they may be unable to decide between two options that they feel describe their state equally well.
- *Problems with the text of an individual question.* Patients may find the question difficult to understand or upsetting.
- *Problems specific to particular subgroups of patients.* Thus it might be found that elderly patients have a higher than average proportion of missing values for questions which they regard as less applicable to them (such as strenuous activities), or which are cognitively demanding.
- *Problems with translation of a question or culture-related difficulties of interpretation.*
- *Problems understanding the structure of the questionnaire.* If a group of consecutive missing responses occur, it can indicate that respondents do not understand the flow of the questions. For example, this might happen following *filter* questions of the form: "If you have not experienced this symptom, please skip to the next section."
- *Problems with a group of related items.* If responses to a group of items are missing, whether or not consecutive questions on the questionnaire, it might indicate that some respondents regard these questions either embarrassing or not applicable.
- *Exhaustion.* This can be manifested by incomplete responses towards the questionnaire's end.

The proportion of missing forms should be reported, too. Again, any information from debriefing forms or any reasons recorded by staff should be described. A high proportion of missing forms might indicate poor acceptability for the instrument. For example it may be too complicated, too lengthy and tedious to complete, or it may ask too many upsetting or irritating questions. Patients may think the layout is unclear. The printing may be too small, or questionnaire may have been printed with an injudicious choice of paper and ink colours.

DISTRIBUTION OF ITEM RESPONSES

The range and distribution of responses to each item should be examined. This might be done graphically, or by tabulating the responses of those questions that have few response categories.

Ceiling effects, in which a high proportion of the total respondents grade themselves as having the maximum score, are commonly observed when evaluating instruments, especially if very ill patients are sampled and frequently occurring symptoms are measured. The presence of ceiling effects (or *floor effects*, with an excess of minimum values) indicates that the items or scales will have poor discrimination. Thus sensitivity and responsiveness will be reduced.

The interpretation of ceiling effects is affected by the distinction between indicator and causal variables. For indicator variables, the response categories should ideally be chosen so that the full range will be used. If the respondents rarely or never use one of the responses to a four-category item, the question becomes equivalent to a less sensitive one with only three categories. If all respondents select the same response option, no differences will be detected between the groups in a comparative study and the question becomes uninformative. An example of such an extreme case might arise when there are questions about very severe states or conditions, with most or even all of the respondents answering "none" or "not at all" to these items. It is questionable whether it is worth retaining such items as components of a larger summated scale, since they are unlikely to vary substantially across patient groups and will therefore tend to reduce the sensitivity of the summated-scale score. Thus an abundance of ceiling or floor effects in the target population could suggest an item should be reviewed, and possibly even deleted.

For causal variables such as symptoms, there are different considerations. In particular it is important to maintain comprehensive coverage of causal items. A symptom may be rare, but if it relates to a serious, extreme or life-threatening state it may be crucially important to those patients who experience it. Such symptoms are important and should not be ignored, even though they manifest floor effects. Equally, a symptom that is very frequent may result in ceiling effects and, in an extreme case, if all respondents report "very much" a problem, the item becomes of limited value for a discriminative purposes in a clinical trial. That item may, however, still be extremely important for descriptive or evaluative purposes, alerting clinical staff to the extensive problems and symptoms that patients encounter.

Questionnaires often use the same standardised responses for many questions. For example, all questions might consistently use four or five response categories ranging from "not at all" through to "very much". Although this is generally a desirable approach, it may be difficult to ensure that the same range of response options is appropriate to all items. Ceiling effects can indicate simply that the range of the extreme categories is inadequate. For example, possibly a four-point scale should be extended to seven points.

ITEM REDUCTION

While items were being generated, there was also the possibility of deleting any that appeared unimportant. However, the number of patients and clinicians included in the initial studies is usually small, and the decision to delete items would be based upon the judgement of the investigator. In later stages of instrument development there is greater scope for using psychometric methods to identify redundant or inappropriate items.

Ideally, a questionnaire should be brief, should cover all relevant issues, and should explore in detail those issues that are considered of particular interest to the study. Clearly compromises must be made: first, between shortening a questionnaire that is thought to be too lengthy, whilst retaining sufficient items to provide comprehensive coverage of QoL (content validity); and second, between maintaining this breadth of coverage whilst aiming for detailed in-depth assessment of specific issues. Sometimes the solution will be to use a broadly based questionnaire covering general issues, and supplement this with additional questionnaires that address specific areas of interest (for example Appendices E12 and E13) in greater depth. This modular approach is also adopted by the EORTC QLQ-C30 and the FACT-G.

Several psychometric methods may be used to indicate whether items could be superfluous. For multi-item scales, multitrait analysis can identify items that are very strongly correlated with other items, and are therefore redundant because they add little information to the other items. It can also detect items that are only weakly correlated with their scale score and are therefore either performing poorly or making little contribution. Cronbach's α can in addition be used to explore the effect of removing one or more items from a multi-item scale. If the α reliability remains unchanged after deleting an item, the item may be unnecessary. However, these methods are inappropriate for *clinimetric scales* or *causal variables*.

Example from the literature

Marx *et al.* (1999) reported the application of clinimetric and psychometric methods in the reduction of 70 potential items to a 30-item instrument. The clinimetric strategy relied upon the ratings of patients to determine which items to include in the final scale. Fifteen items were selected in common by both methods. The clinimetric methods selected a greater number of symptoms and psychological function items. In contrast, the psychometric strategy selected a greater number of physical disability items and factor analysis suggested that the items constituted a single factor.

These results can be explained in terms of causal and indicator variables. The clinimetric strategy favoured the inclusion of causal variables in the form of symptoms. The psychometric strategy favoured the physical disability items because they were measuring a single latent variable and were therefore more highly and more consistently correlated with each other.

As well as seeking to reduce the number of items in a scale, there is also scope for reduction at the scale-level itself. Single-item scales and scale-scores from multi-item scales can be compared, to check whether any are so highly correlated that it would appear they are measuring virtually the same thing.

At all stages, face validity and clinical sensibility should be considered. The principal role of psychometric analysis is to point at potential areas for change, but one would be ill-advised to delete items solely on the basis of very strong or very weak correlations.

CULTURAL AND SUBGROUP DIFFERENCES

There may be subgroups of patients with particular problems. Older patients may have different needs and concerns from younger ones, and may also interpret questions differently. There may be major cultural differences, and a questionnaire developed in one part of the world may be inappropriate in another. For example, respondents from Mediterranean countries can be less willing to answer questions about sexual activity than are those from northern Europe. Subjects from Oriental cultures may respond to some items very differently from Europeans.

The field study should be designed with a sufficiently large sample size to be able to detect major differences in responses according to gender, age group or culture. However, it is difficult to ensure that similar patients have been recruited into each subgroup. For example, in a multi-country field study there might be country-specific differences in the initial health of the recruited patients. Some countries might enter patients with earlier stage disease, and treatment or management of patients may differ in subtle ways. Thus observed differences in, for example, group mean scores could be attributable to "sampling bias" in patient recruitment or management, and it is extremely difficult to ascribe any observed mean differences to cultural variation in the response to questions.

Methods of analysis might include comparison of subgroup means and SDs. However, to eliminate the possibility of sampling bias, differential item functioning (DIF) is an attractive approach for multi-item scales. DIF analysis, which is described in Chapter 6, allows for the underlying level of QoL for each patient, and examines whether the individual item responses are consistent with the patients' QoL.

Example

> There may be different semantic interpretation of words by different cultures. Nordic and northern European countries interpret "anger" as something which is bad and to be avoided; in Mediterranean countries, "anger" is not only acceptable, but there is something wrong with a person who avoids expressing anger. Thus the interpretation of an answer to the question "Do you feel angry?" would need to take into account the cultural background of the respondent.

7.12   CONCLUSIONS

Designing and developing new instruments constitutes a complex and lengthy process. It involves many interviews with patients and others, studies testing the questionnaires upon patients, collection of data, and statistical and psychometric analyses of the data to confirm and substantiate the claims for the instrument. The full development of an instrument may take many years. If at any stage inadequacies are found in the instrument, there will be a need for refinement and re-testing. Many instruments undergo iterative development through a number of versions, each version being extensively reappraised. For example, the Appendix shows version 3.0 of the EORTC QLQ-C30 and version 4 of the FACT-G.

Instruments in the appendices, like many other instruments, will have undergone extensive development along the lines that we have described. How should one select an instrument for use? Assuming that you have formed a shortlist of potentially suitable instruments that purport to address the scientific issues that are relevant to your study, the next step is to check whether the instruments have been developed rigorously. The topics of this and previous chapters provide a basis. Points to consider are the following.

1. Is there formal written documentation about the instrument? Are there peer-reviewed publications to support the claims of the developers? Is there a user manual?
2. Was the instrument developed using rigorous procedures? Are the results published in detail? This should include all stages from identification of issues and item selection through to a large-scale field-testing.
3. Are the aims and intended usage of the instrument clearly defined?

4. What is the target population, and has the instrument been tested upon a wide range of subjects from this population? If your population differs from the target one, is it reasonable to expect the instrument to be applicable, and is additional testing required to confirm this? Will your study include some subjects, such as young children, for whom the instrument may be less appropriate?
5. Is the method of administration feasible? How long does the instrument take to complete? Is help necessary? Is the processing of questionnaires easy, or do items require coding, such as measurement of visual analogue scales?
6. Is the scoring procedure defined? Is there a global score for overall QoL? Are there any global questions about overall QoL?
7. Is there evidence of adequate validity and reliability? Do the validated dimensions correspond to the constructs that are of relevance to your study? How comprehensive has the validation process been, and did the validation studies have an adequate sample size?
8. Is there evidence of adequate sensitivity and responsiveness? How do these values affect the sample size requirements of your study?
9. Are there validated translations that cover your needs, present and future?
10. Are there guidelines for interpreting the scale scores?

Sometimes an existing instrument may address many but not all of the QoL issues that are important to a clinical investigation. In such circumstances, one can consider adding supplementary questions to the questionnaire. These questions should be added at the end, after all the other questions of the instrument, to avoid any possibility of disturbing the validated characteristics of the instrument. Interposing new items, deleting items, and altering the sequence of items may all alter the characteristics of the original questionnaire. The copyright owners of many instruments enforce this principle of new items appearing only at the end of their questionnaire. Ideally, each additional item should itself be tested rigorously, but in practice this is frequently not feasible. For example, a clinical trial may have to be launched by a specific deadline. However, as a minimum, all new items should be piloted upon a few patients before being introduced to the main study. Debriefing questions similar to those we have described should be used.

In summary, our advice is: Don't develop your own instrument—unless you have to. Wherever possible, consider using or building upon existing instruments. If you must develop a new instrument, be prepared for much hard work over a period of years.

C Analysis of QoL Data

8   Cross-sectional Analysis

Summary

This chapter describes the types of analysis and graphical methods appropriate to the comparison of groups of patients with QoL assessment at a common time point. The methods described are thus cross-sectional in nature. We describe some basic ideas for assessing statistical significance when comparing two groups, such as z- and t-tests, and the associated confidence intervals and the extension of these to the comparison of several groups using analysis of variance (ANOVA). These ideas are then generalised to enable differences to be adjusted for covariates, such as baseline patient characteristics (e.g. age and gender), using regression techniques. The relationship between ANOVA and linear regression is illustrated. Modifications to the methods for binary and ordered categorical variables are included, as well as methods for continuous data that do not have the Normal distribution form. Finally some graphical methods of displaying cross-sectional data are introduced.

8.1   TYPES OF DATA

As we have seen, QoL data are usually collected using a self-assessment instrument containing a series of questions. The answers to some of these questions may be analysed directly, or be first combined into a number of scales or domains, such as physical, emotional or cognitive, for the subsequent analysis. The variables from these questionnaires are of various types: they include binary, categorical, ordered categorical, numerical discrete or, less frequently, continuous variables. The statistical methods required for summarising and comparing groups of patients depend on the type of variable of concern.

NOMINAL DATA

Nominal data are data that one can name. They are not measured but simply counted. They often consist of "either/or" type observations; for example, Dead or Alive. At the end of the study, the proportion or percentage of subjects falling into these two binary categories can be calculated. In the SF-36, question 4c asks subjects to answer "Yes" or "No" to: ". . . Were limited in the *kind* of work or other activities".

However, nominal data may have more than two categories—for example, ethnic group or marital status—and the percentages falling into these categories can be calculated. The categories for nominal data are regarded as unordered since, for example, there is no implication that Chinese, Indian and Malayan ethnicity are ranked in order on some underlying scale.

Example

> Liddell and Locker (1997), in investigating attitudes to dental pain, recorded the marital status of subjects and classified them as: Never married, Married/ common law or Separated/divorced/widowed. The Pain Anxiety Symptoms Scale (PASS) was used for measuring QoL, and it may be anticipated that a subject's PASS score will differ in the three marital groups.

Nominal data with more than two categories are occasionally used with QoL variables, but this is more often encountered for covariates such as marital status, place of treatment, living conditions and (for cancer patients) histology.

ORDERED CATEGORICAL OR RANKED DATA

In the case of more than two categories, there are many situations when they can be ordered in some way. For example, the SF-36 question 1 asks: "In general, would you say your health is: Excellent, Very good, Good, Fair, Poor?" In this case there are five ordered categories ranging from Excellent to Poor. The proportion or percentage of subjects falling into these five categories can be calculated, and in some situations these categories may be given a corresponding ranking 1, 2, 3, 4 and 5 which may then be used for analysis purposes. An example is the test-for-trend as alluded to in Table 8.2 (see below). However, although numerical values are assigned to each response, one cannot always treat them as though they had a strict numerical interpretation, as the magnitude of the differences between, for example, Excellent (Rank 1) and Very good (2) may not necessarily be the same as between Fair (3) and Poor (4).

Example from the literature

> Stiggelbout *et al.* (1997) posed three questions assessing fear of recurrence of cancer. Possible responses to the item: "Do you feel insecure about your health?" were: Not at all, Somewhat/to some extent, Rather, Very much.
>
> In this case there are four ordered categories, and 80 (38%), 96 (46%), 29 (14%) and 4 (2%) of the 209 patients gave the respective response. Their ranks would be 1, 2, 3 and 4.

The majority of questions on QoL instruments seek responses of the ordered categorical type.

NUMERICAL DISCRETE/NUMERICAL CONTINUOUS

Numerical discrete data consist of counts; for example, a patient may be asked how many times they vomited on a particular day, or the number of pain relief tablets taken. On the other hand, numerical continuous data are measurements that can, in theory at least, take any value within a given range. Thus a patient completing the

EuroQol questionnaire is asked to indicate: "Your own health today" on a 10-cm vertical scale whose ends are defined by "Worse imaginable health state" with value 0 cm and "Best imaginable health state" with value 10.0 cm.

In certain circumstances, and especially if there are many categories, numerically discrete data may be regarded as effectively continuous for analytical purposes.

CONTINUOUS DATA: NORMAL AND NON-NORMAL DISTRIBUTIONS

A special case of numerical continuous data is that which demonstrates a Normal distribution—see, for example, Campbell and Machin (1999). In this case special statistical methods such as the t-test are available, as we shall describe. Frequently, however, QoL data do not have even approximately a Normal distribution. For example, many items and scales, especially when applied to healthy subjects or extremely ill patients, may result in data with a large number of maximum "ceiling" or minimum "floor" scores, which is clearly not of a Normal distribution form. Then alternative statistical methods, not based upon the assumption of a Normal distribution, must be used.

AGGREGATING CONTINUOUS DATA

The usual method of analysing continuous data involves calculating averages or means, or possibly mean changes or mean differences. This is the standard approach to aggregating continuous data into summary statistics, and is applied to continuous data of nearly all sources, from weights and heights through to blood pressures. However, many regard this as being questionable when applied to QoL data, because it assumes inherently that the scores are on equal-interval scales. In other words, it assumes that since the mean of two patients both scoring 50 on a scale from 0 to 100 equals the mean of two patients scoring 25 and 75, these pairs of patients have, on average, equivalent QoL.

Clearly the data should be analysed and reported in a manner that allows for the distribution of patient responses. If there is concern that low scores are particularly important, overall means may be inadequate to reflect this and, for example, it may be appropriate in addition to consider percentages of patients below a threshold value. When data follow a Normal distribution, the means, SDs and CIs provide an informative way to describe and compare groups of patients, and usually suffice to reflect any overall shift in response levels due to treatment differences. However, when the distributions are non-Normal, and especially when the shape of the distributions is not the same in all treatment groups, care must be taken to describe these distributions in detail as the reporting of a simple mean or median may not be adequate.

8.2 COMPARING TWO GROUPS

The essence of statistical analysis is to *estimate* the value of some feature of the patient population, derived from the data that have been collected. This may be the sample mean $\bar{x}$, the sample proportion p, the slope of a linear regression relationship β, or the difference between two such quantities calculated from distinct groups. In all these circumstances, what we observe is regarded as only an estimate of the true or underlying population value. The precision associated with each estimate is provided by the corresponding standard error (*SE*).

In very broad terms, the majority of statistical significance tests reduce to comparing the estimated value of the quantity of interest with its standard error by use of an expression like

$$z = \frac{\text{Estimate}}{SE(\text{Estimate})}. \tag{8.1}$$

The value of z so obtained is sometimes called a *z-statistic*, and is referred to tables of the Normal distribution (Table T1). Large values lead one to reject the relevant null hypothesis with a certain level of statistical significance or *p*-value. Statistical significance and the null hypothesis have been referred to earlier in Chapter 4; in brief, the *p*-value is the probability of the data, or some more extreme data, arising by chance if the null hypothesis were true.

The associated (95%) confidence interval (*CI*) takes the general form of

$$\text{Estimate} - 1.96 \times SE(\text{Estimate}) \quad \text{to} \quad \text{Estimate} + 1.96 \times SE(\text{Estimate}). \tag{8.2}$$

The general expressions (8.1) and (8.2) will change depending on circumstances, and may have to be amended radically in some situations. Precise details are to be found in general textbooks of medical statistics, including Campbell and Machin (1999) and Altman (1991). Altman *et al.* (2000) focuses on confidence intervals in particular.

BINOMIAL PROPORTIONS

If there are two groups of patients, then the proportions responding to, for example, the SF-36 question 4a, relating to the ". . . kind of work or other activities", can be compared. Thus if there are m and n patients respectively in the two groups, and the corresponding number of subjects responding "Yes" are a and b, then the data can be summarised as in Table 8.1.

Here the "estimate" we are focusing on is a difference in the proportion answering "Yes" in the two treatment groups. This estimate is

$$d = p_I - p_{II} = \frac{a}{m} - \frac{b}{n}, \tag{8.3}$$

and the standard error (*SE*) is

$$SE(d) = \sqrt{\frac{p_I(1 - p_I)}{m} + \frac{p_{II}(1 - p_{II})}{n}}. \tag{8.4}$$

The null hypothesis here is that there is truly no difference between the treatments being compared, and that therefore we expect d and hence z to be close to 0.

Table 8.1 Proportion of patients responding "Yes" to SF-36 question 4a in two treatment groups

Category	Treatment group		Totals
	I	II	
"Yes"	a	b	r
"No"	c	d	s
Totals	m	n	N
Proportion "Yes"	$p_I = a/m$	$p_{II} = b/n$	$p = r/N$

CATEGORICAL DATA

In Table 8.1 there are $R = 2$ rows and $C = 2$ columns, giving the $G = 4$ cells of a 2×2 contingency table. An analysis of such a table can also be conducted by means of a χ^2 test. The general expression for the χ^2 test is

$$\chi^2 = \sum_{i=1}^{G} \frac{(O_i - E_i)^2}{E_i}, \qquad (8.5)$$

where O_i and E_i are the observed and expected number of observations. For the $G = 4$ cells of Table 8.1, the observed values are $O_1 = a$, $O_2 = b$, $O_3 = c$ and $O_4 = d$ with expected values $E_1 = mp = rm/N$, $E_2 = np = rn/N$, $E_3 = m(1 - p) = ms/N$ and $E_4 = n(1 - p) = ns/N$.

This test has now moved away from the format described by equation (8.1) but gives exactly the same results. Although in common use, a disadvantage of the χ^2 approach is that it does not provide the components for calculating a confidence interval in an obvious way.

Example from the literature

Glaser *et al.* (1997), in comparing children who have had central nervous system tumours with a control group, state: "Despite no differences between overall school behaviour . . . they were less likely to express concern for others ($\chi^2 = 8.24$), Fisher's exact $p = 0.02$ . . .".

Use of Table T4 with $df = 1$ and $\chi^2 = 8.24$ leads to a p-value < 0.01. However, since the values in Table T4 with $df = 1$ are in fact equivalent to those of Table T1 squared, a more precise p-value can be obtained. Thus Table T1 with $z = \sqrt{8.24} = 2.87$ gives the p-value = 0.0041. Since a small p-value is taken as an indication that the null hypothesis may not hold, we conclude that there is a difference between the two groups with respect to "overall school behaviour".

In more technical language, the quantity z^2 follows a χ^2 distribution with $df = 1$. In general, a χ^2 test has $df = (R - 1) \times (C - 1)$, where R and C are the numbers of rows and columns of the corresponding $R \times C$ contingency table.

Fisher's exact test, referred to by Glaser *et al.* (1997), is another approach that is appropriate if the total sample size is small. It does not seem essential here, as there are 27 children with central nervous system tumours and a similar number of controls. In broad terms, Fisher's test would be appropriate if any of the four shaded cells of Table 8.1 has an expected value less than 5.

For a categorical variable of k (> 2) categories, there will be a $2 \times k$ table. The corresponding test is χ^2 of the form of equation (8.4), but now there are $G = 2k$ cells, and the calculated value is referred to Table T4 with $df = k - 1$.

Example from the literature

Hopwood *et al.* (1994) summarise the HADS anxiety score of patients with lung cancer during the palliative chemotherapy for their disease. Table 8.2 shows the first post-treatment assessments, categorised as Normal, Borderline or Case. These three categories are indeed ordered and given the ranks labelled $x = 1$, 2 and 3. Thus 15/91 (16%) are regarded as Cases with the two-drug regimen, while the corresponding figure for the four-drug regimen is 3/71(4%).

Ignoring first the fact that anxiety is an ordered categorical variable, direct calculation of equation (8.4) is possible. Here, $k = 3$, $O_1 = 62$, $O_2 = 14$, ... and $O_6 = 3$ and the corresponding expected values (in italics in Table 8.2) are $E_1 = 65.72$, $E_2 = 15.17$, ... and $E_6 = 7.89$. If all these values are substituted in equation (8.4), then $\chi^2_{Homogeneity} = 6.08$ with two degrees of freedom. The corresponding entry in Table T4 for $\alpha = 0.05$ is 5.99 which is close to 6.08; hence the *p*-value is approximately 0.05. This test suggests that there may be real differences in the proportion of Normal, Borderline and Cases within the two treatment groups.

Table 8.2 HADS anxiety score by chemotherapy regimen at the second assessment in patients with small-cell lung cancer (Reproduced by permission from Hopwood *et al.*, 1994)

Anxiety	Rank (x)	Chemotherapy group Two-drug	Four-drug	Totals	q (%)
Normal	1	62 *(65.72)*	55 *(51.28)*	117	53.0
Borderline	2	14 *(15.17)*	13 *(11.83)*	27	51.9
Case	3	15 *(10.11)*	3 *(7.89)*	18	83.3
	Totals	91	71	162	

This *test for homogeneity* asks a general question as to whether there are any differences between the two treatments—it is very non-specific. However, in the situation of an ordered categorical variable as is common with QoL data, a *test-for-trend* with $df = 1$ can supplement the homogeneity χ^2 test of equation (8.5). This makes use of the category ordering by assigning numerical values to the respective ranks as in Table 8.2, and checks if there is any evidence of increasing or decreasing changes over the categories. In terms of Table 8.2 this test checks for trend in the values of q.

Following the necessary calculations (see Altman, 1991, pp. 261–5), $\chi^2_{Trend} = 4.08$. In this case direct use of Table T4 gives the *p*-value < 0.05, rather than the more precise 0.0434 if one had referred $z = \sqrt{4.08} = 2.02$ to Table T1.

One can also check to see whether the assumption that the proportion q changes in a linear way with x is a reasonable assumption. This test for departure from trend compares χ^2_{Trend}, which will always be the smaller of the two, with $\chi^2_{Homogeneity}$. The difference between them $\chi^2_{Homogeneity} - \chi^2_{Trend} = 6.08 - 4.00 = 2.04$ has $df = k - 2 = 3 - 2 = 1$, and from Table T4 the p-value exceeds 0.1. More precisely, since $df = 1$, $z = \sqrt{2.04} = 1.43$ and the p-value is 0.15.

In summary, the overall test for homogeneity is almost statistically significant, suggesting a difference in HADS anxiety in the two treatment groups. However, most of this can be accounted for by a trend to fewer Cases of high anxiety levels with the four-drug regimen, since the test for departure from trend was not statistically significant.

NORMALLY DISTRIBUTED DATA

If the data can reasonably be assumed to have an approximately Normal distribution, then an appropriate summary statistic is the mean. This may be the case for data that are continuous, numerically discrete or ordered categorical. However, before analysis, checks should be made to verify that the assumption of a Normal distribution is reasonable.

Example from the literature

Greimel, Padilla and Grant (1997) state that when their QoL cancer scale (QOL-CA) was applied to 227 cancer patients who had been discharged from hospital: "The overall QOL-CA scores were normally distributed within a range from 22 to 78 (mean, $\bar{x} = 55$, $SD = 11$)".

If the data are indeed Normal, then the mean plus and minus twice (more precisely this should be 1.96) the SD would cover most of the range of the data. In their case, these values are $55 - (2 \times 11) = 33$ to $55 + (2 \times 11) = 77$ and do lie within the range of 22 to 78 as expected. It is prudent to check whether the mean QoL item or scale $\pm 2 \times SD$ has this property. Suppose the mean in the example above had been 15 but with the same SD, then the lower value would be $15 - (2 \times 11) = -7$, which is an impossible value on the scale. This would indicate that the data are distributed close to the end of the scale, and that their distribution is skewed and not of the Normal distribution form.

Assuming the QoL data have an approximately Normal form, the two treatments are compared by calculating the difference between the two respective means $\bar{x}_I$ and $\bar{x}_{II}$. Thus the true difference, δ, is estimated by

$$d = \bar{x}_I - \bar{x}_{II}, \tag{8.6}$$

where

$$SE(d) = \sqrt{\frac{SD_I^2}{n_I} + \frac{SD_{II}^2}{n_{II}}} \tag{8.7}$$

and SD_I and SD_{II} are the standard deviations within each group. Provided SD_I and SD_{II} are not too dissimilar, an approximate test of significance for the comparison of two means is then provided by equation (8.1) as before. However, a better estimate of the SE is obtained by assuming that, although the means may differ, the SDs of each group are both estimating a common value, denoted σ. Therefore the two estimates SD_I and SD_{II} can first be combined to obtain a pooled estimate of σ. This is given by

$$SD_{Pooled} = \sqrt{\frac{(n_I - 1)SD_I^2 + (n_{II} - 1)SD_{II}^2}{(n_I - 1) + (n_{II} - 1)}}. \tag{8.8}$$

The corresponding standard error (SE) is then

$$SE_{Pooled}(d) = SD_{Pooled}\sqrt{\frac{1}{n_I} + \frac{1}{n_{II}}}. \tag{8.9}$$

There will usually be very little difference in the numerical values calculated here from those by equation (8.7).

Hence the test of significance for the comparison of two means is provided by the *t-test*:

$$t = \frac{d}{SE_{Pooled}(d)}. \tag{8.10}$$

This is then referred to Table T1 of the standard Normal distribution to obtain the corresponding significance level or *p*-value.

In order to ascertain the *p*-value in small samples, however, t of equation (8.10) is referred to Table T3 of the *t*-distribution with $df = (n_I - 1) + (n_{II} - 1) = (n_I + n_{II}) - 2$, rather than Table T1. Similarly, the expression for the $100(1 - \alpha)\%$ CI of equation (8.2) replaces $z_{1-\alpha/2}$ by $t_{1-\alpha/2}$ where the particular value of t to use will depend on the degrees of freedom. From Table T1 for $\alpha = 0.05$ we had $z_{0.975} = 1.96$, and this value remains fixed whereas, in small sample situations, $t_{0.975}$ will change with differing df. One recommendation is always to use Table T3 in preference to Table T1 since the final row of the former contains the entries of Table T1. As a rule, if the degrees of freedom are less than 60 then Table T3 should be used.

Example

Smets *et al.* (1998, Table 2) give the mean scores for mental fatigue for 154 disease-free patients as 6.95, $SD = 4.2$ and for 139 subjects from the general population as 8.33, $SD = 4.8$. From these data $d = 8.33 - 6.95 = 1.38$, $SE(d) = 0.5294$. Here the sample sizes are large, so from Table T1 the 95% CI is given by $1.38 \pm (1.96 \times 0.5294)$ or 0.04 to 2.42. The CI does not include the null hypothesis value of $\delta = 0$. Thus there is evidence to suggest that patients have a lower mental fatigue score than the general population.

NON-NORMALLY DISTRIBUTED DATA

In many situations, QoL data do not have even approximately the Normal distribution form.

Example

The HADS data from Julious *et al.* (1997) of Table 8.3 has 22 categories that are formed from the summed responses to seven items on the scale. The data are numerically discrete, with a far from Normal distribution form. Consequently, the median rather than the mean provides a better summary, and differences in the way the statistical tests are calculated then result.

Table 8.3 Frequency of responses on the HADS for depression (Based on Julious *et al.*, 1997)

Category	Depression score	No. of patients
Normal	0	4
	1	16
	2	12
	3	13
	4	12
	5	10
	6	19
	7	13
Borderline	8	11
	9	9
	10	4
Case	11	5
	12	11
	13	4
	14	2
	15	3
	16	4
	17	0
	18	0
	19	1
	20	0
	21	1
Total		154

In these situations the usual procedure is to replace individual data values, which are first ordered or ranked from smallest to largest, by the corresponding rank. Thus each value now has one of the values 1 to N, where N is the total number of observations. If there are two groups of exactly equal size and the null hypothesis of no difference between the groups is valid, then the sums of the sets of ranks for each group would be approximately equal. Otherwise, the sums would differ. This test is termed the *Mann–Whitney test* and is often denoted by U. Full details are provided by Altman (1991).

In contrast, the *test-for-trend* of the data from Hopwood, Stephens and Machin (1994) compares the mean values of the variable x, which can take only the values 1, 2 and 3, in the two treatment groups. Here

$$\bar{x}_{2D} = \frac{(62 \times 1) + (14 \times 2) + (15 \times 3)}{91} = 1.48 \text{ and}$$

$$\bar{x}_{4D} = \frac{(55 \times 1) + (13 \times 2) + (3 \times 3)}{71} = 1.27,$$

where the smaller mean from the four-drug regimen indicates lower anxiety levels in this group. Note here that the medians of both treatment groups are 1 so that this summary measure does not distinguish between the groups.

Although the standard method for comparing two means is the two-sample z- or t-test, this is strictly only the case if the variable (here x, the rank) has an approximately Normal distribution. This is clearly not the case here. As a consequence the Mann–Whitney distribution free test may be preferable for these categorical responses.

Example from the literature

Glaser *et al.* (1997) compare the school behaviour and health status of 27 children after treatment for CNS tumours with school-age controls using, amongst others, teacher assessment by the Health Utilities Index (Mark III).

The authors used the Mann–Whitney U-test and quote: ". . . and were perceived to have impaired emotion ($z = 2.64$, $p = 0.01$)." In their report they have used the notation z in place of U but the latter would usually be preferable as it is then clear exactly which test procedure has been used in the calculation.

Morton and Dobson (1990) show how the differences in the response patterns can be summarised using the average ranks $\bar{R}_I$ and $\bar{R}_{II}$ for groups I and II. Thus

$$\theta = \frac{(\bar{R}_I - \bar{R}_{II})}{\bar{N}}, \tag{8.11}$$

where $\bar{N}$ is the average number of observations per group.

Example

We illustrate the calculation of θ using the data of Table 8.2. All observations from both groups are first numbered from 1 to 162 so that observations in category $x = 1$ have the numbers from 1 to 117, those in category $x = 2$ from 118 to 144 and those in category $x = 3$ from 145 to 162 (Table 8.4). The average rank for category 1 is the average of the smallest and largest numbers for the category; that is, 59.0. Similarly, the average rank for category 2 is 131.0 and for category 3 is 153.5.

Then making use of Table 8.2 the rank total for the two-drug group is $(62 \times 59.0) + (14 \times 131.0) + (15 \times 153.5) = 7794.5$ and its average is $7794.5/91 = 85.6538$. The rank total for the four-drug group is $(55 \times 59.0) + (13 \times 131.0) + (3 \times 153.5) = 5408.5$ and its average is $5408.5/71 = 76.1761$. The average number of subjects in the groups is $(91 + 71)/2 = 81.0$. Therefore using equation (8.11), $\theta = (85.6538 - 76.1761)/81.0 = 0.1170$.

This estimator is a measure of the difference between the two groups. If all the observations in the 4D are larger than any in the 2D group, $\theta = -1$; if all the 2D group observations are larger than the 4D group observations, $\theta = +1$; and if they have similar rankings, $\theta = 0$.

Table 8.4 Ranking of HADS observations from a small-cell lung cancer trial data of Table 8.2 to derive a median for each category

Category	Observation number	Category rank
1	1–117	59.0
2	118–144	131.0
3	145–162	153.5

One possible approach if data do not have a Normal distribution is to use a *transformation*; for example, using the logarithm of the data for analysis rather than the actual data. However, this may complicate interpretation of the results. Bland and Altman (1996) provide further details.

TIME-TO-EVENT

We will see in Chapter 9 that, in certain circumstances, it may be appropriate to summarize longitudinal QoL data such that the repeated values from each subject are reduced to a single measure, such as the *Area Under the Curve* (AUC). Once summarized in this manner, the analysis then proceeds in a cross-sectional manner. In some situations, a disease may reduce the QoL of patients from a baseline of, say, Q_0 to levels far below their age-matched contemporaries, in which case the object of therapy might be to restore the subject to the normative level, say $Q_{Population}$. This leads to assessment of the time taken from start of treatment until the level $Q_{Population}$ is achieved. This is the *time-to-event*, where the "event" is having attained $Q_{Population}$. Thus time-to-event is cross-sectional in nature and may be used to summarise the overall experience of patients within a treatment group.

Often, time-to-event data do not have a Normal distribution and are very skewed, and so the methods described in this chapter are not immediately applicable. Although a logarithmic transformation of the data may improve the situation, it does not provide the solution because time-to-event studies may have "censored" observations. Suppose, in the clinical trial we are conducting, Q_0 is observed, followed at successive and regular intervals by assessments by $Q_1, Q_2, \ldots, Q_T$, and none of these has attained the target $Q_{Population}$. The patient then refuses to complete any further QoL assessments. All we can say about this patient is that $Q_{Population}$ was not achieved in time T. We term such an observation *censored* and denote it by

$T+$. There is always a possibility that the target may be achieved after this time but we will never observe it.

Thus time-to-event studies generate times (often termed *survival times* since the statistical techniques were developed in studies measuring times to death), some which are censored. As indicated, censored values are often denoted by a "+". For example, $T = 26$ days implies the patient reaches Q_N by that time, whereas $T+ = 26+$ indicates that period of observation has gone by without reaching Q_N and, for whatever reason, we have no QoL information for this subject beyond this time. It is beyond the scope of this text to describe the associated statistical techniques for summarising such data, but they can be found in Parmar and Machin (1995).

8.3   ADJUSTING FOR COVARIATES

NORMALLY DISTRIBUTED DATA

In most circumstances the QoL measure of primary interest will be affected by characteristics of the subjects under study. In a clinical trial these could include the treatment under study and the age of the patient. We can relate the value of the QoL observed to one of these variables (for example, age) by the following *linear regression model*:

$$\mathrm{QoL} = \beta_0 + \beta_{Age}\,Age, \tag{8.12}$$

where the constants β_0 and β_{Age} are termed the *regression coefficients*. In particular, β_{Age} is the slope of the regression line that relates QoL to age.

If b_{Age}, the estimate of β_{Age} that is obtained by fitting this model, is close to 0 we conclude that QoL does not change with age. The mean QoL then provides an estimate b_0 of β_0.

Example from the literature

Greimel, Padilla and Grant (1997) use a linear regression model to relate activities-of-daily-living (ADL) scores to various characteristics of 227 cancer patients who had been discharged from hospital. In particular they regressed ADL on patient age and estimated the slope of the regression line as $b_{Age} = -0.006$. They do not give the estimate of β_0.

The negative value of b_{Age} here suggests, as one might anticipate, that the ADL scores decline slowly with age. The decline over the age range in the study of 21 to 88 years is estimated by $-0.006 \times (88 - 21) = -0.402$. This is less than half a point on the ADL scale.

However, such a linear regression model implies that the rate of decline is constant over the more than 60 years age span, which is very unlikely. If this were indeed the case, the "model" of equation (8.12) would not be appropriate to describe these data. A sensible precaution, before embarking on a regression analysis in this and any situation, is to make a scatter plot of ADL against the variable in question. In this example, we would examine how QoL changes with age to verify whether the relationship is, approximately at least, linear.

The analysis for comparing the means of two treatments by the z- or t-tests can also be formulated using a linear regression model of the form

$$QoL = \beta_0 + \beta_{Treatment} v, \tag{8.13}$$

where v is coded 0 for the first treatment group and 1 for the second. Then if $v = 0$ in this equation, $QoL = \beta_0$ and this can be thought of as the true or population mean value of the QoL score for the first treatment group. Similarly, when $v = 1$, $QoL = \beta_0 + \beta_{Treatment}$ represents the population value of the QoL score for the second treatment group. Hence the difference between the groups is $(\beta_0 + \beta_{Treatment}) - \beta_0 = \beta_{Treatment}$. This was estimated by d of equation (8.6). The equivalent null hypothesis of no difference between treatments can be expressed as $\beta_{Treatment} = 0$. This leads to $z = b_{Treatment}/SE(b_{Treatment})$, where $b_{Treatment}$ is the corresponding estimate derived from the data.

The test-for-trend described earlier is equivalent to fitting the linear regression line of QoL on the variable v.

Example

The data of Hopwood *et al.* (1994) in Table 8.2 can also be used to estimate the slope of the relationship. This gives $b = 0.1156$ with $SE(b) = 0.0571$. From these, $z = b/SE(b) = 0.1156/0.0571 = 2.02$ and, using Table T1, the p-value is 0.0434 as before following the χ^2_{Trend} test.

The positive slope, $b = 0.1156$, indicates that the relative proportion of patients receiving two-drug treatment tends to increase as the category changes from Normal through Borderline to Case. This trend suggests that 4D is the better therapy. The corresponding 95% *CI* for the slope using equation (8.2) is 0.003 to 0.228.

Suppose a study were investigating the relative merits of two types of intervention on QoL and the outcome measure was ADL. Since it is known that ADL declines with increasing age, one might ask whether a difference in mean ADL observed between the two intervention groups at the end of the study is explained by a different spectrum of subject ages within each intervention group. This can be assessed by combining equations (8.12) and (8.13) into the multiple regression equation

$$ADL = \beta_0 + \beta_{Treatment} v + \beta_{Age} Age. \tag{8.14}$$

This equation can then be fitted to the data using standard computer packages. The process is best done in two stages.

First we can fit the model $ADL = \beta_0 + \beta_{Treatment} v$, to obtain estimates of β_0 and $\beta_{Treatment}$. Then we fit the full model, equation (8.14), to obtain new estimates of β_0 and $\beta_{Treatment}$ together with an estimate of β_{Age}. If the second value corresponding to $\beta_{Treatment}$ remains effectively unchanged then, despite any imbalance of age within the two groups, the estimate of the difference between treatments remains unaffected. However, if the value corresponding to $\beta_{Treatment}$ is markedly different, then the imbalance of age within the two groups does affect the estimated difference between the interventions. This "adjusted for age" estimate is then a better measure of the treatment difference.

Many clinical trial protocols specify a baseline (time 0) QoL assessment, Q_0, followed by at least one further assessment at a fixed time point following treatment (time 1) to obtain Q_1. Pre-treatment QoL may influence later values, and this study design allows estimation of both the treatment effect upon Q_1 and the association of Q_1 with Q_0. By analogy with equation (8.14), the regression model to describe this situation for two treatment groups is

$$Q_1 = \beta_0 + \beta_{Treatment} v + \beta_{QoL} Q_0. \qquad (8.15)$$

In this model, the effect of treatment on QoL can be assessed while adjusting for Q_0.

An alternative method of analysis is to first calculate for each subject $D_{QoL} = Q_1 - Q_0$ and then fit the following regression equation:

$$D_{QoL} = \beta_0 + \beta_{Treatment} v. \qquad (8.16)$$

This will not give the same values for β_0 and $\beta_{Treatment}$ as equation (8.15) unless $\beta_{QoL} = 1$ exactly.

There is no simple answer as to which is the best approach to adopt, since the first is modelling the actual values of QoL at follow-up whilst the second models the change from baseline. In general, when comparing groups, we would recommend the former as the regression coefficient $\beta_{Treatment}$ then estimates the difference between groups. If the latter is used, then $\beta_{Treatment}$ measures a difference of differences (or changes) which is not so easy to interpret.

If other variables, such as age and gender, also influence QoL, the regression equation (8.14) can be extended to include them:

$$QoL = \beta_0 + \beta_1 v_1 + \beta_2 v_2 + \ldots + \beta_u v_u. \qquad (8.17)$$

These regression models can all be fitted using standard statistical packages. A careful description of multiple regression is given by Altman (1991, Section 12.4).

In randomised controlled trials, through the randomisation process, variables such as age and gender are usually fairly balanced between the treatment groups. It is often more critical to adjust for these factors in non-randomised studies.

Example

Loge *et al.* (1999) compared fatigue in 459 Hodgkin's disease survivors (HDS) and 2214 persons sampled from the general population, using the Fatigue Questionnaire. Table 8.5 shows the regression-adjusted comparison of those controls without specific diseases and the HDS patients. Age did not affect the difference between controls and HDS, although in this example gender appeared to be important.

Table 8.5 Multiple regression analysis of results from a fatigue questionnaire in patients surviving Hodgkin's disease and a control group (Based on Loge *et al.*, 1999)

Variable	*b*	*p*-value
Age	0.01	NS
Gender (M=0, F=1)	0.6	0.005
Educational level	−0.03	0.05
Controls *vs.* HDS	3.0	0.001

NON-NORMALLY DISTRIBUTED DATA

If the data have a binary form, for example if the responses are "Yes" or "No" as is the case from SF-36 question 4c, then the regression methods described require modification. Previously we assumed that the QoL scale was a categorical variable that for practical purposes has a Normal distribution form. This is clearly not the case if the variable is binary. For technical reasons, because the proportion, denoted p, has a restricted range from 0 to 1 and not from $-\infty$ to $+\infty$ as is the case for a variable with a Normal distribution, $\log [p/(1 - p)]$ is used on the left-hand side of the corresponding regression model such as equation (8.12). The right-hand side remains unchanged. The expression $\log [p/(1 - p)]$ is usually abbreviated as logit(p)—hence the terms *logit transformation* and *logistic regression*.

The logit transformation of p leads to summarising the relative merits of two treatments by the *Odds Ratio (OR)* rather than by the difference between two proportions. Thus from Table 8.1, where p_I is the probability of a response "Yes" with treatment I, then $(1 - p_I)$ is the probability of responding "No". This gives the odds of the responses as p_I to $(1 - p_I)$ or $p_I/(1 - p_I)$. For example, if $p_I = 0.5$ then the odds are 1 since the two responses are equally likely. Similarly, for treatment II, the corresponding odds are $p_{II}/(1 - p_{II})$. The ratio of these two odds is termed the OR, that is

$$OR = \frac{p_{II}/(1 - p_{II})}{p_I/(1 - p_I)} \tag{8.18}$$

The value under the null hypothesis of no treatment difference corresponds to $OR = 1$ since the odds will then be the same in both treatment groups. It is estimated, using the notation of Table 8.1, by $OR = (a/c)/(b/d) = ad/bc$.

If we are investigating differences between two treatments in this context, then an equation of the form (8.13) is replaced by the logistic regression equation

$$\text{logit}(p) = \beta_0 + \beta_{Treatment}(v). \tag{8.19}$$

Again if the treatment group is I, $v = 0$ and logit $(p) = \beta_0$; whereas if the treatment group is II, $v = 1$ and logit $(p) = \beta_0 + \beta_{Treatment}$. The difference between these two is $(\beta_0 + \beta_{Treatment}) - \beta_0 = \beta_{Treatment}$. From this the odds ratio is estimated by $OR = \exp(\beta_{Treatment})$. As indicated earlier, the null hypothesis of no treatment difference is expressed through $\beta_{Treatment} = 0$, since $OR_{Equivalence} = e^0 = 1$.

Example

Suppose the principal interest in the trial described by Hopwood *et al.* (1994) is the proportion of patients with Normal (HADS) anxiety in the two treatments. Table 8.2 can be reduced to Table 8.6.

Using the z-test for the difference in proportions with Normal anxiety levels, here 0.6813 and 0.7746 in 2D and 4D respectively, gives $z = 1.32$ and corresponding p-value $= 0.19$. The estimate of $OR = (62 \times 16)/(55 \times 29) = 0.6219$. The corresponding logistic regression model fitted to these data using STATA (1999) is $\text{logit}(p) = -0.2849 - 0.4749v$, so that $b_{Treatment} = -0.4749$ and $OR = \exp(-0.4749) = 0.6219$, which is the same as the value we calculated before.

For this example there is no advantage to the more complex logistic approach. However, in addition to the HADS score itself and the treatment received, patient-specific variables such as age, gender, stage of disease and so on are routinely recorded in such studies. Logistic regression enables their influence on the observed treatment differences to be assessed.

Table 8.6 HADS anxiety by treatment regimen at the second assessment in patients with small-cell lung cancer (Data from Hopwood *et al.*, 1994)

Anxiety	Treatment group		Totals
	Two-drug	Four-drug	
Normal	62 (68.1%)	55 (77.5%)	117
Borderline/case	29	16	45
Totals	91	71	162

8.4 ANALYSIS OF VARIANCE

We have described the test for the comparison of two means in two equivalent ways: the z- or t-test (depending on the sample size), and a regression analysis approach. A third equivalent way is by means of *analysis of variance* (ANOVA). Thus calculations summarised by equations (8.9) and (8.10) can be cast into an ANOVA format as in Table 8.7. Here the variance, V, is merely the SD squared.

In this table, $g = 2$ is the number of treatment groups, T_I is the sum of all the n_I observations of treatment I, T_{II} is the sum of all the n_{II} observations of treatment II, and $T = T_I + T_{II}$ is the sum of all the $N = n_I + n_{II}$ observations. It should also be noted that V_{Within} is the square of SD_{Pooled} used in equation (8.8), while $V_{Between}$ is proportional to d^2. The final column gives the value of Fisher's F-test; this requires two sets of degrees of freedom, one for the Between groups with $df_{Between} = g - 1$, and one for Within groups with $df_{Within} = N - g$. This is often expressed using the notation $F(df_{Between}, df_{Within})$. It can be shown in this situation when we are comparing two groups that $F = t^2$, the square of equation (8.10), so that the two procedures lead to exactly the same test.

The ANOVA of Table 8.7 refers only to a single QoL observation per patient with no repeats. It can be compared with the rather more complex Table 3.11 that was used to estimate the intraclass correlation and used repeated measures of QoL from

Table 8.7 Analysis of variance (ANOVA) table to compare $g = 2$ means

Source of variation	Sums of squares	Degrees of freedom (df)	Variances	Variance ratio
Between treatments	$S_{Between} = \dfrac{T_I^2}{n_I} + \dfrac{T_{II}^2}{n_{II}} + \dfrac{T^2}{n}$	$g - 1$	$V_{Between} = \dfrac{S_{Between}}{g - 1}$	$F = \dfrac{V_{Between}}{V_{Within}}$
Within treatments	$S_{Within} = S_{Total} - S_{Between}$	$(n_I - 1) + (n_{II} - 1)$	$V_{Within} = \dfrac{S_{Within}}{(n_I - 1) + (n_{II} - 1)}$	
Totals	$S_{Total} = \sum x_i^2 - \dfrac{T^2}{N}$	$n_I = n_{II} - 1 = N - 1$		

each patient. In Table 3.11 it was possible to divide the total variation into three component parts—between patients, between repeats within patients, and error (or residual variation) with corresponding division of the df. In that situation, if a statistical test of differences between patients is required, the F-ratio $= V_{Patients}/V_{Error}$ would be referred to Table T5 with df's of $(p-1)$ and $(rp-r-p+1)$ corresponding to v_1 and v_2 in Table T5. For comparison of repeats within patients, $F = V_{Repeats}/V_{Error}$ with $v_1 = (r-1)$ and $v_2 = (rp-r-p+1)$.

The ANOVA of Table 8.7 can be extended to $g > 2$ groups. For example, if there are $g = 3$ groups, then an extra term T_{III}^2/n_{III} will be added to $S_{Between}$, and $n_{III} - 1$ added to the degrees of freedom for S_{Within}. However, in this case F is not simply t^2 and Table T5 is required to obtain the corresponding p-value.

Example from the literature

Greimel, Padilla and Grant (1997) used the ANOVA to compare comorbidity (total score) between three age groups among cancer patients who had been discharged. Table 8.8 gives the mean comorbidity score for each age group. The resulting significance test, calculated using ANOVA, gave $F = 13.7$.

Here $N = 227$ patients and there are $g = 3$ groups; thus $df_{Between} = g - 1 = 2$ and $df_{Within} = N - g = 224$. This latter figure is large and one therefore uses the entries corresponding to $df = \infty$ in Table T5. Thus with $df_{Between} = 2$ and $df_{Within} = \infty$ in Table T5, the critical value for $\alpha = 0.05$ is $F(2, \infty) = 3.00$, for $\alpha = 0.01$ it is $F(2, \infty) = 4.61$ with p-value < 0.01.

The authors concluded: "The results showed that patients older than 65 years of age have a significantly higher level of comorbidity than patients 65 years of age and younger. . . ."

Table 8.8 Age differences in co-morbidity in patients who have been discharged following treatment for cancer (Based on Greimel ER, Padilla GV and Grant MM (1997). Physical and psychosocial outcomes in cancer patients: a comparison of different age groups. *British Journal of Cancer*, **76**, 251–255, by permission of the publisher Churchill Livingstone)

	Age (years)				
Total comorbidity score	<45	45–65	>65	F	p-value
N	37	106	84		
Mean	3.0	4.3	5.2	13.7	< 0.01
SD	0.9	2.2	2.1		

Doubtless the results do indicate such a conclusion, but ANOVA is not the best approach for analysis of these data. ANOVA is more appropriate when comparing three or more treatment groups, or perhaps several categorical groups, rather than groups defined arbitrarily from what is a continuous variable such as age. For example, Schag *et al.* (1992) use ANOVA to compare the QoL of four patient groups all with HIV infection using the HIV Overview of Problems–Evaluation System (HOPES). Grouping age as in Table 8.8 tends to suggest there is a jump in comorbidity score at each age group boundary, whereas there is more likely to be a gradual and smooth change with age. A scatter plot of comorbidity against age will reveal the shape of this change. Since age is continuous, a regression approach to the analysis would be more statistically efficient.

Example from the literature

Smets *et al.* (1998, Table 3) investigated the influence of gender and educational level on levels of mental fatigue, in 154 disease-free cancer patients treated with radiotherapy. The *F*-tests following ANOVA are $F(1, 150) = 8.08$ for gender differences and $F(3,148) = 2.11$ for educational level. From Table T5, the corresponding *p*-values are <0.01 and approximately 0.1, suggesting a gender difference in mental fatigue score but not one by educational level.

When comparing two groups we can use either an ANOVA or a regression approach to the analysis. However, in the case of more than two treatment groups ANOVA is easily extended whereas some care has to be taken with equation (8.13). Thus we cannot merely regard treatment as variable v in equation (8.13) and give it values (say) 0, 1 and 2, as this would imply that the three treatments (I, II and III) were of an ordered nature—although if they were, this is precisely what we should do. Instead, when comparing three (unordered) treatments, we have to express the regression model in the following way:

$$\text{QoL} = \beta_0 + \gamma_1 v_1 + \gamma_2 v_2. \tag{8.20}$$

The variables v_1 and v_2 are termed dummy variables. In this model, $v_1 = 1$ if the treatment group is I but $v_1 = 0$ if the treatment group is not I; and $v_2 = 1$ if the treatment group is II but $v_2 = 0$ if the treatment group is not II. In this way the three treatment groups correspond to different pairs of values of (v_1, v_2) in the following way. The pair $(v_1 = 1, v_2 = 0)$ defines treatment I patients. Similarly the pair $(v_1 = 0, v_2 = 1)$ defines treatment II patients. Finally, the pair $(v_1 = 0, v_2 = 0)$ defines treatment III since the values of v indicate neither a treatment I patient nor a treatment II patient.

In this model there are therefore two regression coefficients, γ_1 and γ_2, to be estimated for the treatment effects. The null hypothesis of no treatment differences corresponds to testing whether the regression coefficients are simultaneously zero; that is, if $\gamma_1 = \gamma_2 = 0$. Extending this approach, if there are g treatment groups then g—1 dummy variables will need to be created.

The advantage of the regression model approach of equation (8.20) over the ANOVA of Table 8.7 is that covariates can be more readily added to the model so that the final treatment comparisons can be adjusted for the (possible) influence of these variables. In some studies ANOVA can also be adjusted for covariates (ANCOVA), but this is not as flexible as the regression approach. Therefore we recommend the use of regression techniques for QoL analysis.

CHECKING FOR NORMALITY

When analysing QoL scale data it is often advantageous to be able to assume that the data have an approximately Normal distribution shape. We have suggested that comparing the magnitudes of the mean and *SD* may lead one to suspect a rather skew distribution, which can be confirmed by a histogram of the data. For small samples, it may be difficult to judge the degree of non-Normality of the data, and Altman (1991) describes how a *Normal plot* aids this process. When data are clearly not from a Normal distribution, statistical procedures based on the ranks are available.

NON-NORMALLY DISTRIBUTED DATA

Although the ANOVA described earlier relates to a QoL variable that can be assumed to have a Normal distribution form, the method of analysis can be extended to continuous data that are skewed. In this case, the individual values of the QoL measure are replaced by their ranked values. For example, if five patients recorded pain on a VAS as 2.2, 2.3, 2.4, 3.6 and 7.8 cm, then these indicate a rather skew distribution. These are then replaced by their ranks 1, 2, 3, 4 and 5 respectively. The ANOVA, termed *Kruskal–Wallis*, then proceeds as we have previously described but now utilising the rank values rather than the individual observed values. It should be emphasised that the ranking is made by first combining all the N observations from the three or more (treatment) groups. The ranks are then summed for each of the g different groups separately; the corresponding test statistic is

$$KW = \frac{12 \sum n_i \left(\bar{R}_i - \frac{(N+1)}{2} \right)^2}{N(N+1)} \tag{8.21}$$

where there are n_i observations and $\bar{R}_i$ is the mean of the ranks in the ith group. If the null hypothesis is true then the test statistic KW follows the χ^2 distribution of Table T4 with $df = (g - 1)$.

This method can also be applied to ordered categorical data, but difficulties arise if there are (and there usually will be) many tied observations—as is the case with HADS anxiety scores of Table 8.3.

8.5   ANOVA MODELS

RELATIONSHIP WITH REGRESSION

In equation (8.12) we described the linear regression equation of QoL on age, and we repeat this equation here with one adjustment; we add the so-called *error term ε*.

$$Q = [\beta_0 + \beta_{Age} Age] + \varepsilon. \tag{8.22}$$

With this equation we are stating that a particular observed value of QoL for a subject with a certain age will be equal to $[\beta_0 + \beta_{Age} Age]$. However, at the same time, we recognise that there may be other factors associated with QoL, which we are not considering here. For example, there may be additional variation owing to differences between subjects, such as gender, ethnic origin or stage of disease, as well as more random differences for which there is no obvious explanation. As a consequence, the model will not be perfect and so there may be (and usually will be) some departure in the observed QoL value from that predicted by the model were we to know β_0 and β_{Age} precisely. This departure is termed the "error component" in the model that we have denoted by ε in equation (8.22). Once the model is fitted to the data, it can be estimated as

$$e = Q - [b_0 + b_{Age} Age]. \tag{8.23}$$

Here b_0 and b_{Age} again represent the estimates of β_0 and β_{Age} respectively; and e, the estimate of ε, is often termed the *residual* (from the fitted model). The true value ε may be positive, zero or negative. It is usually taken to be random and to average out to zero over all the subjects in a particular study. It is also assumed that the particular value of ε for one subject will not be influenced by the value in any other subject; and that the ε's are therefore uncorrelated. In technical terms ε is often assumed to have a Normal distribution with mean zero and a constant standard deviation σ across all age groups.

For notational convenience, and since in general we will not be confined to age as the covariate, we rewrite equation (8.22) as

$$Q_j = \alpha + \beta x_j + \varepsilon_j, \tag{8.24}$$

where α replaces β_0, β replaces β_{Age}, and x_j replaces Age. The j refers to the individual subjects in the study. If there were two treatment groups then x_j takes the value of 0 or 1 depending on which treatment the patient is given.

We have also pointed out that the approach to the analysis for comparing groups can be made either by ANOVA or by linear regression techniques. Regression methods are (statistical) model-based approaches and so, since the methods are equivalent, ANOVA too is model-based. However, the model is usually formulated in a slightly different way.

The object of the ANOVA is to ascribe some of the variation in QoL observed amongst the n subjects to specific factors—for example, treatments. The remaining (unexplained) proportion of the variation in QoL is then described as random variation. The ANOVA model takes the following form:

$$Q_{ij} = (\mu + \pi_i) + \varepsilon_{ij}. \tag{8.25}$$

Here i corresponds to the different treatment groups and j to the different patients. Those of treatment 1 will take the value π_1 in the above model and those of treatment 2 take the value π_2. Thus $\mu + \pi_1$ corresponds to α of the regression model (8.24), when $x_i = 0$. Similarly, $\mu + \pi_2$ corresponds to $\alpha + \beta$ in the same model, when $x_i = 1$. If we take $\pi_1 + \pi_2 = 0$, then this implies $\pi_1 = -\pi_2$, which we can label simply π. This is equivalent to stating that treatment 1 is above the mean μ by $+\pi$ and treatment 2 is below the mean by $-\pi$, implying $\beta = 2\pi$ and $\alpha = \mu - \pi$. Thus there is a direct relationship between μ and π, and between α and β. Consequently the ANOVA model of equation (8.25) is equivalent to the linear regression equation (8.24) although it is written in a somewhat different format.

In the situation of no differences between treatments, $\pi = 0$, while μ is estimated by the overall mean of the data, $\bar{Q}$. The term in brackets on the right-hand side of equation (8.25) is that part of the variation in Q explained by the model. In contrast, ε_{ij} is the remaining or residual variation in Q that we have not been able to explain. As already noted, for the purposes of brevity we did not include this term with the corresponding regression equations but it is there just the same. It implies that the models we are discussing are not perfect descriptors of how the QoL measure behaves for a patient. Here in the ANOVA model format, as well as the regression format, this residual variation is assumed to follow a Normal distribution with a mean of zero and a constant standard deviation, σ, which is estimated by $\sqrt{V_{Within}}$ of Table 8.7.

8.6   GRAPHICAL SUMMARIES

Analysis of QoL data from clinical trials and other studies can be classified into two broad categories: *confirmatory data analysis*, and descriptive or *exploratory data analysis*.

Confirmatory data analysis is used when a number of hypotheses are to be tested. These should have been formulated before the study was commenced and should be specified in the clinical trial protocol. The testing of hypotheses can be based largely upon standard statistical significance testing, although there may be practical problems arising from the multidimensional nature of QoL assessments, the "longitudinal" nature of the repeated measurements over time, and the occurrence of missing data for individual patients.

Exploratory and descriptive data analyses, as their names suggest, are used to explore, clarify, describe and interpret the QoL data. Frequently these analyses will reveal unexpected patterns in the data, for example suggesting differences in QoL with respect to treatment or other factors. However, exploratory analyses often consist of a large number of individual comparisons and significance tests, and some apparently strong effects may in fact arise out of chance fluctuations in the data. Thus exploratory analyses may result in the generation of new hypotheses that should then be explored in subsequent studies.

Because exploratory analyses are less concerned with significance testing, graphical methods may be especially suitable. These largely visual methods have a number of advantages over purely numerical techniques. In particular, judicious use of graphics can succinctly summarise complex data that would otherwise require extensive tabulations. At the same time, graphics can be used to emphasise the high degree of variability in QoL data. Graphical techniques can highlight changes in QoL which are large and clinically significant, whilst making it clearer to readers which changes are unimportant even though some clinically unimportant changes may represent statistically significant departures from zero.

HISTOGRAMS AND BAR CHARTS

The simplest summaries are *histograms* and *bar charts*, which show the frequency distribution of the data. These are often used to establish basic characteristics of the data. For example, prior to using a *t*-test one ought to check whether the data are distributed symmetrically and whether they appear to have a Normal distribution.

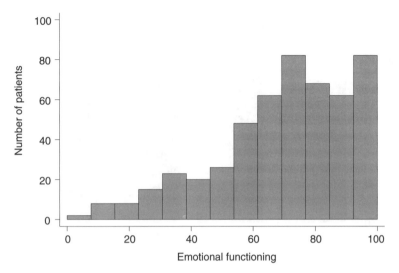

Figure 8.1 Histogram of baseline emotional functioning (EF) in patients with multiple myeloma (Data supplied by Wisløff *et al.*, 1996)

Example

Wisløff *et al.* (1996) evaluated QoL in 524 multiple myeloma patients from a randomised clinical trial that compared the use of melphalan–prednisone alone (MP) against MP with alpha-interferon (IFN + MP). They reported EORTC QLQ-C30 scores at baseline, and then at 1, 6, 12, 24, 36 and 48 months.

Figure 8.1 shows the histogram of baseline emotional functioning (EF) scores of patients with multiple myeloma. In this case the data are concentrated at the higher levels and the shape does not conform to that of the Normal distribution.

Most clinical trials compare two or more treatments, and many other investigations and analyses are also of a comparative nature. Thus graphs comparing two groups are particularly common in publications. One useful way of displaying the differences between groups of patients is a bar chart.

Example

Figure 8.2 displays the mean EF scores for males and females, according to age group. The reported EF is consistently higher (better) in males than in females.

ASSOCIATION OF VARIABLES

When showing the association between two variables the simplest and most informative graphic is the *scatter plot*. An example is shown in Figure 8.3.

A convenient compromise between the use of the bar diagram of Figure 8.2, which gives no indication of the variability, and the scatter diagram of Figure 8.3 is to use a

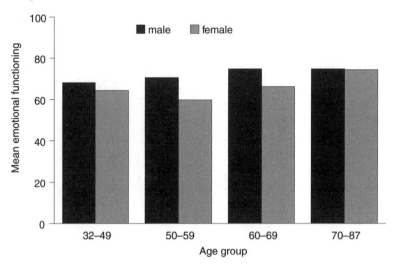

Figure 8.2 Bar chart illustrating the baseline EF scores from multiple myeloma patients of different ages (Data supplied by Wisløff *et al.*, 1996)

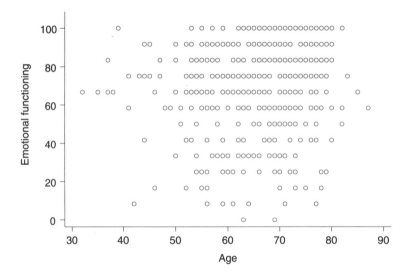

Figure 8.3 Scatter plot of the baseline EF in patients with multiple myeloma at different ages (Data supplied by Wisløff *et al.*, 1996)

series of box-and-whisker plots. A *box-and-whisker plot* indicates the median value at the centre of the box, and the 25th and 75th percentiles are indicated by the edges of the box. The "whiskers" each side of the box extend to the largest and smallest observed values within 1.5 box lengths, and the outliers are indicated by open circles. The width of the individual boxes is proportional to the inverse of the *SE* of the patient ages within the corresponding age interval, and so the wider the box the more information it contains. Since $SE = SD/\sqrt{N}$, the box width is also proportional to the square-root of the number of patients within each group.

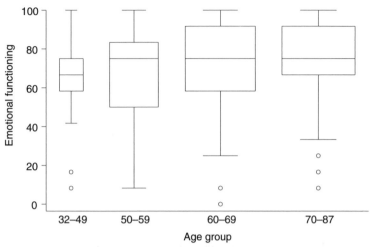

Figure 8.4 Box-and-whisker plot of the baseline EF in patients with multiple myeloma at different ages. The box widths are proportional to inverse *SE* (Data from Wisløff *et al.*, 1996)

Example

Figure 8.4 shows the same data as Figures 8.2 and 8.3, using a series of box-and-whisker plots. From this one can see that the median EF varies little with age, except perhaps in the youngest age group (which is also the smallest group of patients). There is, however, considerable variability within each age group.

PATIENT PROFILES

One form of presentation that is particularly useful in QoL analyses is the *profile plot*. This attempts to display many dimensions simultaneously, divided on the basis of a grouping variable. Profile plots are convenient ways to summarise changes in many dimensions, but can handle only a single, grouped explanatory variable. They may be particularly useful when a consistent and unambiguous pattern is seen across successive groups.

Example

Figure 8.5 summarises the mean score profiles of patients after one month of treatment either with or without IFN. The bold line indicates the patients allocated to IFN, and shows that at one month the IFN group tended to report worse functioning and more symptoms for nearly all scales of the EORTC QLQ-C30. Wisløff *et al.* (1996) reported that many of these differences during the first year of treatment were statistically significant.

One disadvantage of profile plots is that there may be a tendency to assume that the different dimensions can be compared. However, items on QoL questionnaires

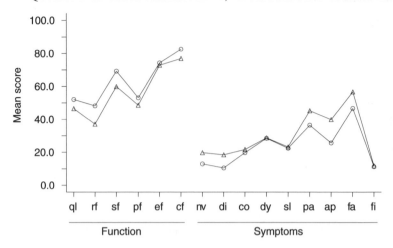

Figure 8.5 Profile of function and symptom values at one month after commencing treatment with or without interferon in patients with myeloma (Data supplied by Wisløff *et al.*, 1996)

are rarely scaled uniformly, and so it is usually meaningless to describe whether one item or scale takes higher (or lower) values than other items and scales.

8.7   ENDPOINTS

In this chapter we have not taken particular note of which of the often numerous QoL items or scales we have chosen for analysis. However, in practice it is important to identify the key components of the QoL instrument that are the most relevant for the study concerned. These components should be identified clearly as the main study endpoints. Their number should be few, no more than two or three. In designing a study and determining sample size it is imperative that the key endpoints are so identified. The same is true at the analysis stage. In any event, it is not usually possible to explore in great detail all QoL items or scales on an instrument. It is better to select the important ones in advance of conducting the study, and these would also shape the form of the analysis, be it cross-sectional, graphical or longitudinal in nature.

8.8   CONCLUSIONS

In any analysis attempting to summarise a QoL study there are many issues that need addressing. Fundamental to these is the choice of variables for analysis, the form the analysis will take, and whether the underlying (statistical) assumptions are satisfied with these data. It is often useful to commence with some initial graphical displays of the data. There are usually many QoL items and scales for examination but the main focus should remain with the previously identified primary endpoints. In most circumstances, the final analysis may be best approached using regression techniques since these are generally the most flexible.

9 Exploring Longitudinal Data

Summary

The majority of studies involving QoL assessment include repeat assessments over time. Thus in a randomised trial and other studies there may be a baseline assessment, followed by a series of further assessments during the active treatment period, followed by (often less frequent) further assessments. QoL data are therefore longitudinal in form, the analysis and presentation of which is relatively straightforward if the number of observations per patient is equal. However, for QoL assessment this will seldom if ever be the case. The final dataset will usually be very ragged with the numbers of assessments available for analysis differing from patient to patient. In this chapter we introduce a summary of such data by means of the area under the QoL curve. However, the main focus is on how such longitudinal data can be represented in a graphical format.

9.1 AREA UNDER THE CURVE

In describing the cross-sectional analyses in Chapter 8 we considered a single aspect of the QoL assessment for a particular instrument, measured at one particular time. For example, if we had been describing an analysis from the HADS we might be referring to depression at a fixed time from commencement of treatment, with no reference to depression levels at earlier or later assessment times. Such an analysis will rarely encapsulate all the features of the total data collected. Thus usually we will wish to examine the QoL profiles of patients over time, to summarize these for the individual patients, to describe collectively all those receiving the same treatment, and finally to compare treatments.

Example

Figure 9.1 shows the pain profile of two patients assessed on a daily basis during hospitalisation for severe burns. Both completed all the assessments although, since the duration of hospitalisation for the two patients differs, the number of assessments cannot be the same.

Even when QoL data have a longitudinal format it is often advisable to summarize them by extracting key elements from the patient profile. Examples are the patients' QoL at a fixed time after the active treatment period has been completed, or perhaps a measure such as the time from randomisation until QoL is

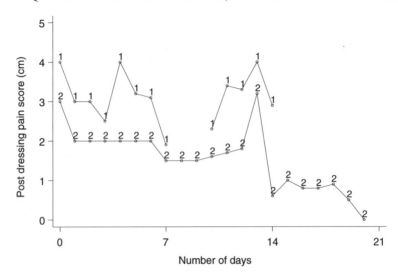

Figure 9.1   VAS pain profiles of two patients with severe burns (data from Ang *et al.*, unpublished)

improved by a pre-specified amount. Another such measure, but one that uses all the QoL data of each available assessment, is the *Area Under the Curve (AUC)*. In Figure 9.1 the *AUC* is the area between the pain profile of each patient and the horizontal axis representing zero pain. Once calculated, the *AUC* for pain may be used as a summary value for each patient.

To calculate the *AUC* the data points are first joined by straight lines as in Figure 9.1. These then describe the shape of the "curve". The area is calculated by adding the areas under the curve between each pair of consecutive observations. For the first two QoL assessments, taking values QoL_0 and QoL_1 of one patient at consecutive times t_0 and t_1, the corresponding area is:

$$A_1 = \frac{(\mathrm{QoL}_1 + \mathrm{QoL}_0)(t_1 - t_0)}{2}.$$

Similarly

$$A_2 = \frac{(\mathrm{QoL}_2 + \mathrm{QoL}_1)(t_2 - t_1)}{2},$$

and if there are $k + 1$ assessments in all:

$$A_k = \frac{(\mathrm{QoL}_k + \mathrm{QoL}_{k-1})(t_k - t_{k-1})}{2}.$$

After calculating the corresponding areas we have

$$AUC = (A_1 + A_2 + \ldots + A_k)/T. \tag{9.1}$$

The final divisor T is the duration of time from the first or baseline assessment (time 0) until the final assessment (assessment $k + 1$). This takes into account the possible and usual different times and periods of assessment of each patient.

The AUC is calculated individually for each patient and these can then be averaged across all patients within each separate treatment group. The corresponding treatment means may then be compared using z- or t-tests, ANOVA or regression techniques as appropriate, and as outlined in Chapter 8.

We can calculate the AUC even when there are missing data (see Chapter 11). Thus patient 1, in Figure 9.1, does not complete assessments on days 8 and 9. The observations at days 7 and 10 have not been joined to emphasise this missingness. However, the calculation proceeds without these, as there is no requirement in equation (9.1) that the time intervals be equal between successive observations. Therefore, in situations where despite a fixed schedule being specified, there are some deviations from the observation schedule for virtually every patient, the calculation of AUC can still be made.

This type of calculation may not be appropriate if the final observation anticipated is missing. However, in studies in which patients with an ultimately fatal disease are assessed until as close to death as is reasonable, the "final" QoL observation may be assumed to be the worst possible QoL value for that item or scale. This then provides the final value, and so an AUC can then be calculated using equation (9.1). In this situation T will correspond to the time from baseline assessment to patient death.

With the AUC we have summarised each patient's longitudinal experience as a single quantity, and so the analysis once more becomes cross-sectional in nature and the methods of Chapter 8 may again be applied. Lydick *et al.* (1995) have discussed methodological problems associated with the use of AUC in the context of patients with episodic diseases.

Example from the literature

Bailey, Parmar and Stephens (1998) report the AUC calculated from patients with non-small-cell lung cancer recruited to a randomised trial of conventional radiography versus Continuous Hyperfractionated Accelerated Radiotherapy (CHART). The patients completed the RSCL, and 78 CHART and 50 conventional radiotherapy patients answered the question relating to "Decreased sexual interest" with respective median AUCs of 1.15 and 0.98. These medians were then compared using a Mann–Whitney test, resulting in a p-value of 0.481.

9.2 GRAPHICAL PRESENTATIONS

A fundamental decision to be made when graphing aggregated longitudinal data from QoL instruments is what measure to plot against time. The four principal choices are: the percentage of patients with values exceeding a certain level; median scores of items and scales; mean scores of items and scales; individual data points. Which to choose may be determined by the context.

PERCENTAGES

Example from the literature

> The Medical Research Council Lung Cancer Working Party (1992) conducted a randomised trial of palliative radiotherapy with two fractions (F2) or a single fraction (F1), in poor-performance patients with inoperable non-small-cell lung cancer. Of particular concern was the distress caused by dysphagia with this disease.
>
> The percentage of patients reporting dysphagia "mild soreness when swallowing" or worse on a daily basis is shown in Figure 9.2. This basic plot shows that there is a large difference in the percentage of patients reporting dysphagia between the F1 and F2 regimens. This is particularly noticeable in the second and third weeks post-randomisation.

The difficulty with this form of presentation is that it does not indicate the reducing number of patients (and hence how precisely the associated percentages are estimated) in the plot as time progresses from diagnosis. A sensible addition to this (and many plots) is to include the number at risk by treatment group at various points beneath the time axis. In this example assessments are made daily so that patient numbers would be given only at convenient intervals. If there is a less frequent or irregular schedule it is important to give numbers observed on these occasions.

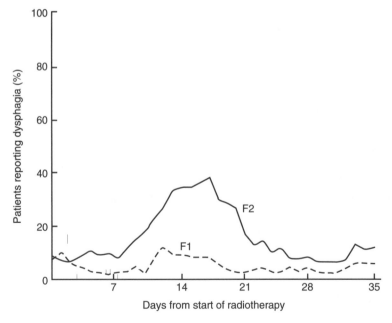

Figure 9.2 A trial comparing two radiotherapy regimens for non-small-cell lung cancer, which used a daily diary card to assess QoL (After Medical Research Council Lung Cancer Working Party, (1992). A Medical Research Council (MRC) randomized trial of palliative radiotherapy with 2 fractions or a single fraction in patients with inoperable non-small-cell lung cancer and poor performance status. *British Journal of Cancer*, **65**, 934–941, by permission of the publisher Churchill Livingstone)

There may be more than two response possibilities (that is, more than Present or Absent categories), and the concept of percentage plots can be extended to handle these. Thus, in the example of reported dysphagia levels, this might be done by superimposing plots corresponding to the cumulative percentage of patients in the successive categories. These categories could correspond to "no soreness when swallowing", "mild soreness when swallowing", "quite a bit of soreness when swallowing" and "very much soreness when swallowing". The cumulative total of these is then 100% at each assessment time point. However, with such a plot it is not so easy to include two (or more) patient groups within the same panel as the likelihood of superimposed data points is high and any substantial overlap can obscure the underlying patterns.

MEANS VERSUS MEDIANS

The RSCL and the HADS are typical QoL instruments that, like many others, use raw items with four-point categories, often with labels such as "not at all", "a little", "quite a bit" and "very much" for the respective categories which are then scored 1 to 4. Also, many QoL items have strongly skewed distributions in the associated responses. Thus for items representing rare symptoms and side-effects or infrequent problems, the majority of patients may report "not at all"; that is, the minimal response for the QoL item. In contrast, with items concerning more common problems there may be a large proportion of patients reporting "very much"; that is, the maximum response for the item. As a consequence, it is not unusual for as many as half the patients to report the maximum for some items, and the minimum for others. In these cases, the medians for the QoL items would be these *floor* or *ceiling* values of either 1 or 4. Such medians carry limited information when presented in graphical format, and it becomes better to plot mean values rather than medians. Analytical problems associated with floor and ceiling values have been referred to earlier in Chapters 5 and 7.

ALL AVAILABLE DATA

Since QoL measurements are usually collected repeatedly over time, it is almost inevitable that there will be a lot of incomplete data. In fact if it weren't for this the presentation and analysis of QoL data would be greatly simplified and would not differ substantially from methods used in many other applications. One can rapidly assess the magnitude of the "missing" problem by a plot of all available data at each time point. Such a plot is useful in examining simultaneously both attrition and departures from the assessment schedule. This plot is likely to be only useful for QoL scales, as individual items will usually have too few categories for the technique to be helpful.

Example from the literature

Figure 9.3 shows a scatter diagram of the HADS depression scores reported by patients with small-cell lung cancer recruited to a randomised trial of the

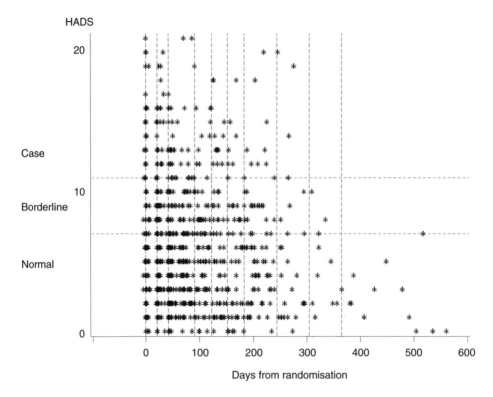

Figure 9.3   Scatter plot of the HADS depression scores against day of assessment for patients with small-cell lung cancer (From Machin and Weeden, 1998)

MRC Lung Cancer Working Party (1996), plotted against the actual date of assessment. The critical values defining clinical depression "cases" and "border-line" scores have been indicated to aid interpretation. Although ten QoL assessments were scheduled to be completed within one year, several patients returned assessments much later.

To further examine the adherence to the schedule of assessments, Machin and Weeden (1998) provided a multi-panel form of the data in Figure 9.3. It is clear from this multi-panel plot (Figure 9.4) that an increasing proportion of patients depart from the fixed schedule as time goes on. The increasing scatter of the QoL assessments relative to the scheduled assessment times indicates the increasing departures from the protocol schedule. Even the baseline QoL assessments were not all made immediately prior to randomisation and start of treatment (day 0).

Figure 9.4 takes up considerable space on the printed page. However, to illustrate the patterns within both treatment groups would require even more space, unless of course different plotting symbols or colour codes are used within each panel. This is not usually practicable as many points may be obscured due to coinciding values at some times. Nevertheless, the plots of Figures 9.3 and 9.4 do indicate the attrition following the baseline QoL values since the number of observations in the successive clouds of points reduces as time progresses.

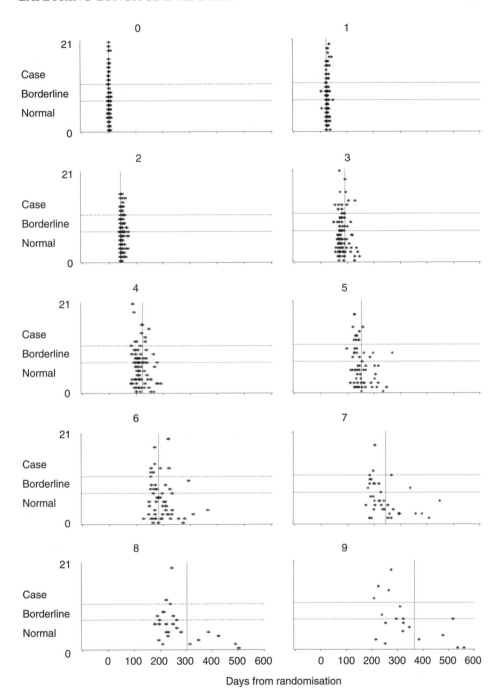

Figure 9.4 Scatter plot of the HADS depression score at each assessment against day of assessment for patients with small-cell lung cancer (From Machin and Weeden, 1998)

INDIVIDUAL PROFILES

It is also clear from Figure 9.3 that the behaviour of individual patients is not indicated over time. Once again, if the numbers of patients were very small, individual plotting symbols or a different colour for each patient could be used. These would then identify the individuals and the respective patterns could be examined to give some idea of the variation between and within individual profiles. A compromise is to select "typical" patients from all those in the study and graph their profiles only. These profiles then give an indication of the potential variation, but cannot provide a complete picture.

Example from the literature

Machin and Weeden (1998) give the HADS depression profiles of eight patients superimposed on the cloud of all the data points from the patients with small-cell lung cancer. This is reproduced in Figure 9.5.

The patients chosen for illustration were the first patients in the data file who had completed only baseline HADS; baseline and only the first (post-randomisation) HADS; baseline, only the first and second post-randomisation HADS; and so on. The plotting symbols 0, 1, 2, . . ., 9 respectively indicate this. With this number of profiles within the same plot it is quite difficult to follow the individual patterns. A further compromise, in this example, would be to plot those corresponding to 1, 3, 5, 7 and 9 in Figure 9.5.

There is considerable variation in the successive values of HADS anxiety for each patient. In addition, their profiles are quite different and so are some of the completion times of the respective assessments, albeit supposedly carefully scheduled.

HISTOGRAMS AND BOX PLOTS

If the variation about the schedules is not regarded as serious, then each QoL assessment can be taken as if it had occurred at the scheduled time. This effectively imposes acceptable *windows* of variation for this purpose. These windows are intervals surrounding the schedule dates, defining those assessments that can be included in the analysis. Assessments lying outside the window will not be included in the summary or analysis. Once the windows are imposed, the data can be summarised as a series of histograms, one for each scheduled assessment point. However, a more compact presentation can be given by using box-and-whisker plots similar to Figure 8.4.

Example from the literature

Machin and Weeden (1998) give the successive box-and-whisker plots for each of 10 HADS depression assessments in patients with small-cell lung cancer. This is reproduced in Figure 9.6, which includes the numbers of patients completing each assessment, the divisions of borderline and case referred to

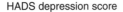

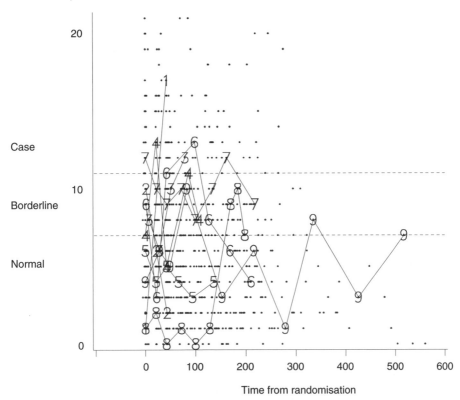

Figure 9.5 Individual profiles of HADS depression score in selected patients with small-cell lung cancer (From Machin and Weeden, 1998)

earlier, and the successive median values joined to describe the summary profile. However, care needs to be taken with the interpretation of this profile as patient attrition may remove those patients with (say) the worst (highest) HAD scores. The data are plotted separately for the two randomised treatment regimens, a two-drug (2D) and a four-drug (4D) regimen as described by MRC Lung Cancer Working Party (1996).

In constraining the data into windows we are assuming that the variation in day-to-day values over the short spans of time are regarded as minor. Nevertheless, there may be circumstances when this is clearly not the case. In these situations the windows need to be selected with care. For example, if the study schedule defines QoL assessments immediately after receiving chemotherapy in patients with cancer, it would not be appropriate to include assessments before that cycle of treatment. In addition, the window should not go too far beyond the cycle as the immediate impact of treatment on QoL may have diminished by that time. A wide window could lead to a rather false impression of the true situation. It is better if windows are defined before the study begins, as later choices may be rather subjective and possibly introduce bias into the analytical procedures.

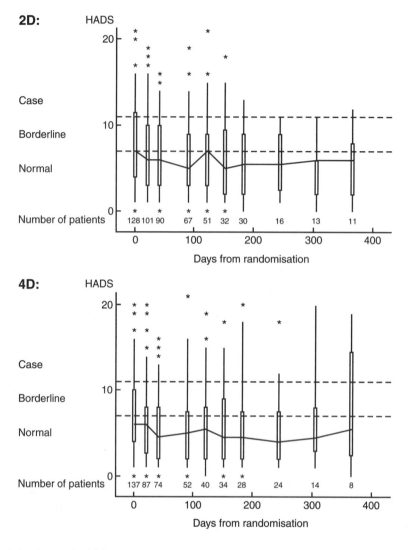

Figure 9.6   Box-and-whisker plots of HADS depression scores for the 10 scheduled assessments of patients with small-cell lung cancer recruited to the MRC Lung Cancer Working Party trial (From Machin and Weeden, 1998)

If there remain data outside the selected windows then these could be added to the equivalent of Figure 9.6. Their clouds would occupy the gaps between the successive box-and-whisker plots. In this way all the information collected is summarised even though little analytical use may be made of the clouds of points between the box-and-whisker plots.

SUMMARY PROFILES

Although it is not possible with large numbers of patients to examine all the individual patient profiles, it is nevertheless important to evaluate changes in QoL over time. However, it must be recognised that those patients with the fewest assessments available may be the most severely ill. This may be particularly so towards the end of the time course of a study, when patients may possibly be close to death, and this would almost certainly have affected their QoL were we able to assess it. These data "omissions" may result in the assessments that we are able to observe seriously misrepresenting the "true" patterns of the overall patient group.

One method of examining this situation in detail is to present, group-by-group, the summary profiles comprising all the patients in "duration of follow-up groups". This suggestion replaces the individual profiles summarised in Figure 9.5 by the mean profiles of all the patients who fall into each of the respective groups 0 to 9. For example, one of these summaries would be provided by data from those patients completing baseline plus four consecutive HADS (indicated by the plotting symbol 4 in Figure 9.5). These data are then summarised at each scheduled assessment by the corresponding mean QoL score.

If these profiles are similar in shape and have similar mean values over the comparable assessment schedule times, then it may be reasonable to summarise all the data at each schedule over all the available patients. This then provides a single summary profile. This profile, despite the absent data, may provide a reasonable description of QoL changes over time. On the other hand, if the shapes of the profiles are very different then it may be inadvisable to collapse the data further. This might also be the case, if the profiles are similar in shape but are parallel to each other rather than superimposed. In this case, treatment and follow-up influence QoL in a similar way but initial values are a strong indicator for prognosis.

A final step in this graphical analysis will be to divide the data into treatment groups and plot the corresponding means at each assessment point for each treatment group separately.

Example from the literature

Hopwood, Stephens and Machin (1994) utilised this approach with part of the data from the MRC Lung Cancer Working Party (1996) trial. They considered the HADS anxiety rather than depression assessments. They excluded all data from patients having gaps in their assessment profiles as they were describing a methodology rather than the actual results of the clinical trial. Figure 9.7a shows the mean HADS for each follow up profile. Since the plots appeared fairly consistent it was concluded that there were no major differences in these subgroups so that the combined (all-patient) profile of Figure 9.7b could be calculated. This is divided by treatment group in Figure 9.7c.

The purpose of this step-by-step approach is to see, at least informally, whether or not it is justified to summarise all the available data as a single block. If one could, this is effectively concluding that the "missing" data (were we to know them) would not materially change the estimates of the corresponding means. Their absence of course means that the estimates we do have will have less precision, since they will be based on fewer observations than those that were potentially available. However, provided these estimates are not biased, between-treatment comparisons may still reflect the true situation. A more formal approach to this can be made through statistical modelling, aspects of which are described in Chapter 10.

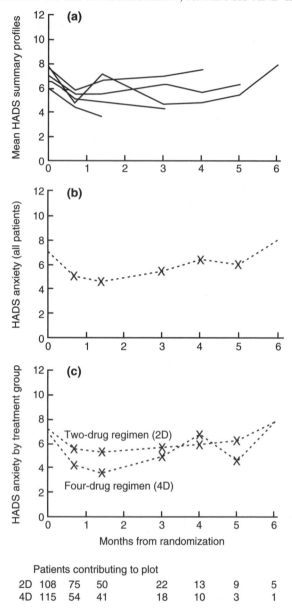

Figure 9.7 Profiles of HADS anxiety score for patients with small cell lung cancer (a) according to number of assessments completed, (b) by all patients, (c) by treatment group (Based on Hopwood *et al.*, 1994, Figures 2, 3 and 4)

REVERSE PROFILES

Sometimes different approaches to graphical summary may be preferable. For example, the mean profiles like those of Figure 9.7a might have been similar but shifted along the time axis depending on the number of QoL assessments made.

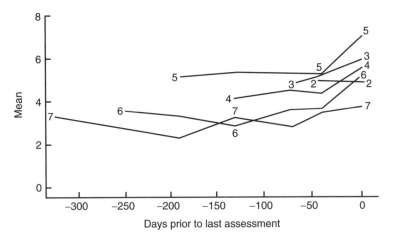

Figure 9.8 Mean HADS depression score in patients with small-cell lung cancer, reverse plotted from date of last assessment (From Machin and Weeden, 1998)

This could occur if the QoL profiles of patients tended to be similar at critical stages, for example similar for all patients close to death. In this case placing the origin as the date of last assessment and plotting backwards in time, rather then forwards from baseline, may result in similar profiles which could then be averaged.

Example

> Figure 9.8 shows a reverse profile plot of HADS depression score in patients with small-cell lung cancer, calculated from date of last assessment as the reference point. In these patients this time was usually when the patient was close to death. These data suggest that HADS depression levels rise as death approaches. The integers used as plotting symbols indicate the number of assessments completed by that particular group of patients.

VARIABLITY

One advantage of the repeated box-and-whisker plots in Figure 9.6 is that they not only summarise the changing median QoL levels with time, but also summarise and quantify the associated variability. This variability is described by both the inter-quartile range and the whiskers themselves. The number of patients contributing to each point in this graph can be added beneath the time axis, displaying in a compact form all the principal features of the data.

It is unlikely that any approach to data presentation will be entirely appropriate or optimum for all situations. Indeed what may seem the best for one QoL item or scale in a particular instrument may not be optimal for another. However, some compromise is needed. What we suggest is that the method of presentation should be that which satisfies best the needs of the most important QoL scale in the context of the particular study—once determined, this presentation would be carried throughout. It would be perplexing for the reader if each QoL variable were to be presented in its own unique way. If a comparison is to be made between the current study and work conducted previously by others, then choosing the same style of presentation clearly facilitates the comparison even in situations where the method of presentation may not be optimal. However, one must avoid repeating poor methods of presentation.

For studies describing a single group of patients, it may be useful to add 95% confidence intervals for the mean at each scheduled QoL assessment. These emphasise the increasing uncertainty attached to the values at later times with increasing patient attrition. However, care should be taken not to clutter the graphical presentation. For example, it would be difficult to add confidence intervals to the box-and-whisker plot of Figure 9.6 but would be quite feasible for the mean profile of Figure 9.7b. For graphical presentations intended to illustrate the comparison between groups, confidence intervals for each mean would not be appropriate to add to the graphical presentation as it is the difference between groups which is if interest. Any confidence interval should then be for the differences observed, and it may not be easy to include these into the graphical presentation. They may need to be provided in a separate tabular format.

MISSING DATA

We have focused above on data that are incomplete through patient attrition. In many examples this attrition may be caused by the death of the patient, in which case there is no way that the *absent data* could ever have been collected. It is then often useful to include a summary of the survival experience of the patients in the study. This may be done by presenting the Kaplan–Meier survival curve (Parmar and Machin, 1995). Survival curves give a ready appreciation of the reason for absent data through patient attrition.

It is also common for patients in QoL studies to have *missing data* at one or more scheduled times in an otherwise complete set of QoL reports. In this case, attempts are often made to impute their value (see Chapter 11). Such imputed values should not be added to the clouds of data points such as those of Figure 9.4 even though they may be used to estimate the mean QoL at each scheduled assessment time.

9.3   TABULAR PRESENTATIONS

Much of the information summarised in graphical form above could have been presented in tabular format, perhaps even in a more compact way. However, in reporting longitudinal QoL studies it is important to convey the extent of attrition (and hence absent data) and this can usually be best illustrated graphically. Such detail can really only be given for a limited number of scales from each QoL instrument used in the study; the remaining variables will have to be presented in tabular format. Such tables should indicate the numbers of subjects providing information for each item or scale, the proportion of missing as opposed to absent values, a summary statistic such as the mean or percentage, and a measure of the variability. The tables should also highlight the principal endpoints of the investigation in some way.

Example from the literature

Wisløff *et al.* (1996) give a tabular summary of the symptom and toxicity aspects of their trial in the tabular format of Table 9.1, in which for each assessment the mean score is given for each treatment and this is repeated for each symptom. One way in which this tabulation could be modified would be to rank the symptoms in terms of frequency of occurrence from month 0 onwards—starting with "muscle pain", "joint pain", "night sweats", and so on until "hair loss". The reason that "joint pain" precedes "night sweats" in this ranking, although they are numerically equal at month 0, is that there is more of the former at month 1. The rows of the table would then follow this ranking. In this way it would be a little easier to follow the patterns of the major symptoms as they would be grouped close together.

Table 9.1   Means of toxicity and symptom scores* in the melphalan–prednisone (MP) and melphalan–prednisone + interferon (IFN) arms, prior to and at various times during therapy (From Wisløff *et al.*, 1996)

	Month after start of therapy											
	0		1		6		12		24		36	
	MP	IFN	MP	IFN	MP	IFN	MP	IFN	MP	IFN	MP	IFN
No. of patients[a]	271	253	255	232	218	206	196	181	142	144	67	74
No. of drop-outs[b]	24	33	5	8	6	4	4	4	3	5	0	0
Symptoms												
Night sweats	21	23	19	20	15	14	14	13	15	12	17	16
Fever	5	11	6	12	3	8	4	6	3	5	5	6
Chills	6	10	11	17	8	13	8	12	8	11	9	14
Dizziness	15	14	14	18	13	17	11	16	9	17	14	15
Hair loss	4	4	6	7	11	22	10	13	8	9	12	12
Headache	12	14	12	15	13	12	13	11	12	13	14	12
Sore mouth	8	8	10	11	8	13	7	10	8	11	13	6
Muscle pain	28	31	26	31	25	27	24	26	25	24	30	29
Joint pain	21	23	21	24	21	20	23	23	25	21	26	24
Dry skin	17	20	20	27	16	28	17	23	21	22	20	22
Coughing	16	16	16	18	16	14	19	16	15	13	14	13

* Scores range from 0 to 100, higher scores representing higher levels of symptoms or toxicity.
[a] Patients completing the questionnaire at each time point.
[b] Patients who are alive and who have completed all previous questionnaires, but not the one at this time point.

One difficulty with a tabular format such as Table 9.1 is that the times of QoL assessment, although clearly indicated here, are often not equally spaced. As a consequence, it is often difficult to appreciate the true shape of the changes with time by scanning entries in a table. This is also a difficulty with successive bar charts that are presented equally spaced on the printed page rather than at locations determined by their relative positions in time. Although this may be easy to rectify using other forms of plot, as we do in Figure 15.2b later, unequally spaced columns would not be a practical format for tabular display.

Although we recommend that some measure of variability should be included in a tabular display, it is difficult to see how this could be added to all the entries of Table 9.1 without making it unacceptably complicated. A compromise is to identify the "major" symptoms of concern at the protocol development stage and provide the variability measure for these only. This could be done by listing these "major" symptoms first in Table 9.1 and in the order of importance as specified by the protocol (not by the results). The measure of variability would then be added alongside or beneath the corresponding mean. Following a break in the table, the remainder of the symptoms could then be listed in rank order of observed importance at baseline assessment in the manner that we have previously indicated.

9.4   REPORTING

From the previous sections it is clear that the process of examining longitudinal QoL data in detail may be a complex and lengthy one. Seldom will the patterns revealed be simple, and indeed they may be very intricate, so their summary will usually be daunting. However, by first focusing on the few major questions posed by the study and reporting these in careful detail, it may not be so important to report with the same level of detail the other endpoints. The guidelines for reporting outlined in Chapter 15 set out some vital aspects that we will concentrate upon. It is inevitable in reporting any study that compromises have to be made as journal editors and readers will wish for clear messages uncluttered by detail.

COMPLIANCE WITH SCHEDULE AND ATTRITION

As we have indicated, if the study involves repeated QoL assessments on patients whose ability to complete the questionnaire is likely to be compromised, for example by death itself, as time goes on it is useful to summarise the survival experience by a Kaplan–Meier survival curve. A single survival curve may suffice if there is no major difference in survival between the therapeutic groups, but only if there is also no major difference in compliance. If there is a marked difference in survival and/or if the pattern or rate of non-compliant patients differ substantially, then treatment-specific detail must be provided.

Example

Figure 9.9 shows the survival over 48 months of patients with myeloma treated in the randomized study of the Nordic Myeloma Study Group (1996), whose QoL data were described by Wisløff et al. (1996).

One advantage of this plot is that it also enables the QoL assessment schedule to be indicated by marking the time axis in an appropriate way. It is customary in reporting survival curves that the numbers of patients at risk be indicated at key points beneath the time axis. These numbers can be supplemented by the compliance, possibly for each group, especially at key stages such as when important patient management events take place. Examples of critical events include the time active (protocol) therapy ceases, the time of disease response assessment, or the anticipated time of discharge to community care. When the principal QoL endpoint under consideration is one that poses personal difficulties with respect to the ability or willingness to respond for many subjects, it may sometimes be appropriate to

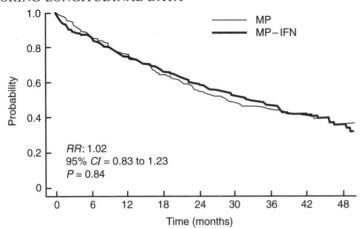

Figure 9.9 Kaplan–Meier estimates of the survival curve of patients with myeloma (From Nordic Myeloma Study Group (1996). Interferon-alpha2b added to melphalan-prednisone for initial and maintenance therapy in multiple myeloma. *Annals of Internal Medicine,* **124,** 212–222)

count these patients as "non-compliant" even though they may have completed the other assessment items. It will be a matter of judgement which figures to report.

The upper panel of Table 9.1 provides a tabular alternative to the graphical format of Figure 9.9. This shows the number of patients completing the QoL questionnaire at each scheduled assessment together with the number of patients who were alive at that time but who did not complete the questionnaire. The total of these two gives the numbers still alive at the respective assessment points and declines quite rapidly over the three years of the study. This tabular format is more compact than the corresponding graphical alternative.

However, these methods of presentation may reflect not the compliant but the "off-schedule" patients. As we have indicated, a convenient method of dealing with these is to impose acceptable windows. If the QoL assessment returned falls within the respective window for that schedule, it is included; but otherwise it is excluded from analysis. Once again if this is a minor proportion of the total anticipated QoL assessments this causes no major problem. However, in other circumstances the departure from schedule (being outside the windows) may be of major concern and also differ between the treatment groups. In this case, if the QoL variable is numeric with a reasonable range of values we recommend that the format of Figure 9.3 be utilised. Separate panels may or may not be required for each treatment group depending on the context. If keeping to schedule slips as patients progress through the trial, as in Figure 9.4, then it may be important to add a comment to this effect. For example one might state: "Although compliance with schedule is within the stipulated window for 98% of the patients at the baseline assessment, this reduces to 50% at the one-year assessment and is only 25% at two years. There were no substantial differences in this trend between the treatment groups."

TREATMENT COMPARISONS

In randomised trials the main focus is to make comparisons between treatments, and it will often be useful to provide a graphical summary similar to Figure 9.7c (another example is given in Figure 15.2b) after going through the stages we have described. Whether such a plot provides an unbiased summary of the QoL changes over time and between treatments will depend to a large extent on the pattern and proportion of compliant patients. Again, it is a matter of judgement as to whether this is indeed the case in a particular situation. Any concerns in this respect should be included in the accompanying text. Indications of the associated variability can be added to this graph at each assessment point. If the summary measure plotted is a mean, then a horizontal line spanning two standard deviations above and below the mean can be indicated. For the two treatments at each QoL assessment point the two corresponding lines can be displaced slightly horizontally so as not to overlap directly. Judgement again will have to be made as to whether a single-panel (Figure 9.7c) or a double-panel format (Figure 9.6) is the more suitable. What is *not* recommended is to include the 95% confidence interval (*CI*) for the difference between treatments at each assessment point, since these tend to encourage point-by-point comparisons which introduce problems similar to those of repeated statistical tests. However, if the protocol had stipulated that a major endpoint was the QoL at a particular time point, then it would be appropriate to give an indication of the 95% CI for that comparison only.

On the other hand, if longitudinal data have been summarised for each patient by a single quantity, then the longitudinal component of the presentation disappears and one is left with a cross-sectional analysis to report. Thus if the *AUC* is used, then each treatment group will have a corresponding mean, $\overline{AUC}$, and standard error, *SE(AUC)*. The *AUC* data can then be presented graphically by either box-and-whisker plots or histograms, one for each treatment group. However, it is essential that the difference in means be quoted and the corresponding 95% *CI* stated. Because this measure is derived from the original and multiple QoL responses it may less easily convey its own meaning to the reader. Thus it may be best to provide the combination of a tabular format to summarise the component data for this derived measure with a graphical display of the resulting distributions, such as the distributions of the *AUC*s.

Example

Figure 9.10 shows the histograms of the *AUC*, here denoted AUC_{36}, calculated for the assessment of fatigue over the whole 36 months from the date of randomisation in the trial described by Wisløff *et al.* (1996). The corresponding numbers of patients for the MP and INF treatment groups are 238 and 213 with respective means 43.5 (*SD* = 22.3) and 47.5 (*SD* = 16.0). The difference between these means of 4.0 (95% *CI*: 0.02 to 8.02) is suggestive of more fatigue reported by those patients receiving IFN ($p = 0.049$).

Just as for any other endpoint, it should have been indicated in the protocol that AUC_{36} is an important one that will be the focus of analysis. In fact, repeating the *AUC* calculations for this trial but using only the first 24 months' data (AUC_{24}) and again using AUC_{12} produces *p*-values of 0.003 and 0.001 respectively. These indicate that the excess symptom levels reported with IFN are greater in the early part of the

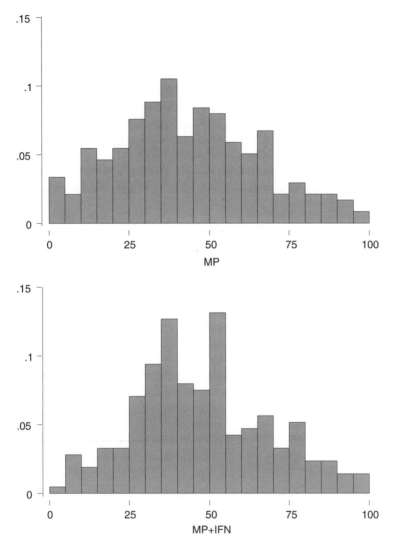

Figure 9.10   Histograms of AUC_{36} for patients with myeloma, by treatment received (Data supplied by Wisløff *et al.*, 1996)

treatment period. Any investigator, albeit pre-specifying that AUC_{36} was the key variable, would be foolish not to explore the data in detail, and once the phenomenon is noticed should report it as an observation requiring confirmatory study on another occasion. Thus in future trials earlier endpoints, for example AUC_6, might replace AUC_{36} as the major endpoint.

9.5   CONCLUSIONS

Longitudinal data, especially when there is attrition due to missing data and death, presents a number of problems in analysis and interpretation. These difficulties are further compounded by unequally-spaced scheduled assessment times, and variability in the time of the actual assessment. For these reasons the initial exploration of the data should place emphasis upon summary tabulations and graphical methods. Summary measures, such as the *AUC* or the percentage of time that a patient has QoL levels above a specific threshold, can reduce longitudinal data to a single summary score for each patient. This has the advantage that the methods of Chapter 8 can then be applied, for example to provide significance testing of treatment differences. *AUC* is one method of combining QoL values over time. An alternative method, using QALYs, is described in Chapter 12; this weights different health states according to patients' values or "utilities". However, the modelling methods described in Chapter 10 may also be applied, so as to explore the data in greater depth and in particular to estimate the magnitude of the treatment effect and test its significance.

10 Modelling Longitudinal Data

Summary

In Chapter 9 emphasis was placed on describing in graphical form changes in QoL with time and their summary across groups of patients. However, these comparisons were not quantified to any extent. This chapter describes a modelling approach to the description of longitudinal data, which permits both estimation of effect sizes and statistical tests of hypotheses. These models are an extension of the linear regression and ANOVA techniques described in Chapter 8. In particular, they take account of the fact that successive QoL assessments by a particular patient are likely to be correlated. The alternative approaches are classified as repeated measures, general estimating equations and multi-level models. They all require the specification of an auto-correlation structure and this is described. Some of the statistical assumptions underpinning the techniques for fitting these models to QoL data are complex, so we have focused more on interpretation than on technical aspects. Although the mathematical details of some models might appear complex, the aim is only to find a model that describes the data well and thereby enables a simple estimate of the treatment effect.

10.1 PRELIMINARIES

In Chapter 9 we used graphical approaches for exploring QoL data to provide a visual summary that is relatively easy to interpret while taking account of the possible impact of missing data through attrition. However, such approaches do not permit formal statistical comparisons to be made. Tabular presentations, including confidence intervals for between-group summary differences, can to some extent be useful for this purpose although these too may not necessarily give a complete or appropriate summary of the situation. Just as the use of a regression model was the more powerful analytic tool when investigating the role of age on QoL in Chapter 8, so modelling is also important here. However, modelling longitudinal data with missing observations is a relatively complex process and it will usually benefit from a detailed examination of the data by the methods of Chapter 9 before proceeding to this stage.

One important aspect of longitudinal data is that the observations may not be independent. This contrasts with cross-sectional data in which there is, for the particular QoL item under consideration, a single variable whose value in a subject will not depend on the magnitude of the corresponding value in other subjects. In longitudinal analysis we have repeated measures on the same subject, and so successive observations are unlikely to be independent. This is one reason why care in analysis and presentation are important.

10.2   AUTO-CORRELATION

Section 4.3 introduced the use of the correlation coefficient in several situations, and defined the correlation coefficient with equation (4.1). We repeat that equation here, introducing some notational differences with x_1 and x_2 replacing the variables x and y respectively of the former equation. Thus

$$r_T(1,2) = \frac{\sum(x_1 - \bar{x}_1)(x_2 - \bar{x}_2)}{\sqrt{\sum(x_1 - \bar{x}_1)^2 \sum(x_2 - \bar{x}_2)^2}}. \tag{10.1}$$

Here x_1 and x_2 represent the values of two successive assessments of the same QoL item or scale, from the same instrument, made by the same patient. For example, these may be their emotional functioning (EF) values at the time of randomisation and one month later. Previously x and y had represented two different QoL measures from the same or different instruments, reported at a single time—for example, EF and performance status (PS) values immediately before treatment commences.

Equation (10.1) is termed the *auto-* or *serial-correlation* and measures the strength of the association between successive (longitudinal) measurements of a single QoL variable on the same patient.

This will be a Pearson correlation if x_1 and x_2 have the Normal distribution form, or the Spearman rank correlation if they do not. The expression is symmetric in terms of x_1 and x_2, and hence $r_T(1,2) = r_T(2,1)$. The notation for correlation coefficients such as $r_T(1,2)$ is reduced to r_T if the context is clear.

AUTO-CORRELATION MATRIX

Suppose QoL is assessed on numerous occasions and the measurements at different times are $Q_{j0}, Q_{j1}, \ldots, Q_{jT}$ for patient j in the study. Then equation (10.1) can be utilised, one pair of these observations at a time, with the respective Q replacing the x values. The resulting correlations are the auto-correlations that we denote by, for example, $r_T(0,3)$. We use T to emphasise the time element, and the 0 and 3 indicate that we are correlating the baseline and third follow-up QoL assessments. If there are assessments at $T + 1$ time-points, there will be $(T + 1)T/2$ pairs of assessments leading to separate auto-correlation coefficients. For example, for $T = 5$ there are $(6 \times 5)/2 = 15$ auto-correlation coefficients that may be calculated, from $r_T(0,1)$ through to $r_T(4,5)$.

Example

Figure 10.1 shows the scatter plot of EORTC QLQ-C30 emotional functioning (EF) scores at baseline (pre-treatment) assessment (EF_0) against the corresponding scores one month after starting treatment (EF_1), for 457 patients with multiple myeloma. The Pearson auto-correlation coefficient between these two assessments (1 month apart) is 0.61. The Spearman auto-correlation coefficient with the same data gives 0.58—a very similar figure.

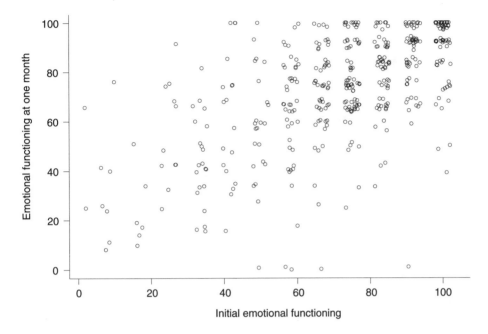

Figure 10.1   Scatter plot of emotional functioning (EF) for multiple myeloma patients, prior to treatment and one month after starting treatment (Data supplied by Wisløff *et al.*, 1996)

In fact QoL assessment in this example was also carried out at 6, 12, 24, 36 and 48 months during therapy. Thus Table 10.1 summarises the resulting 15 auto-correlation pairs for the assessments until month 36, while Figure 10.2 gives a panel of the corresponding scatter diagrams.

It can be seen from Table 10.1 that the auto-correlation coefficients are moderately large (between 0.39 and 0.65) and that once on-treatment (month 1 onwards) the auto-correlations are above 0.54 for all pairs of measurements up to two years apart.

Table 10.1   Matrix of Pearson auto-correlation coefficients for emotional functioning (EF) of multiple myeloma patients immediately prior to and during the first 36 months of therapy (Data supplied by Wisløff *et al.*, 1996)

	0	1	6	12	24	36
0	1					
1	0.61	1				
6	0.44	0.54	1			
12	0.46	0.57	0.65	1		
24	0.39	0.54	0.55	0.60	1	
36	0.47	0.47	0.49	0.57	0.54	1

It should be noted from Figure 10.2 (and similarly for Table 10.1) that the scatter plots are only given beneath the leading diagonal since the plot of, for example, x_1

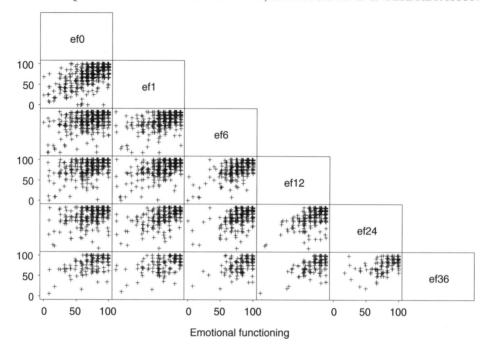

Figure 10.2 Pairwise scatter diagrams for emotional functioning (EF) of multiple myeloma patients immediately prior and during the first 36 months of therapy (Data supplied by Wisløff *et al.*, 1996)

against x_2 provides the same information as x_2 against x_1 and so has the same value for the correlation coefficient.

AUTO-CORRELATION PATTERNS

The pattern of an auto-correlation matrix, such as that of Table 10.1, gives a guide to the so-called *error structure* associated with the successive measurements.

Example from the literature

Cnaan, Laird and Slasor (1997, Table IV) give the correlation matrix after fitting a statistical model to patients assessed by the total score from the Brief Psychiatric Rating Scale (BPRS). One correlation matrix was calculated after fitting a statistical model that included the variables: baseline BPRS, treatment, centre and week. These correlations are given in the lower left half of Table 10.2.

Examination of these values suggests an underlying pattern of decreasing correlation as the observations become further apart. For example, $r_T(2,3) = 0.76$ whereas $r_T(2,6) = 0.60$. The time difference or lag between the observations are $3 - 2 = 1$ week and $6 - 2 = 4$ weeks respectively.

Table 10.2 Auto-correlation matrices derived from patients with schizophrenia assessed with the BPRS calculated after fitting two statistical models (Based on Cnaan *et al.*, 1997, Tables IV and V)

Week	1	2	3	4	5	6
1	1	*0.61*	*0.50*	*0.27*	–	*0.32*
2	0.63	1	*0.75*	*0.59*	–	*0.60*
3	0.52	0.76	1	*0.73*	–	*0.67*
4	0.34	0.64	0.77	1	–	*0.77*
5	–	–	–	–	1	–
6	0.35	0.60	0.72	0.85	–	1

Although in this example no assessment was made at week 5, we have included the corresponding row and column in Table 10.2 to emphasise this gap in observations. In general QoL assessments will not be evenly spaced and this may obscure the underlying patterns somewhat. Thus it is more difficult to examine the patterns given in Table 10.1 as the time intervals between successive assessments are mostly unequal and of quite different periods. A further problem arises if patients depart from the prescribed QoL assessment schedules, although this may be partially overcome by identifying acceptable windows as outlined in Chapter 9.

Several underlying patterns of the auto-correlation matrix are used in modelling of longitudinal QoL data. These include *independent, exchangeable, multiplicative, unstructured,* and *user-fixed.* Burton, Gurrin and Sly (1998) give a detailed description.

The error structure is *independent* (sometimes termed *random*) if the off-diagonal terms of the auto-correlation matrix are zero. The repeated QoL observations on the same subject are then independent of each other, and can be regarded as though they were observations from different individuals.

On the other hand, if all the correlations are approximately equal then the matrix of correlation coefficients is termed *exchangeable,* or *compound symmetric.* This means that we can re-order (exchange) the successive (timed) observations in any way we choose in our data file without affecting the pattern in the correlation matrix. It may be reasonable to suppose that this is the underlying pattern suggested by the correlation matrix of Table 10.1 in which the values of the auto-correlations fluctuate around approximately $r_T = 0.5$.

Frequently, as the time or lag between the successive observations increases, the auto-correlation between the observations decreases. Thus we would expect a higher auto-correlation between QoL assessments made only two days apart than between two QoL assessments made one month apart. In such a situation one may postulate that the relationship between the size of the correlation and the "lag", that is the time between t_1 and t_2, may be of the form

$$\rho_T(t_1, t_2) = \rho^{\varphi|t_2 - t_1|}. \tag{10.2}$$

The $|t_2 - t_1|$ implies that if the difference between t_2 and t_1 is negative the sign should be ignored, and φ takes a constant value that is usually less than one. A correlation matrix of this form is called *multiplicative* or *time series.*

Example

> Suppose the true auto-correlation between the first two of many successive but equally spaced QoL assessments is $\rho_T(0,1) = \rho_T = 0.546$. Then, on the basis of equation (10.2) with $\varphi = 0.6$, the auto-correlation between the baseline ($t = 0$) and the second follow-up assessments ($t = 2$) is anticipated to be $\rho_T(0,2) = \rho^{0.6 \times |2-0|} = 0.546^{0.6 \times 2} = 0.484$. Further, that between baseline and third assessment, $\rho_T(0,3) = \rho^{0.6 \times |3-0|} = 0.546^{0.6 \times 3} = 0.336$ and is clearly smaller.

Finally, the *unstructured* auto-correlation matrix presumes no particular pattern or "structure" to the correlation matrix, while one that is *user-fixed* has, as the term indicates, values that are specified by the user.

The auto-correlation pattern materially affects the way in which the computer package estimates the regression coefficients in the corresponding statistical model, and so it should be chosen with care.

10.3   REPEATED MEASURES

ANOVA

In some situations QoL assessment may be made over a limited period rather than over an extended time span. In this case it may be reasonable to assume that all subjects complete all the assessments. Thus instead of having a ragged data file with the number of observations for each subject varying from subject to subject, the file has a "rectangular" shape. This enables an ANOVA approach to be considered.

The rationale for repeated-measures ANOVA is to regard time also as a factor in addition to, for example, treatment. In a two-treatment randomised clinical trial, the treatment factor has two levels and each patient is randomised to one of the treatment options, or factor levels. However, although time may also be considered a factor with T levels it is not randomised as successive QoL assessments necessarily follow one after the other. As a consequence, the structure of the underlying statistical model has to be modified to take account of this.

This structure is a "split-plot" design, where the term "plot" arises as the particular design was first introduced in agricultural research and the "plot" referred to a small piece of ground. In our situation each "plot" is a subject and the "sub-plot" is the time of the QoL assessment.

For the case of g treatments being compared in a clinical trial having T QoL assessments on each of m patients per treatment group, the ANOVA corresponding to Table 8.7 is extended to take the form of Table 10.3.

The sub-plot nature of this design results in two residual or error variance terms in Table 10.3. One assesses the between-patient variability within treatment groups and is used to test the hypothesis of no differences between treatments using the F-ratio of Table T5 with $(g - 1)$ and $g(m - 1)$ degrees of freedom. The second is used to test the hypothesis of no change in QoL over time using the F-ratio with $(T - 1)$ and $g(m - 1)(T - 1)$ degrees of freedom. The F-ratio is used also to test for the interaction between Treatment and Time. If an interaction is present, this suggests that any differences in treatments observed do not remain constant over time. We discuss this in detail below.

Table 10.3 Layout for the repeated-measures ANOVA for comparing g treatments, in m subjects per treatment with QoL observed on T successive occasions

Source of variation	Sums of squares	df	Mean squares	F
Between treatments	S_{Trt}	$g - 1$	$M_{Trt} = S_{Trt}/(g - 1)$	$F_{Trt} = M_{Trt}/M_{Pat}$
Patient residual	S_{Pat}	$g(m - 1)$	$M_{Pat} = S_{Pat}/g(m - 1)$	
Between times	S_{Tim}	$T - 1$	$M_{Tim} = S_{Tim}/(T - 1)$	$F_{Tim} = M_{Tim}/M_{TimResid}$
Interaction	$S_{Trt*Tim}$	$(g - 1)(T - 1)$	$M_{Trt*Tim} = S_{Trt*Tim}/(T - 1)$	$F_{Trt*Tim} = M_{Trt*Tim}/M_{TimResid}$
Time residual	$S_{TimResid}$	$g(m - 1)(T - 1)$	$M_{TimResid}/[(m - g)(T - 1)]$	
Total	S_{Total}	$gmT - 1$		

Repeated-measures ANOVA is an attempt to provide a single analysis of a complete longitudinal dataset. In such studies, the patients are often termed "Level 2" units and the repeated QoL assessments the "Level 1" units. This terminology leads to the more general "*multi-level*" models that we return to later.

Diggle, Liang and Zeger (1994) point out that the use of the repeated-measures ANOVA implies an *exchangeable* auto-correlation between any two observations on the same patient. This may not always be appropriate for QoL assessments.

MODELLING

The main difficulty with repeated-measures ANOVA, in the context of QoL research, is that there are seldom equal numbers of QoL assessments recorded per patient or subject. Although ANOVA methodology can be extended to handle some "unbalanced" situations, in the standard format shown in Table 10.3 the number of assessments must be equal for all patients. However, we mentioned in Chapter 8 that ANOVA was a model-based form of analysis and this remains so in the repeated-measures situation. It is therefore possible—and usually simpler—to use a regression-modelling approach rather than repeated-measures ANOVA. The regression model corresponding to the analysis of Table 10.3 can be described as follows:

$$Q_{jit} = \alpha + \tau x_i + \beta t + \omega_{jit}. \tag{10.3}$$

Here Q_{jit} is the QoL assessment of patient j at assessment t and who is receiving treatment i, and $x_i = 0$ corresponds to the patient receiving one of the treatments whereas $x_i = 1$ if it is the other. The ω_{jit} is the *error* or *residual term* similar to that introduced in equation (8.22). However, as shown in Table 10.3, there are two residual terms corresponding to "Patient Residual" and "Time Residual". This implies that each ω_{jit} really has two parts, one a between-patients component the other a within-patient component. We have been investigating the within-patient component when examining the patterns in the auto-correlation matrices.

Use of the basic model (10.3) implies that QoL changes in a linear way with time; that is, the scatter diagrams of QoL profiles of patients against time should appear, at least approximately, as straight lines and have the same slope from patient to patient. A second assumption is that, if there is a difference in QoL values between patients on the two treatments, then it is the same value at each assessment time.

Once we specify the form of the model and the pattern of the auto-correlation, this model can be fitted using, for example, STATA (1999).

Example

Wisløff *et al.* (1996) describe a randomised clinical trial in which the fatigue (FA) of patients with myeloma receiving either MP or MP+IFN was assessed on several occasions over a four-year period. If we assume the exchangeable pattern for the correlation matrix, then the bold entries of Table 10.4 give a summary of the results of fitting equation (10.3) to part of the data. The numbers in parenthesis represent the respective *SE*s.

Table 10.4 Analysis of fatigue (FA) levels in patients with myeloma receiving either MP or MP+IFN. Patients with complete information on assessments from month 1 up to and including month 36 (Data supplied by Wisløff *et al.*, 1996)

Model	Regression coefficient	Type of auto-correlation matrix			
		Exchangeable	Independent	Unstructured	Multiplicative
I	Constant, α	38.21	38.21	36.60	39.35
	Treatment, τ	5.26 (2.40)	5.26 (1.54)	5.30 (2.40)	5.10 (2.24)
II	Constant, α	**41.41**	41.40	41.73	42.23
	Treatment, τ	**5.26 (2.40)**	5.26 (1.53)	5.18 (2.40)	5.10 (2.23)
	Time, β	**−0.30 (0.06)**	−0.30 (0.09)	−0.30 (0.07)	−0.25 (0.08)
III	Constant, α	39.02	39.02	39.32	39.85
	Treatment, τ	10.05 (2.76)	10.05 (2.45)	9.97 (2.82)	9.86 (2.92)
	Time, β	−0.07 (0.09)	−0.07 (0.13)	−0.09 (0.10)	−0.04 (0.12)
	Interaction, γ	−0.45 (0.13)	−0.45 (0.18)	−0.43 (0.13)	−0.42 (0.17)
IV	Constant, α	22.36	22.36	21.43	22.36
	Treatment, τ	9.25 (2.49)	9.25 (2.45)	9.07 (2.47)	9.05 (2.65)
	Time, β	−0.07 (0.09)	−0.07 (0.12)	−0.01 (0.12)	−0.05 (0.11)
	Interaction, γ	−0.45 (0.13)	−0.45 (0.16)	−0.43 (0.13)	−0.42 (0.16)
	Baseline FA, φ	0.35 (0.04)	0.35 (0.03)	0.37 (0.04)	0.37 (0.04)

Considering the on-treatment data from month 1 to month 36, the results of fitting this model are shown as model II of Table 10.4, in which

$$FA = 41.41 + 5.26x_i - 0.30t.$$

From this model one deduces that as time goes by, that is as t increases, reported FA decreases while those patients also receiving IFN score approximately 5.3 units higher on each occasion. For example, at $t = 1$, the first assessment post-commencement of treatment, those who received MP alone had $FA_{MP} = 41.41 - 0.30 = 41.11$, whilst those also receiving IFN had $FA_{IFN} = 41.41 + 5.26 - 0.30 = 46.37$. The contribution due to time, −0.30, is in both expressions, as is the constant term 41.41, and so the difference $FA_{IFN} - FA_{MP} = 5.26$ remains the same at each assessment. Using equation (8.1) the ratios $z = -0.30/0.06 = -5.0$ and $z = 5.26/2.40 = 2.2$ imply, from Table T1, *p*-values of <0.0001 and 0.026 for the time and treatment effects respectively. These suggest a statistically significant decline in FA with time but higher levels of FA in those receiving IFN.

In the model indicated by bold numbers in Table 10.4 we have not considered the interaction component of Table 10.3, and so the comparison with repeated-measures ANOVA is not quite complete. However, before discussing the interaction we show the basic steps involved in constructing statistical models.

MODEL BUILDING

The major research question in the context of a clinical trial is the treatment effect, and so of primary interest is the following model:

$$Q_{jit} = \alpha + \tau x_i + \omega_{jit}. \tag{10.4}$$

This is a simplified version of equation (10.3), setting $\beta = 0$ so that the time element is not included. Fitting this model, again using the exchangeable auto-correlation matrix, gives (model I of Table 10.4) FA = 38.21 + 5.26x_i. The treatment effect is significant since $z = 5.26/2.40 = 2.2$, $p = 0.026$. Although this is statistically significant, the model building process asks if there are other and additional variables that might also explain some of the variation in QoL. In our context, the next model to consider is equation (10.3) which, once fitted, confirms the statistical significance of the treatment effect but also suggests that time plays a role ($z = -0.30/0.06 = -5.0$, $p < 0.0001$).

AUTO-REGRESSION

Although we have already introduced an auto-regression model in equation (10.3) as a means of effecting a repeated-measures ANOVA, we now examine a rather simpler model so as to explain the role of β. Since in longitudinal studies there are not only observations on many subjects but also repeating observations over time on the same subjects, we may wish to investigate changes in QoL over time, using a linear regression model. Thus we might propose that QoL changes with time according to the following expression:

$$Q_t = \alpha + \beta t + \omega_t. \tag{10.5}$$

This has much the same form as equation (8.24) but t, denoting time, replaces x_j and we write ω in place of ε. With this expression we are saying that the QoL of *an individual patient* changes with *time* according to this linear model. Now, in contrast to equation (8.24), the observations are all made on the same subject and so the ω cannot be assumed to be independent or uncorrelated.

Example from the literature

Hart *et al.* (1997) investigated the value of homeopathic arnica C30 for pain in patients after total abdominal hysterectomy. They presented individual plots to demonstrate the variety of pain score changes against time after operation. One of these profiles, for a patient receiving arnica as opposed to placebo, is reproduced in Figure 10.3. The profile chosen is approximately linear over the study period so that equation (10.5) may be a reasonable description in this case.

In general we will have more than a single subject and so the more general form of equation (10.5) for subject j is

$$Q_{jt} = \alpha + \beta t + \omega_{jt}. \tag{10.6}$$

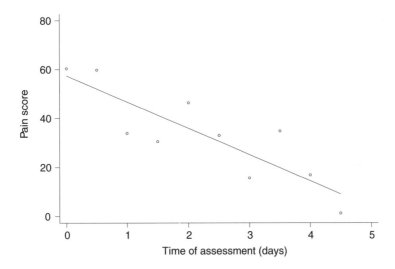

Figure 10.3 Pain score changes for a patient receiving arnica following total abdominal hysterectomy (Data from Hart *et al.*, 1997, Figure 2)

INTERACTIONS

A plot of the Wisløff *et al.* data is shown in Figure 10.4, and this suggests that it is unrealistic to assume that the mean difference in QoL values between the two treatments remains constant over time. The graph suggests a treatment difference at month 1 and which has largely disappeared by month 36. This is a Treatment × Time *interaction*. The corresponding statistical test using the repeated-measures ANOVA of Table 10.3 compares $F_{Trt*Tim}$ with an *F*-ratio with $(g - 1)(T - 1)$ and $g(m - 1)(T - 1)$ degrees of freedom.

To model the interaction a further regression coefficient, γ, has to be added to equation (10.3). This is attached to the multiple of x_i and t, giving

$$Q_{jit} = \alpha + \tau x_i + \beta t + \gamma\, x_i t + \omega_{jit}. \tag{10.7}$$

Using the example data, this is shown as model III in Table 10.4. The corresponding $z = -0.45/0.13 = -3.5$, which from Table T1 gives $p = 0.0023$ and is statistically significant.

It is important to note that there is a large change in the regression coefficient for treatment, from 5.26 with model II to 10.05 with model III. This arises because there is also a change in the interpretation of τ. In model II, τ represents the average treatment effect, averaged over the observations at 1, 6, 12 and 24 months. Inspecting Figure 10.4, at month 1 the difference is of the order of 10 units of FA, while at month 24 it is close to zero, with intermediate values at months 6 and 12. These provide an average value of approximately 5 units of FA. In contrast, the τ in Model III is interpreted as the estimated difference between treatments were observations to be made at $t = 0$, just after treatment commenced, rather than at baseline which is just before treatment commenced. Hence the estimate of τ as 10.05. At $t = 0$ the contribution of the interaction term of equation (10.6) is zero,

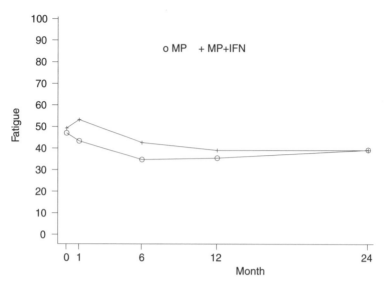

Figure 10.4 Mean levels of fatigue in patients with multiple myeloma, before and during treatment with MP or MP + IFN (Data supplied by Wisløff *et al.*, 1996)

whereas at later QoL assessments the interaction term enters the model given by equation (10.6) and reduces the value of the estimated treatment effect. Thus for IFN at $t = 1$ (the first post-treatment QoL assessment), $x_i = 1$, $\gamma x_i t = -0.45 \times 1 \times 1 = -0.45$. This reduces the estimated effect of treatment to $10.05 - 0.45 = 9.60$ units of FA. By 12 months, at $t = 12$, we have $\gamma x_i t = -0.45 \times 1 \times 12 = -5.40$ and so the treatment effect is reduced to $10.05 - 5.40 = 4.65$. The estimates that are provided by model III are hence close to those suggested by Figure 10.4.

PAIRED DATA

We have discussed a special case of equation (10.6) in Chapter 8 when the baseline QoL measure ($t = 0$) is compared with a later value at some fixed time (this can be arbitrarily labelled $t = 1$). Using equation (10.6) at $t = 0$ and $t = 1$ we have for subject j, $Q_{j0} = \alpha + \omega_{j0}$ and $Q_{j1} = \alpha + \beta + \omega_{j1}$ respectively. Their difference is $D_j = Q_{j1} - Q_{j0} = \alpha + \beta + \omega_{j1} - \alpha - \omega_{j0}$, that is

$$D_j = \beta + (\omega_{j1} - \omega_{j0}).$$

The null hypothesis of no difference between baseline and subsequent QoL corresponds to $\beta = 0$. Each subject has his or her own error term, here $(\omega_{j1} - \omega_{j0})$, which comprises the residuals from both the time 0 (baseline) and time 1 observations. The value that this difference takes for a particular patient will be independent of the values taken by other subjects in the study. They are thus uncorrelated.

The data in this situation are termed "paired". For a particular study with n subjects observed at baseline and at one further occasion, the estimate of β is $b = \bar{D}$ with $SE(b) = SD/\sqrt{n}$, where SD is the standard deviation obtained from the differences D_j. This in turn leads to the paired z-test of equation (8.1), or a paired t-test if the study is small, for testing the differences in QoL on these two occasions. Thus, for two QoL assessment times, longitudinal data can be reduced to single measurements per patient (change in QoL), so that no new principles are involved and the analysis has become cross-sectional in nature.

BETWEEN- AND WITHIN-SUBJECT VARIATION

Earlier we examined the possible forms of the error term in the regression model of equation (10.3), and there were several options available. The model described a particular subject j but we may wish to extend this to a group of n subjects. In doing this there are several further choices to make. One possibility is to assume that all subjects have the same QoL profile with respect to time, apart from random variation. In this case the model remains as equation (10.6) but the error must now contain components that include random fluctuations accounting for both within- and between-subject variation. We shall explore this using generalised estimating equations.

GENERALISED ESTIMATING EQUATIONS (GEE)

Repeated-measures ANOVA is a form of "fixed effects" model, and it also implies that the auto-correlation structure is of the exchangeable form. Applying this methodology to some of the data of Wisløff et al. (1996) gave the model introduced in bold in Table 10.4. However, models using the other forms of auto-correlation matrix, independent, unstructured or multiplicative, can be fitted using so-called generalised estimating equations (GEE). This methodology is implemented for example in STATA (1999).

Example

> Applying the GEE methodology to the FA data of Wisløff et al. (1996), assuming independent, unstructured and multiplicative forms of the auto-correlation matrix, gives the results summarised in Table 10.4. Focusing on model III as this seems most appropriate for these data, the estimated regression provided by the exchangeable and independent models are the same, but the SE associated with the treatment effect is smaller whilst that for time and the interaction somewhat larger. Both the corresponding estimates of the regression coefficients and their SEs of the unstructured and multiplicative auto-correlation models differ from one another and from both the exchangeable and independent models. Thus the results change with the underlying auto-correlation structure assumed. Nevertheless, the models are in broad agreement, suggesting a statistically significant Treatment effect and an interaction, Treatment × Time.

In practice it is often difficult to choose whether exchangeable, unstructured or multiplicative auto-correlation structure is appropriate. As a consequence, when examining the initial and subsequent (after model fitting) correlation matrices, if the choice is still not clear, models may be developed using each of the alternatives and these are then compared. If the models are all similar both with respect to the variables included and the corresponding regression coefficients, then there is little difficulty about which to choose for interpretation. Conversely if there are major differences this is an indication for further investigation.

The general methodology of GEE is very flexible and in principle can deal with all the observed data from a QoL study. The subjects are not required to have exactly the same numbers of assessments, and the assessments can be made at variable times. The latter allows the modelling to proceed even if a subject misses a QoL assessment. This assumes that the probability of being missing is independent of any of the random terms (the residuals) in the model. However, care is still needed here, as this assumption may not hold. The very fact that the data are "missing" may itself be informative (see Chapter 11). In this circumstance, taking no particular note of its absence may result in incorrect conclusions being drawn from the data.

Although the detail need not concern us too much, the process of fitting GEE models begins by assuming the independence form of the auto-correlation matrix. Thus it begins by fitting the model as if each assessment were from a different patient. Once this model is obtained the corresponding residuals—see equation (8.23)—are calculated and these are then used to estimate the auto-correlation matrix assuming it is the exchangeable type. This matrix is then used to fit the model again and the residual once more calculated and the auto-correlation matrix obtained. This process is repeated until the corresponding regression coefficients that are obtained in the successive models differ little on successive occasions; that is, they converge. This process is termed *iteration*.

Example

The lower diagonal of Table 10.5 shows the independence form of the auto-correlation matrix of the Wisløff *et al.* (1996) data prior to fitting a GEE model of treatment, time and their interaction.

Table 10.5 Matrices of auto-correlation coefficients for fatigue (FA) of multiple myeloma patients during the first 24 months of therapy. The lower diagonal gives the independence matrix before model-fitting whilst the upper gives the exchangeable form after model-fitting (Data supplied by Wisløff *et al.*, 1996)

	1	6	12	24
1	1	0.40	0.40	0.40
6	0.62	1	0.40	0.40
12	0.48	0.61	1	0.40
24	0.39	0.47	0.56	1

Thus while the model-fitting values of r_T average approximately 0.5, the final exchangeable value is lower at 0.4. It will usually be the case that after model-fitting the auto-correlations will appear to have been reduced.

FIXED AND RANDOM EFFECTS

Although we may postulate that the slope of the regression line β can be assumed the same for all subjects, each may have a different starting point. This can be expressed by modifying α of equation (10.6) to α_j to give

$$Q_{jt} = \alpha_j + \beta t + \omega_{jt}. \tag{10.8}$$

Again there are options here. One is to assume that α_j (the intercept) is unique for each of the n subjects and so there are n of these to estimate. An alternative is to assume that the subjects chosen for study are a random sample of subjects from a population that has mean α and a standard deviation σ_α. In fitting this latter model we estimate for the first term of equation (10.8) only the two parameters, α and σ_α, rather than n individual values for α_j. The first of these models is termed a *fixed-effects* model, the second a *random-effects* model.

It is important to note a possible confusion of terms arises here as *random* is used in two contexts. Here, it describes a property of the regression coefficients, α_j, in the model of equation (10.8), whereas in Table 10.2 it refers to the error part of the model, ω_{jt}. We will use *random-effects* for the former and *independent* for the latter.

In the random-effects model, one is effectively modelling α by means of the following equation:

$$\alpha_j = \alpha + v_j, \tag{10.9}$$

where α is the fixed part of this model and v_j is the residual, error or random part which is assumed to have a mean of zero and standard deviation σ_α. In this case the format of equation (10.8) changes to

$$Q_{jt} = \alpha + \beta t + v_j + \omega_{jt}. \tag{10.10}$$

Thus we are introducing a second component to the residual variation which now comprises both v_j and ω_{jt}. These are analogous to the variance components referred to when describing the intraclass correlation coefficient (*ICC*) in Table 3.11 and equation (3.8).

One can go a step further than having a random-effects model for the intercept α alone, by also postulating that the slope β can be dealt with in a similar way, so that different patients can have different slopes. This leads from equation (10.8) to

$$Q_{jt} = \alpha_j + \beta_j t + \omega_{jt}. \tag{10.11}$$

In this situation, the β_j can be estimated from a fixed-effects model, or regarded as having mean β and a standard deviation σ_β in a random-effects model. The latter can be expressed as $\beta_j = \beta + \eta_j$, where η_j is the corresponding residual which is assumed to have a mean of zero and standard deviation σ_β.

Finally, in order to make use of regression techniques to compare two treatments with respect to longitudinal QoL measures, we have to extend the above models to include a regression coefficient for treatment. Thus we write, for example:

$$Q_{jit} = \alpha_j + \tau x_i + \beta_j t + \omega_{jit}. \tag{10.12}$$

This model can specify either fixed- or random-effects for either or both of α and β. Models that contain both fixed and random effects are termed *mixed*.

The advantage of the random-effects model is that there are fewer regression parameters to estimate. It is based upon the assumption that the subjects in the study are chosen at random from some wider patient population. This will seldom be true, at least in the context of a clinical trial for which trial patients are screened for eligibility and entered only after giving informed consent. Thus although the treatment assigned is at "at random", this is a very different use of the word random, and does not imply that random-effects models are necessarily appropriate; once again, there is multiple use of the same word describing different situations. However, it is usually reasonable to assume that the trial patients have been chosen at random from a large number of potentially eligible patients, and that they represent a random selection from this artificial population. Thus a random-effects model is frequently applied whenever a study includes large numbers of patients.

MULTI-LEVEL MODELS

If we assume a random-effects model is appropriate, then models can be fitted using multi-level modelling statistical software which is implemented in MLwiN (Goldstein *et al.*, 1998) for example. In this process the repeated QoL assessment within a patients are the "Level 1" units and the patients themselves are the "Level 2" units. Use of multi-level modelling as opposed to GEE allows examination of the "error" parts of the model in more detail.

Example

Applying the multi-level methodology to the selected FA data from Wisløff *et al.* (1996) gives the results summarised in model III of Table 10.6. Here the mixed model includes treatment (τ) as a "fixed effect" while the intercept (α) and time (β) as "random effects". This can be compared with the model III results summarised in Table 10.4. The model suggests a statistically significant treatment effect and a strong Treatment × Time interaction as we had observed before. The regression coefficients and standard errors do not differ materially from those of Table 10.4.

It should be noted that because of the presence of a strong Treatment × Time interaction, the 95% confidence interval of 4.43 to 15.69 is relevant only to the comparison between groups at $t = 0$.

COVARIATES

All the models can be extended further to include covariates, in a similar way to that we have described in equation (8.17), as it is recognised that patient-specific details may influence subsequent patient outcome measures. In the context of QoL studies, the pre-treatment QoL or baseline assessment may be particularly critical. For

Table 10.6 Multi-level modelling analysis of fatigue (FA) levels in patients with myeloma receiving either MP or MP+IFN. Patients with complete information on assessments up to and including month 24 only (Data supplied by Wisløff *et al.*, 1996)

Regression coefficient	Model III			Model IV		
	Estimate (*SE*)	*p*-value		Estimate (*SE*)	*p*-value	
Constant, α	39.01			21.56		
Treatment, τ	10.06 (2.87)	$p = 0.0004$		9.22 (2.44)	$p = 0.0002$	
95% CI	4.43 to 15.69			4.43 to 14.00		
Time, β	−0.08 (0.10)	$p = 0.47$		−0.08 (0.10)	$p = 0.47$	
Interaction, γ	−0.45 (0.15)	$p = 0.002$		−0.45 (0.13)	$p = 0.002$	
Baseline, φ	–	–		0.37 (0.04)	$p < 0.0001$	

example, this is likely to be the case in circumstances where these baseline levels determine to some extent the pattern of subsequent "missing" data.

Example

Adding the baseline FA measure to the random-effects model previously discussed for the data of Wisløff *et al.* (1996) gives the model IV summarised both in Table 10.4 and the final columns of Table 10.6. The regression coefficient of baseline FA (FA_0) is statistically significant, suggesting its major influence on subsequent reported levels.

If baseline variables or other "prognostic indicators" are important predictors of outcome, they may be expected to account for some of the otherwise unexplained variability in the data. As a consequence, some of the *SE*s for other coefficients may become smaller when these strong predictors are included. This means both that we have better estimates of the coefficients—including those for the treatment effect— and that their *p*-values may become more highly significant. However, if we include unnecessary variables in the model, such as those baseline characteristics that are irrelevant to subsequent outcome, we are in effect adding more noise and this will weaken the estimation of treatment effect. One should resist the temptation to add a large number of covariates just because "they may be important".

In a randomised trial the baseline (pre-randomisation) characteristics may be anticipated to be broadly similar in the different groups of patients because of the randomisation procedure itself, and so the estimate of the treatment effect is unlikely to be biased. However, as in this example, including covariates can alter the estimate of the treatment effect. Thus there is a suggestion that perhaps the true difference between the treatments may be a little bit smaller than when we ignored the baseline FA score (for example, 9.25 instead of 10.05 if we assume exchangeable or independent auto-correlations).

Example from the literature

Cnaan, Laird and Slasor (1997) describe the application of general linear mixed models to a randomised clinical trial of patients with schizophrenia assessed by the total score from the BPRS. There were four treatments: three doses (low, medium, and high) of an experimental drug and a control drug. Patients were evaluated at baseline, 1, 2, 3, 4 and 6 weeks. However, of 245 patients randomised only 60% completed the 6-week assessment. The results of part of their analysis using the random-effects model is summarised in Table 10.7.

The corresponding algebraic model, for a patient receiving low-dose treatment, at week w is:

$$\text{BPRS} = \alpha + \tau_L + \beta_L(w - 3) + \beta_Q (w - 3)^2 + \varphi \, \text{BPRS}_0, \quad (10.13)$$

where w is the week number and BPRS_0 is the baseline value. The corresponding fitted equation is

$$\text{BPRS} = 1.90 + 2.04 - 1.52 \, (w - 3) + 0.37 \, (w - 3)^2 + 0.65 \, \text{BPRS}_0.$$

At week 3, this reduces to $\text{BPRS} = 3.94 + 0.65 \, \text{BPRS}_0$. Thus for patients with $\text{BPRS}_0 = 40$, the predicted score at week 3 with low-dose treatment is $3.94 + (0.65 \times 40) = 29.94$ or approximately 30.

Table 10.7 Random-effects model for changes in BPRS in patients with schizophrenia (Based on Cnaan et al., 1997)

Variable name	Parameter	Estimate	SE
Intercept	α	1.90	2.51
Low dose	τ_L	2.04	1.06
Medium dose	τ_M	-1.64	1.03
High dose	τ_H	-0.13	0.05
Week	β_L	-1.52	0.25
Week * Week	β_Q	0.37	0.09
Baseline BPRS	φ	0.65	0.07

There are several details in this last example that require further explanation. The first is that there are four treatments involved (doses, in this example), rather than the two different treatments of equation (10.3). This implies that the τx_i part of that equation has to be expanded to $\tau_L x_{Lj} + \tau_M x_{2j} + \tau_H x_{3j}$. A patient j receiving the control treatment is indicated by $x_{Lj} = x_{Mj} = x_{Hj} = 0$. For a patient receiving a low dose, $x_{Lj} = 1, x_{Mj} = x_{Hj} = 0$; for one receiving a moderate dose, $x_{Lj} = 0, x_{Mj} = 1, x_{Hj} = 0$; and for one receiving a high dose, $x_{Lj} = x_{Mj} = 0, x_{Hj} = 1$. The variables x_{Lj}, x_{Mj}, and x_{Hj} are called *dummy variables*.

Secondly, time in weeks occurs twice in equation (10.13). The first term with regression coefficient, β_L, is the linear and the second, β_Q, the time-squared or quadratic part. Together they express the fact that, in contrast to the example of Figure 10.3, the change in the QoL score over time may not be linear but may be somewhat curved. This can be interpreted as a decrease in BPRS scores with time, but the decrease is larger initially and then levels off. Further, the equation includes $(w - 3)$ rather than w, but subtracting the 3 is merely a convenience device to ease the computational problems as squared terms tend to get large and this makes the fitting process less stable.

Finally, there is a covariate term with regression coefficient φ. This is included here since it is well known that the initial BPRS is an important predictor of future values irrespective of the treatment given. Thus any treatment comparisons need to be adjusted for variation in the baseline values for the patients.

CHOOSING THE AUTO-CORRELATION STRUCTURE

Although we have illustrated this chapter with the auto-correlation matrix calculated from successive observations of FA in patients with myeloma, the actual matrix we really wish to examine is that obtained from the residuals. As we have noted, the residual is the difference between the actual observed QoL value and the one predicted from the fitted model; that is a quantity w which estimates the respective ω. However, we cannot determine this without first fitting the model, leading to some circularity. The usual procedure is to make an initial assumption about the auto-correlation structure, often as in our example based upon the auto-correlations of the observed values; then fit the model, and examine whether this structure from the residuals has the form that we assumed in the first place. If so, we may accept the assumption as reasonable; if not, we may try an alternative.

Example from the literature

The model of equation (10.13) led to the lower diagonal auto-correlation matrix of Table 10.2 (Cnaan, Laird and Slasor, 1997). The upper and italicised corner was calculated using the same model but with a further covariate (patient status) added. It can be seen that the values of the auto-correlation coefficients are smaller in the upper corner than the corresponding values in the lower corner. For example, the first model gives $r_T(1,6) = r_T(6,1) = 0.35$ and the second model 0.32. This will generally be the case if one model contains one or more extra variables over and above those already contained in the first model. The extra variables help explain some of the "unexplained" variation, and so the size of the ω values will in general be smaller leading to smaller correlation coefficients.

10.4   OTHER SITUATIONS

LOGISTIC MODELS

So far we have assumed that the QoL variable under study is a continuous or scale variable that can be assumed to have a Normal distribution. However, the methodology is not confined to this situation. For example, the QoL variable could be an item with binary responses, in which case allowance would be made in the model-fitting process. This is done by specifying a *link function*. If the basic distribution is Normal the link is known as an *identity link*, which means the QoL variable is not changed for the fitting process. On the other hand, if the QoL item is binary, the basic distribution is often taken as binomial and the corresponding link is the *logit* transformation. This transformation was introduced when describing the logistic item response or Rasch models in Chapter 6. Then the left-hand side of the above equations will be of the form $\log_e[Q/(1 - Q)]$, with equation (10.14) corresponding to equation (10.3):

$$\log_e[Q_{ji}/(1 - Q_{ji})] = \alpha + \tau x_i + \beta t + \omega_{jit}. \tag{10.14}$$

The technical details of the methods for fitting the above models become complex, but the processes are implemented in most statistical packages that provide GEE or multi-level models. The theoretical approach is a very general one, and other distributions can be accommodated by specifying suitable link functions; statistical packages incorporating these methods usually provide a number of choices.

MANOVA

In the previous sections we have assumed that we are dealing with a single scale or item from a QoL instrument. However, most instruments comprise several items and scales that are assessed concurrently, ranging, for example, from two for HADS (anxiety and depression) to 15 with the EORTC QLQ-C30 (five functional scales, one global health status, three symptom scales and six items). Thus the complete analysis of QoL data from a clinical study may seek to summarise multiple features, even though sensible study design should have specified in advance the one or two aspects of QoL that are of principal interest. The "all features" analysis poses major problems for the investigator in terms of the magnitude of the task and of the complexity of the eventual summary. In principle at least, such a multivariable analysis can be drawn into a single one by extending the repeated-measures ANOVA to *multivariate analysis of variance*, or MANOVA.

MANOVA leaves unchanged the right-hand side of equations such as (10.5), which contain the "independent" or "explanatory" variables. However, the left-hand side now reflects all the QoL measures and not just the single "dependent" variable that we have so far included. This poses some immediate problems as the variables may not all be of the same type; that is, some may be binary, some ordered categorical and others continuous with a Normal distribution. However, MANOVA is not applicable unless all of the outcome variables can be assumed to have the same form, or all are reduced to, say, binary form despite the resultant loss of information. This makes the methodology less attractive. Another major difficulty is that some but not all of the responses at a particular assessment may be missing; that is, some of the items within an otherwise complete QoL assessment are not available as opposed to the whole form being missing. The resulting patterns of items missing from forms and whole missing forms can be very complex.

In theory, a single MANOVA, perhaps focusing on a between-treatments comparison, reduces the number of statistical significance tests conducted on the data and so avoids some of the difficulties associated with multiple testing (see Chapter 15). Goldstein *et al.* (1998, Chapter 4) describe how the multi-level modelling approach can be extended to include this multivariate situation, which then removes the constraints of equal numbers of observations per subject but does not necessarily overcome difficulties associated with the pattern of missing values.

Perhaps the single greatest difficulty with the use of MANOVA arises when summarising what has taken place. This approach is not easy to explain and the results are difficult to interpret, which detracts from its routine use.

MISSING DATA

For reasons of clarity when describing the techniques included in this chapter we have purposely omitted detailed reference to missing data but have recognised that the numbers of observations per subject may not be equal owing to attrition. For example, in a trial with patients in advanced cancer the attrition may be caused by the death of the patient. We have assumed that prior to this the QoL assessments are all complete although not necessarily on schedule. In practice, there will be missing data and, depending on their type and volume, this may have serious impact on the analysis and interpretation. The GEE and multi-level methodologies can be applied when some data are absent, but for every missing observation there is a reduction in the statistical power of the analysis and, perhaps more importantly, the possibility of bias leading to incorrect conclusions.

10.5 CONCLUSIONS

It should be mentioned that, as pointed out by Cnaan *et al.* (1997), a wide variety of names are used in the statistical literature to describe versions of the same model. These names include mixed linear; two-stage random-effects; multi-level linear; hierarchical linear and random regression coefficient models. Some of these differ only by the technical way in which the standard errors are estimated.

One difficulty associated with powerful statistical packages which can fit numerous and complex statistical models almost instantaneously is that they may be used as a "black box" by the unwary. All of the models used in these procedures make assumptions about the nature of the data, and these assumptions are then reflected in the resulting output. In some situations, visual inspection of the data will indicate what is and what is not sensible in relation to the non-error part of the model. For example, Figure 9.7c would suggest that baseline values are very similar across the treatment groups, but it may not be sensible to assume QoL changes linearly with time. An appropriate model would attempt to describe the early advantage in the reduction of HADS anxiety of the four-drug regimen. In addition, there is the problem of specifying the appropriate auto-correlation structure.

There is a further difficulty. We have stated repeatedly that the major endpoint measures for any study of QoL must be pre-specified in the protocol, and this should also be true of the models proposed to describe these data. Our experience is that this is rarely done, one reason being the paucity of previous experience of analysing QoL data in a truly longitudinal manner using the now available methodologies. This lack of experience suggests that the major analyses should rather be of a simple cross-sectional nature, with any statistical modelling that is reported being regarded as tentative and exploratory. They can then form the basis for a better understanding of the processes in future studies.

11 Missing Data

Summary

This chapter describes problems that arise through missing QoL assessment data. Situations are outlined where values are missing from otherwise complete questionnaires or where entire forms are missing. The main difficulty with either type of missing data is the bias they may introduce at the analysis stage. We distinguish QoL data that are "missing" through attrition because the patient has died, from that which could be anticipated but was not returned.

We describe how missing values may be estimated, often termed as *imputed*, to ease the statistical analysis, but stress that imputing values is no substitute for collecting "real" data.

11.1 INTRODUCTION

Difficulties with data collection and compliance are major barriers to the successful implementation of QoL assessments in clinical trials. The principal problem is that bias may be introduced through data that are missing because patients either drop out of the trial completely, or do not participate comprehensively in the QoL assessment. The issue is whether the data actually collected are representative of the QoL of all study patients, including those without data, so that the analysis can be taken as a reliable reflection of the study outcome. If the missing data can be regarded as absent at random, they will on average be similar to the available data. If not, the summary derived only from those who provide data may no longer be representative. In this case the available patient data will give a biased view that will not reflect the true situation.

Considerations of potential bias raises the questions of whether the missing data are missing at random or not at random, and what proportion of missing data is acceptable in a trial or study. In the context of a randomised trial, there is the question of the impact of ignoring missing data. For example, what are the implications of assuming that if the patterns of missing data are similar in all treatment groups, then treatment comparisons will be unbiased? If the impact of missing data cannot be ignored, how can one estimate or allow for the missing data when analysing the trial?

In some situations the fact that data are absent may be "informative", in that this tells us something about the patient from whom they are missing. We need to take note of this information. For example, suppose the likelihood of a missing assessment is high when a patient's health deteriorates just prior to death. Then any analysis of QoL should take account of this pattern, and should recognise that missing values immediately prior to death are more likely to be associated with poor QoL. These values are likely to be different from those that are missing at times distant from death, when patients are expected to be healthier and when the reason for their being missing is more likely to be accidental.

QoL data are usually collected using a self-assessment questionnaire containing a series of questions. Although some other types of clinical data may often be collected retrospectively from, for example, the patient's medical charts, once a patient has missed a QoL assessment the retrospective collection of the patient response is not usually possible.

There is a clear distinction between data that was anticipated but missing, and data that are absent because they cannot be collected. In the context of a clinical trial in a life-threatening disease, QoL may be assessed at monthly intervals. However, data can be expected—and hence have the potential to be "missing"— only for the period while the patient is alive. In this situation, we do not anticipate equal numbers of observations per patient. Nor is it sensible to impute values of QoL items in the period after death.

COMPLETE CASE ANALYSIS

The simplest approach to analysis when some data are missing is to remove all patients with incomplete data from the analysis. Then standard complete-data methods can be used. However, this leaves only those patients for whom the relevant QoL information is entirely complete. In studies of advanced disease, where the assessment just prior to death may be difficult, this generally means deleting an unacceptable number of patients. In addition, during follow-up of patients, those who are in good condition might be expected to have less missing information than those who are not so well. Consequently, QoL as summarised from the "complete-data" patients may be overestimated, particularly at later time points. Therefore complete case analysis has two distinct disadvantages: it reduces the sample size by excluding patients with incomplete data, and may produce misleading results. We do not recommend it unless the proportion with missing data is very small, perhaps fewer than 5% of patients.

AVAILABLE CASE ANALYSIS

Suppose we wish to compare two treatments with respect to QoL at specific time points, using standard statistical tests such as the t-test or the Mann–Whitney test. One possibility is to include in the comparison all the QoL information available at that assessment time point. Although the sample size may then vary at each assessment time point, this method makes use of all available data.

The main disadvantage of this method is that different sets of patients contribute information at different time points depending on the pattern of missing data. Additionally, an overall comparison of treatments is usually preferable to simple cross-sectional comparisons at specific time points, since overall tests allow general statements about treatment effects, are statistically more powerful, and safeguard against multiple testing.

SUMMARY MEASURES

As discussed in Chapter 9, a widely used method for analysis of data collected serially over time is to reduce the data on each patient to a single summary statistic, such as the *AUC*. In trials where a treatment is provided with the intent of palliating a certain symptom, another useful summary statistic may be the patient's worst QoL score for that symptom. Alternatively, a certain change score from baseline may be defined as clinically or subjectively important, and the time taken to reach this change score may be calculated. The summary for all patients is then analysed using an appropriate univariate test.

However, such an approach does not necessarily circumvent the presence of missing values as the key response, perhaps the worst QoL score for that symptom, may be the very item that was missing.

IMPUTED MISSING DATA

To avoid the problems with respect to "complete-case" and "available-case" analyses, an option frequently used is to replace the missing values by imputed values, estimated using the available data and other information about the patient. The imputed values are inserted in the data file, making a now augmented (and complete) file on which the analysis is then undertaken. However, to "impute" data several considerations need to be reviewed.

11.2 TYPES OF MISSING DATA

In QoL situations there are two main types of missing data. These are termed *unit* non-response and *item* non-response respectively. The first refers to a whole QoL assessment missing when one was anticipated from the patient; the second refers to one or several items not completed within an otherwise complete QoL questionnaire.

There are several types of unit non-response, including those arising from *intermittent missing* forms, patient *dropout* from the study, or patient *late entry* into the study. Consider a clinical trial where QoL is assessed every month for two years but a patient completed QoL assessments only at months 0, 2, 3, 5 and 6. There are intermittent missing questionnaires at months 1 and 4. At month 7 the patient dropped out of the study and therefore no additional QoL assessments were received. In contrast, suppose a patient was randomised into this trial in, say, September 1999 and an interim analysis of the ongoing trial was performed at the beginning of December 1999. In this case, the patient would have completed QoL assessments only at months 0, 1 and 2. This is a case of late entry into the trial since one could not expect more questionnaires for this patient at this time.

In some clinical trials of chronic diseases, QoL assessments continue for the remaining life of the patient. However, especially in advanced disease, it is evident that not all patients will complete the same number of assessments, sometimes for medical reasons but ultimately because of death.

Example

Curran *et al.* (1998b) give the Kaplan–Meier plot (Figure 11.1) of time on protocol treatment for breast cancer patients with newly diagnosed bone metastases. The median time on treatment was 6.4 months. The patients were requested to complete a QoL questionnaire pre-treatment, monthly for the first seven months and three-monthly thereafter until progression.

As may be seen, there is substantial attrition of patients, mainly due to progression of their disease. By month 13 only about 12 patients were still on protocol treatment.

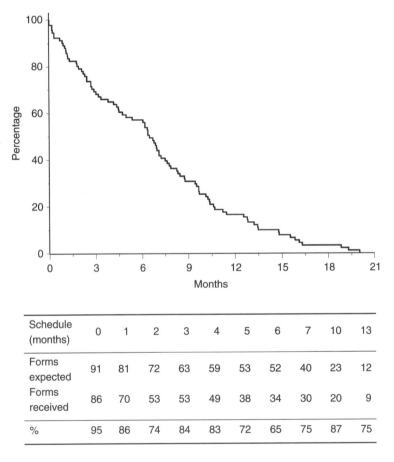

Schedule (months)	0	1	2	3	4	5	6	7	10	13
Forms expected	91	81	72	63	59	53	52	40	23	12
Forms received	86	70	53	53	49	38	34	30	20	9
%	95	86	74	84	83	72	65	75	87	75

Figure 11.1 Kaplan–Meier estimate of the time to progression for patients with metastatic breast cancer (Based on Curran *et al.*, 1998)

11.3 WHY DO MISSING DATA MATTER?

BIAS

The main cause for concern is that missing data may result in bias, and that the apparent results of a clinical trial will not reflect the true situation. That is, we will not know if the difference we observe between treatments is a truly reliable estimate of the real difference. If the proportion of anticipated data missing is small then, provided the data are analysed appropriately, we can be confident that little bias will result. However, if the proportion of data missing is not small then a key question is: "Are the characteristics of patients with missing data different from those for whom complete data are available?" For example, it might be that the more ill patients, or patients with more problems, are less willing or less able to complete the questionnaires satisfactorily. Then the missing QoL assessments (had we been able to receive them) might have indicated a poor outcome whereas those that were completed may reflect a better QoL.

Alternatively, perhaps patients without problems are less convinced about the need to return comprehensive information. In that case, the questionnaires that have been completed may reflect a worse QoL. In practice, there may be a mixture of these two possibilities within a particular trial. There may also be different patterns amongst patients receiving the different protocol treatments within one trial. Any analysis that ignores the presence of missing data may result in biased conclusions about both the changing QoL profiles over time and the between-treatment differences.

Consider a randomised clinical trial where we wish to estimate the overall QoL scores of patients at one time point and compare these between treatments. If we first consider one of the treatment groups, suppose that of the N patients recruited to that treatment $M(< N)$ fail to complete the key QoL assessment. The proportion of missing data is $P = M/N$ and the proportion of patients with complete data is therefore $1 - P$. We assume that the responding and the non-responding patients do have different mean QoL values and these are $\mu_{Responding}$ and $\mu_{NotResponding}$ respectively. The patients recruited to the trial comprise a mixture of those who ultimately do respond and those who do not. The combined mean, were we able to observe it, for all patients is

$$\mu = (1 - P)\mu_{Responding} + P\mu_{NotResponding}. \tag{11.1}$$

But here we are assuming that we do have responses from the non-responders. However, since one clearly cannot observe the non-responders, we cannot estimate μ with the QoL data recorded but only $\mu_{Responding}$. Thus the bias, B, will be

$$\begin{aligned} B &= \mu - \mu_{Responding} \\ &= (1 - P)\mu_{Responding} + P\mu_{NotResponding} - \mu_{Responding} \\ &= P(\mu_{NotResponding} - \mu_{Responding}). \end{aligned} \tag{11.2}$$

The bias will be zero if the mean scores of responders and non-responders are in fact equal. However, since the non-responders do not record their QoL we have no means of knowing if this is indeed the case. If there are no missing data, $P = 0$ and there will be no bias.

In a clinical trial comparing two treatments there will be a potential bias of the form of equation (11.2) for each treatment. The aim of a clinical trial is to estimate the difference in QoL between treatments. Thus the bias of this difference, for a trial comparing a test and control therapy, will therefore be

$$B_{Difference} = B_{Test} - B_{Control}. \qquad (11.3)$$

The treatment comparison will be unbiased only if the bias happens to be the same in both treatment arms, but again we have no means of knowing this.

There can be considerable bias in the estimated treatment difference if the proportion of missing assessments differs substantially between the treatment arms. Information regarding the reason for non-response, if known, may be useful in determining whether the analysis is biased or not. Additionally, if the probability of completing the QoL assessment is associated with patient characteristics measured at entry into the trial, such as their age, performance status or clinical stage of disease, then it may be possible to reduce the bias by adjusting for these factors. It is important to note that the bias of equation (11.2), and hence (11.3), depends upon the proportion of missing data, and not the number of observations. Bias cannot be reduced by increasing the total sample size.

Example

In the example given by Curran *et al.* (1998b), patients completed the EORTC QLQ-C30 (see Appendix E6). Physical functioning (PF) was assessed using items Q_1 to Q_5. In this study the QLQ-C30 (version 2) was used, and these items were scored 1 (No) or 2 (Yes). Thus the minimum sum-score is 5 and the maximum 10, which is then scaled to range from 0 to 100. There were 86 patients completing the first or baseline assessment. However, following recruitment, some patients dropped out before the next QoL assessment was made, and the remainder carried on until the next monthly assessment, following which others dropped out.

Figure 11.2 presents the mean PF score by time of dropout either by death or failure to complete the QoL assessment. Each profile was calculated from the patients completing all QoL assessments up to the specified number of months. As may be seen, those patients who provided information on all five PF assessments tended to have a higher baseline mean PF score than the other groups of patients. Thus there is an intrinsic bias that tends to include only the better patients into the QoL analysis at later time points. Care should therefore be taken in interpreting any graphs or tabular displays that include mean scores calculated from all the data available regarded as if all from one group, albeit comprising subjects for whom differing numbers of QoL assessments are available. The overall mean PF score, the bold broken line of Figure 11.2, rises steadily from 55.4 at baseline to 70.8 at the last assessment, suggesting an overall improvement in PF. This contrasts with the decline in PF that has occurred in, for example, those patient groups with three and four assessments in which the last observed mean PF dropped below previous levels. Since only a few patients dropped out at each month, the overall mean score is dominated by the patients who completed all five assessments.

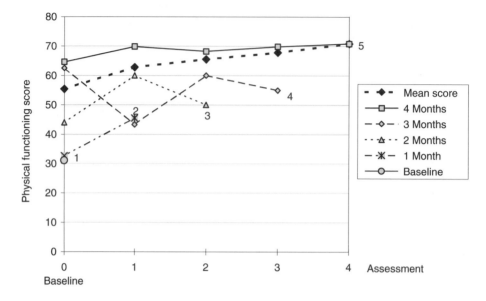

Figure 11.2 Mean physical functioning (PF) score stratified by time of dropout due to death or non-compliance in patients with metastatic breast cancer (Based on Curran *et al.*, 1998)

11.4 MISSING ITEMS

THE PROBLEM

Experience reported for a variety of clinical trials suggests that, for most single items, between 0.5% and 2.0% of values will be missing from returned questionnaires. Thus, overall, the problem of missing items might seem relatively unimportant. However, for a questionnaire that contains about 30 questions, a 1% missing rate for items would, if it occurred at random, imply that about a quarter of patients could have a missing item on their initial QoL assessment. Even a missing rate of 0.5% could result in 14% of patients with items missing. Furthermore, at each subsequent assessment there may be additional missing data and many patients are likely to have some degree of missing QoL data.

Example

A review of 7000 forms in six UK Medical Research Council randomised trials in cancer described by Fayers, Curran and Machin (1998a) indicates that 92% of forms contained complete information with regard to 29 out of the 30 questions in the first section of the RSCL. However, one question "(to what extent you have been bothered by) Decreased sexual interest" presented particular problems. The proportion of forms with missing data varied considerably from trial to trial, ranging from 4% to 14%.

Thus even when there is only a small proportion of missing values for each item, a substantial proportion of patients may have at least one or more missing items during their follow-up period. Analyses based solely upon those patients for whom complete data are available may find that the cumulative exclusion of patients results in too few patients remaining in the final analyses, and hence a severe loss of statistical power. In addition, there is a process of selection of patients into the analysis since only those with complete data are retained. The subsequent subset of patients who have complete data may not be representative of all the patients in the trial.

Analysis of the patterns of missing QoL items suggests that they do often occur at random. Thus although those patients who, perhaps through carelessness, omit answers to one question are more likely to omit answers to other questions, the reason for their so doing may be unrelated to the (unrecorded) level of the particular QoL item. Also, although missing items within forms may take the pattern of a run of adjacent questions, often the questions are unrelated, implying oversight rather than intentional omission. In both these circumstances it is reasonable to assume the data are *Missing Completely At Random* (MCAR). In formal terms, an item is MCAR if the probability of having a missing item is independent of scores on previous observed questionnaires and independent of the current and future scores had they been observed.

In contrast, as already indicated, some QoL items may present particular difficulties; for example, the question concerning "sexual interest" on the RSCL. This question is frequently unanswered. One plausible assumption is that patients experiencing problems are likely to be more reticent concerning this question, and that therefore missing items occur more frequently when there are indeed sexual problems. Thus missing might imply "very much a problem". Alternatively, for those patients who are no longer sexually active, failure to respond may imply "not applicable". In either case imputation should take this into account, as simply ignoring the presence of missing scores for these patients can result in misleading conclusions about the severity of problems. Such data are classified as *Not Missing At Random* (NMAR), because the missing data depend on the value of the unobserved scores and so the missing data mechanism cannot be ignored.

In QoL studies it is likely that there are a number of non-ignorable mechanisms responsible for NMAR data. If sufficient data are collected concerning why QoL questionnaires have not been completed, one may be able to distinguish the missing data mechanisms. In some cases it may be possible to retrieve the QoL scores of a random sample of patients by using alternative modes of administration such as telephone interview or by obtaining proxy scores from members of the patient's family or the responsible medical team. Then the reasons for missing items can be explored.

In some situations, the likelihood of having a missing score may depend on known factors and scores recorded at an earlier QoL assessment, but is independent of the current (not recorded) score. Such data are termed *Missing At Random* (MAR). An example might be age group; older people are more likely to have a higher rate of missing items, and are also likely to have poorer physical functioning scores. Within any particular age group the data are MCAR, but when considering all patients together the data are MAR because those with missing values are likely to have lower true levels of PF than those with complete data.

11.5 METHODS FOR MISSING ITEMS WITHIN A FORM

When individual items from a multi-item scale are missing there are problems in calculating scores for the summated scale. In such cases methods have been developed to impute the most likely values for these items. Such methods are no substitute for real observations but merely a device to facilitate analysis. The objective of imputation is to replace the missing data by estimated values which preserve the relationships between items, and which reflect as far as possible the most likely true value. If properly carried out, imputation should reduce the bias that can arise by ignoring non-response. By filling in the gaps in the data, it also restores balance to the data and permits simpler analyses. There are several approaches that can be used for imputation but the final choice is likely to depend on the particular context.

TREAT THE SCORE FOR THE SCALE AS MISSING

If any of the constituent items are missing, the scale-score for that patient is excluded from all statistical analysis. When data are MCAR, this reduced dataset represents a randomly drawn sub-sample of the full dataset and inferences drawn can be considered reasonable. This exclusion method is the simplest approach to the analysis, but results in overall loss of data and so loss of statistical power in the analysis since the scores based upon several items are excluded whenever even a single item is missing. Far more importantly, however, it may lead to serious bias when there is an informative reason for the item being missing.

SIMPLE MEAN IMPUTATION

For those QoL instruments that use unweighted sum-scores, the missing scale-score can be estimated from the mean of those items that are available. This process is usually restricted to cases where the respondent has completed at least half of the items in the scale.

If no items are missing, the *Raw Score* (*RS*) is calculated as the average of the items:

$$RS = \frac{\sum_{i=1}^{L} Q_i}{L} \qquad (11.4)$$

where the Q_i are the individual response to the L items in the domain. This is then transformed to the *Standardised Score* (*SS*) over the range 0 to 100 by

$$SS = \left\{ 1 - \frac{(RS - Minimum)}{(Range)} \right\} \times 100, \qquad (11.5)$$

where the *range* is the difference between the largest (*maximum*) and smallest (*minimum*) scores possible.

If no more than half the items are missing, then the *RS* is still calculated from equation (11.4) but with L replaced by the number of items available, and only the

	Not at all	A little	Quite a bit	Very much
21. Did you feel tense?	1✓	2	3	4
22. Did you worry?	1	2	3	4
23. Did you feel irritable?	1	2✓	3	4
24. Did you feel depressed?	1	2✓	3	4

Figure 11.3 The emotional functioning scale of the EORTC QLQ-C30

corresponding QoL item values actually observed in the numerator. The corresponding value of RS is then substituted directly into equation (11.5) to obtain the SS.

Example

The emotional functioning (EF) scale of the EORTC QLQ-C30 is formed by summing responses to the $L = 4$ items of Figure 11.3. These items are all on four-point scales scored from 1 to 4, and hence the *range* = 4 − 1 = 3. One patient indicated $Q_{21} = 1$, $Q_{23} = 2$ and $Q_{24} = 2$ but left Q_{22} as missing. Taking account of the missing response:

$$RS = (Q_{21} + Q_{21} + Q_{21})/3 = (1 + 2 + 2)/3 = 1.6677$$

and $SS = \{1 − (1.6667 − 1)/3\} \times 100 = 77.8$.

One disadvantage of simple mean imputation is that, as in this example, it can result in some "strange" scores, such as 77.8, that are intermediate between the scale scores calculated for patients with complete data. This can be inconvenient when tabulating summary scores against treatment or other factors.

HIERARCHICAL SCALES

Simple mean imputation is a very easy method to implement. However, there are a number of situations in which this may result in misleading values of the resulting QoL scores. For example the EORTC QLQ-C30 scale for PF is *hierarchical* in that it contains an implicit ordering of responses. Thus, if a patient replies "Yes" to Q_3 about difficulties with a short walk but does not answer Q_2, it would not be sensible to base an imputed value for this missing response on the average of all the answered items. Clearly those who have difficulty with short walks would have even greater problems with a long walk. In this case the structure of the QoL questionnaire may imply that the replies to some questions will restrict the range of plausible answers to other questions. Thus if we assume the response to "long walk" is missing but the patient responds as having difficulty with short walks, then it would seem reasonable to assume that long walks would also cause difficulty and so we would accordingly impute a value of 2. On the other hand, if the response to "short walk" is missing but the subject responds indicating no difficulty with long walks, then we may assume there is unlikely to be difficulty with short walks and would impute a value of 1.

In contrast, simple mean imputation may still be more appropriate for the other two possible situations—that is, no difficulty with short walks, but long walk missing; and difficulty with long walk with short walks missing.

REGRESSION IMPUTATION

Regression imputation replaces missing values by predicted values obtained from a regression of the missing item variable (Q_{Miss}) on the remaining items of the scale. The data used for this calculation are from all those subjects in the study with complete information on all variables within the scale. More generally, regression imputation is a modelling technique. Fairclough and Cella (1996) describe the method as follows: First estimate the relationship of the missing item to the other items in the subscale using regression and the data from other subjects. The values of the non-missing items within the scale for the subjects with the missing response are then substituted in this regression equation to predict the value of the missing item.

Example

Suppose the missing item is Q_{22} from the emotional functioning scale of Figure 11.4 but the patient completed questions Q_{21}, Q_{23} and Q_{24}. Then the corresponding multiple regression equation required is

$$Q_{22} = \beta_0 + \beta_1 Q_{21} + \beta_3 Q_{23} + \beta_4 Q_{24}, \qquad (11.6)$$

where the β_0, β_1, β_3 and β_4 are the regression coefficients. This equation is then fitted to the data obtained from those patients who have complete data on all items.

Suppose equation (11.6) has been estimated using data from the other patients, giving $Q_{22} = 0.1 + 1.1Q_{21} + 0.8Q_{23} + 0.9Q_{24}$, and that the current patient had responded with $Q_{21} = 1$, $Q_{23} = 2$ and $Q_{24} = 2$. Substituting in these values, we have the imputed value for $Q_{22} = 0.3 + (0.5 \times 1) + (0.4 \times 2) + (0.6 \times 2)$ = 2.8. In practice, this imputed value will be rounded to *3*, the nearest integer, so that finally the scale score for this patient is imputed as $1 + 3 + 2 + 2 = 8$.

Mean imputation of equation (11.4) can be regarded as a special case of regression imputation in which $\beta_0 = 0$ and, for the above example, $\beta_1 = \beta_3 = \beta_4 = 1/3$. In general, if L items in a scale are all scored with the same range and one item is missing then, apart from $\beta_0 = 0$, the remaining βs will all equal $1/(L - 1)$.

Regression imputation has the advantage that it can easily be extended to allow other predictive factors to be added to the equation—for example, age, gender or stage of disease.

SCORE DEPENDS UPON EXTERNAL VARIABLES

The value of an item may be more strongly associated with variables external to the scale—for example, clinical or demographic variables of the patient—than with other items within the scale. In this case, rather than use the associated QoL variables on the right-hand side of regression equation (11.6) it may be more appropriate to predict the missing item by using the clinical or demographic variables.

INFORMATIVE CENSORING

In situations where the fact that the item is missing may be informative, it would not be appropriate to assume that the average value (or a regression model) of the other items should be used to impute the missing score. If "missing" tends to imply that the patient has problems, the estimated score should in some way reflect this. The term "censoring" here indicates that the item is missing albeit in circumstances when it was anticipated since the QoL assessment was essentially complete except for this item. The presumption of "informative" implies that this item was deliberately skipped rather than merely overlooked. If those who have sexual problems were embarrassed and likely to skip questions about decreased interest, missing would be informative and might imply likely problems.

ITEM "NOT APPLICABLE"

It is questionable how to estimate scale scores when some constituent items are missing through not being applicable. For example, patients may return missing for Q_1 in the EORTC QLQ-C30 PF scale because they never try to perform strenuous activities. It is debatable as to how best to allow for these non-applicable items, and the decision will partly depend upon the scientific question being posed. However, in the example cited, it might be argued that if "not applicable" implies limitations in terms of PF it would be reflected by the other items in the scale, in which case regression imputation could still be appropriate.

11.6 MISSING FORMS

THE PROBLEM

Missing forms tend to be a far more serious problem than missing items. Forms are more frequently missing, and if a form is missing, so are all the constituent items on it. Forms may be essentially MCAR if, for example, the patient was inadvertently not asked to complete the QoL assessment for a reason unrelated to his or her health status. On the other hand they may be missing at critical stages depending on the relative health of the patient at the scheduled assessment time. For example, they may be missing just before death. Intermittent forms may also be missing because the patient feels too ill and so unable to complete the questionnaire, or perhaps feels so well that the assessment no longer seems relevant. Hospital staff may also avoid giving the form during a period of severe illness of the patient. Such patients may, however, complete the succeeding form as their relative health state may have changed by that time. These types of missing form will not usually be

MCAR or MAR and are termed *Missing Not At Random* (MNAR).

Randomised phase III trials in cancer patients normally require several hundreds of patients to be recruited, and thus such trials are frequently organised on a multi-centre basis. Whereas a single-centre trial may be able to assemble an enthusiastic team that is committed to assessing QoL, there may be severe problems in motivating some participants of larger multi-centre trials. This can lead to major problems in compliance. In general, multi-centre trials are the most demanding environment for conducting QoL assessments.

Examples from the literature

> Ganz *et al.* (1988) using the FLIC scale, in a study of patients with lung cancer, reported that while 87% of patients returned a baseline questionnaire, overall only 58% of expected forms were completed. Hürny *et al.* (1992), with similar patients, reported a compliance rate of about 50% when using the EORTC QLQ-C30 with a linear analogue scale (LASA) and a mood-adjective checklist (BF-S). They noted that institution, not the patients, appeared to be the major variable contributing to high or low compliance rates. Geddes *et al.* (1990), on behalf of the UK Cancer Research Campaign, reported 68% compliance again in patients with lung cancer. They opined that patients find it difficult to continue completing the assessment when they become ill with progressive disease, "and this poses a methodological problem for investigators who wish to assess effects throughout an entire treatment programme".

11.7   METHODS FOR MISSING FORMS

Statistical methods have been developed to impute the most likely values for missing data when whole QoL assessments are missing. We have shown how values may be calculated for missing items within a form, and how these methods may or may not make use of other information collected on the same form. In contrast, when a whole QoL assessment is missing the imputation procedure must use information from other "similar" patients, values from previous and/or later assessments by the same patient, or a mixture of both. We note that if items are used only as components of a scale, it may not be necessary to impute values for those items, only for the scale score itself. As with missing items, once values have been imputed for the particular missing assessments they may then be stored with the remaining data to give the appearance of a full dataset.

LAST VALUE CARRIED FORWARD

One straightforward imputation technique is the *Last Value Carried Forward* (LVCF) method. The values that were recorded by a patient at the last previously completed QoL assessment are used for items on the current (missing) QoL assessment. Thus, for example, if a patient completes the first assessment but fails to complete the second one, the patient's score from the first assessment would be used as the imputed value for the second (missing) assessment.

Example

> Curran *et al.* (1998a) describe an example in which the EORTC QLQ-C30 PF
> scale was used to assess QoL in post-orchidectomy patients with poor-
> prognosis metastatic prostate cancer. The individual items were summed and
> then transformed to range from 0 to 100. These scores were then used to define
> four categories or states, coded as 1 = Good PF (score $\geq$ 60), 2 = Poor PF
> (score < 60), 3 = Progression, and 4 = Death.
>
> A typical patient might therefore have a sequence of states as shown below:
>
> $$1 \quad 1 \quad 2 \quad 1 \quad - \quad - \quad 2 \quad 2 \quad 3 \quad 3 \quad 4.$$
>
> This patient initially has Good PF (state 1), drops temporarily to Poor (state 2),
> and then improves. There are then two missing QoL assessments, after which
> the patient is in state 2, has disease progression (state 3) and eventually dies
> (state 4). Note that once a patient enters state 3 (progression) or state 4 (death)
> the patient cannot return to one of the previous states.
>
> Using LVCF, the first missing value would be replaced by a state 1. This
> gives a still incomplete sequence, and so the LVCF method can be applied a
> second time to obtain:
>
> $$1 \quad 1 \quad 2 \quad 1 \quad \mathit{1} \quad \mathit{1} \quad 2 \quad 2 \quad 3 \quad 3 \quad 4$$

A key disadvantage of the LVCF method is that it assumes the patient's score
remains essentially constant over time. In the above example, we may be reasonably
confident of the imputed value for the first missing state but perhaps not so certain
of the second imputation, as that (missing) assessment was followed by a worsening
state 2. An imputation method that took account of what *follows* might have
imputed 2 here rather than 1.

It should be noted that had the second incidence of state 3 been missing in the
above sequence, then if the patient were known to be alive at that time, the only
possible option for the LVCF or any other method would be 3. Rarely will such
certainty regarding the true value be justified.

SIMPLE MEAN IMPUTATION

In the context of a missing form, simple mean imputation is usually the replacement
of missing QoL scores by the mean score calculated from those patients who did
complete the QoL assessment.

Example

> At a particular assessment time the mean QoL score (on a scale 0 to 100) was
> $\bar{Q} = 20$ for those patients who were assessed. Thus for those patients for
> whom the assessment is missing, the corresponding score will be imputed as
> $Q = \bar{Q} = 20$.

A feature of mean imputation is that the estimate of the mean of the augmented dataset remains the same as the mean $\bar{Q}$ that was calculated for the original non-missing data. In contrast, the estimate of the SD will be reduced artificially as the imputed values are all placed at the centre (mean) of the distribution. This can lead to distorted significance tests and falsely narrow CIs. However, the SD can be corrected by two equivalent methods.

If there are N patients for QoL assessment of whom M have missing values, the mean $\bar{Q}_{N-M}$ from the $N - M$ patients with QoL observations is used for imputation. Then either the SD of the $N - M$ non-missing values is retained and used, or the SD of the now complete set of observations is corrected by multiplying by f, where

$$f = \sqrt{\frac{N - 1}{N - M - 1}}. \tag{11.7}$$

Example

> At the time of a particular QoL assessment there were $N = 10$ patients, but two of these failed to complete the assessment. The eight observed and ordered QoL values were 1, 1, 2, 2, 2, 2, 3, and 3, with mean = 2.0 and SD = 0.7559.
>
> The $M = 2$ missing values are both imputed as $\bar{Q} = 2.0$, giving the full ordered dataset of 1, 1, 2, 2, *2*, *2*, 2, 2, 3, 3. The mean of the resulting ten values remains as 2, but the corresponding SD is reduced to 0.6667. However, $f = \sqrt{(10 - 1)/(10 - 2 - 1)} = 1.1339$ and the adjusted SD = $1.1339 \times 0.6667 = 0.7560$. This also equals the SD of the eight observed values.

As we have indicated, the two methods are equivalent. In some situations, particularly if the dataset is large, it is easiest to add the imputed values to the data file merely to facilitate analysis by standard computer packages. Then the adjustment method may be the most convenient to apply. It is also important to note that the correlation between different scores (or items) may be affected by the imputation. Imputing a missing value by the corresponding mean value of the remainder of the data will tend to reduce the size of the observed correlation coefficient if the calculation is carried out on the augmented dataset.

The simple mean imputation method that we have described here uses the full dataset from all available patients, but a modification is to take only the mean score of a subset of patients. Patients with similar characteristics to the patient with the missing data would be chosen. The presumption here is that matched patients will behave in a similar way.

HORIZONTAL MEAN IMPUTATION

Unlike the LVCF method, mean imputation takes no account of the longitudinal nature of QoL data. Thus an alternative to simple mean imputation is to impute the missing value from the mean of the patient's own previous scores. This method is termed *horizontal* as it takes into account the longitudinal nature of the QoL data. It reduces to the LVCF method if there is only one previous assessment available or if there has been no change in QoL score over the assessments to date.

Example

> For the sequence 1, 1, 2, 1, –, –, 2, 2, 3, 3, 4 discussed previously, horizontal mean imputation would give 1, 1, 2, 1, *1.25*, *1.25*, 2, 2, 3, 3. Here 1.25 is the mean of the first four item values in the sequence. In practice these values could be rounded to the nearest integer before being added to the augmented dataset.

Horizontal mean imputation is not recommended if there is evidence of a systematic decline or fall in patient QoL scores over time.

Example

> For the sequence 1, 1, 1, 1, 2, 2, 2, 2, 3, –, 4, horizontal mean imputation would result in 1, 1, 1, 1, 2, 2, 2, 2, 3, *1.67*, 4. Here *1.67* (rounded to 2 before addition to the dataset) is the mean of the first nine item values in the sequence. This is clearly not a good estimate in this situation.

STANDARDISED SCORE IMPUTATION

This method adjusts for any shift or trend in the general levels of QoL in the patient population over time. Suppose there are only two assessments and all N patients complete the first assessment but one patient fails to complete the second. Also, suppose that at the first assessment this patient scored Q_1 and the overall mean and SD for the N patients were $\bar{Q}_1$ and SD_1. Then the standardised value for this first observation is given by

$$Z_1 = (Q_1 - \bar{Q}_1)/SD_1.$$

If this patient's score were exactly equal to the mean, Z_1 would be 0, whereas if the score were exactly one SD above the mean, Z_1 would equal +1.

Now suppose the corresponding values of the mean and SD at the second QoL assessment obtained from $N - 1$ patients are $\bar{Q}_2$ and SD_2. If we denote the missing value as Q_2, we can use the standardised value Z_1 from the first QoL assessment to impute the missing value as follows. The method assumes the patient would have the same standardised score at this second assessment (had it been completed) as he or she had at the first; that is:

$$(Q_2 - \bar{Q}_2)/SD_2 = Z_1.$$

This equation can be rearranged to give the imputed missing value as

$$Q_2 = \bar{Q}_2 + Z_1 SD_2. \tag{11.8}$$

Although the method assumes that the standardised score for the missing assessment will be the same as that of the preceding assessment, the mean levels, $\bar{Q}_1$ and $\bar{Q}_2$, at the two assessments may be quite different.

Example

> For the first QoL assessment, the mean and *SD* for a particular domain on the scale 0 to 100 were 30 and 15 respectively. One patient who scored 21 on the first assessment failed to complete the second assessment, but the mean and *SD* of the remainder who did were 34 and 14 respectively.
>
> Here $\bar{Q}_1 = 30$, $SD_1 = 15$, $\bar{Q}_2 = 34$ and $SD_2 = 14$. Thus the mean QoL score has increased, perhaps suggesting a general improvement in QoL over time. From the first assessment of the patient who did not complete the second QoL assessment, $Q_1 = 21$ and $Z_1 = (21 - 30)/15 = -0.6$. This suggests that this patient tends to score beneath the mean compared with other patients. Since Q_2 is missing, it is estimated from equation (11.8) by $Q_2 = 34 + (-0.6 \times 14) = 25.6$, which is approximately 26 whereas the LVCF is 21.

This method assumes that the patients' scores for this assessment form an approximately Normal distribution. This may not be true for all scores obtained from a QoL assessment.

MARKOV CHAIN IMPUTATION

In the methods described so far, the imputed values will be the same for any two patients with the same profile of successive non-missing values. Such methods are termed *deterministic*. Another approach to imputation is to use the concept of a so-called Markov chain. This reflects the possibility that the two patients with missing assessments may have differing QoL profiles had they been recorded. This method assigns, for a patient in a particular QoL state at one assessment, probabilities of being in each of the possible states, including the same, at the next assessment. These probabilities are termed "transition probabilities" and are often described in percentage terms.

Example

> In the prostate cancer example described earlier (see page 237), suppose that at one QoL assessment there are 100 patients in state 1 and that at the next assessment 65 of these remain in state 1. Of the remaining patients, 20 move to state 2, 12 to state 3 and 3 to state 4. The corresponding transition probabilities are 65/100 = 0.65, 20/100 = 0.20, 12/100 = 0.12 and 3/100 = 0.03, or 65%, 20%, 12% and 3% respectively.

Example

> In fact the observed transition probabilities for the prostate cancer trial are shown in Table 11.1. These were constructed from all the data available from QoL assessments four, five and six combined together. This table is referred to as a *matrix of transition probabilities*. Thus at this stage of the trial a patient with Good PF has a transition probability of 76% for remaining in the same

state, whereas the transition probability for Progression is 12.6%. For a patient already in Progression, the probability of remaining in that state is 91.4% and the transition probability of Death of 8.6%. These probabilities can be used to impute missing QoL data.

Table 11.1   Transition probabilities between states (Based on Curran *et al.*, 1998a)

| | Resultant state | | | |
	1 = Good PF	2 = Bad PF	3 = Progression	4 = Death
Initial state				
1 = Good PF	76.0	11.4	12.6	0.0
2 = Bad PF	11.1	75.0	13.9	0.0
3 = Progression			91.4	8.6
4 = Death				100.0

Example

In the patient sequence given above, the fifth and sixth QoL assessments were missing:

$$1 \quad 1 \quad 2 \quad 1 \quad - \quad - \quad 2 \quad 2 \quad 3 \quad 3 \quad 4.$$

The state observed immediately before the first missing QoL value was 1. Taking into account the fact that the patient was in state 2 at the next observed value, we know that the missing states must be replaced by either a 1 or a 2 since a patient cannot return to state 2 from either Progression or Death. Thus the only possible transitions from the fifth to the sixth QoL assessment are, from Table 11.1, $1 \rightarrow 1$ (76.0%) and $1 \rightarrow 2$ (11.4%). However, these transition probabilities total 87.4% rather than 100%. Therefore we divide each of the two possible transition probabilities by 87.4 to obtain: 76.0/87.4 = 0.87 or 87% and 11.4/87.4 = 0.13 or 13%.

To impute the missing values, we make use of these transition probabilities together with a table of random numbers or a computer random number generator, giving random numbers from 0 to 100. If the random number so generated is less than or equal to 87 we impute for the missing QoL state as state 1, otherwise we impute state 2.

Example

Suppose the first random number is 10, which is ≤ 87. Then state 1 is imputed, giving:

$$1 \quad 1 \quad 2 \quad 1 \quad \textit{1} \quad - \quad 2 \quad 2 \quad 3 \quad 3 \quad 4.$$

Since the fifth assessment was imputed as state 1, the transition probabilities for the sixth assessment remain as 87% and 13%. Thus to complete the sequence the same procedure is followed. If the second random number is 68 and is thus ≤ 87, state 1 is again imputed and we have:

$$1 \quad 1 \quad 2 \quad 1 \quad \textit{1} \quad \textit{1} \quad 2 \quad 2 \quad 3 \quad 3 \quad 4.$$

This is the same sequence that was generated using the LVCF method. However, this need not have been the case necessarily had other random numbers been drawn. Thus all the alternatives to *1 1* are possible; that is, *1 2, 2 1* and *2 2*. As a consequence, a second patient with exactly the same QoL profile may have a randomly different missing sequence imputed.

In the method just described we used the knowledge that the missing values could not have been either state 3 or state 4. Thus we restricted our transition matrix accordingly. We have therefore improved the imputation process by taking into account the specific value of the observation following the missing values.

If there are more than one successive missing items, an alternative method of imputation is to calculate probabilities for the possible sequences that may be imputed for the missing sequence. The sequence chosen to impute the missing sequence is itself chosen at random in proportion to the corresponding probability.

Example

In the incomplete patient sequence given above, the last value before the missing value was state 1 and the first value after the missing sequence was state 2. The four possible intermittent sequences of 1 1, 1 2, 2 1 and 2 2 for the missing values are given in Table 11.2, with the associated transition probabilities. The probability of each sequence occurring is then calculated by multiplying the corresponding transition probabilities. Thus for first sequence– that is, *1 1* (moving from state 1 to 1, then 1 again, and ending in 2)—the probability is: $0.870 \times 0.870 \times 0.130 = 0.098$. Once the probabilities for all possible sequences are calculated they are then adjusted to ensure that they sum to 1 or 100%. Thus the adjusted probability for the first sequence is $0.098/(0.098 + 0.099 + 0.002 + 0.099) = 0.329$. Finally to facilitate the choice of sequence using random numbers, the cumulative probability is then calculated by adding the probabilities of the individual sequences.

Using random number tables, we select a number from 000 to 999. If this number is in the range from 001 to 329, sequence 1 1 is imputed. Similarly, if from 330 to 661, the sequence is 1 2; if from 662 to 668, the sequence is 2 1; and if from 669 to 999 or equal to 000, the sequence 2 2 is chosen.

Suppose the random number generator gave 831. This is in the range 669 to 999 and so 2 2 is chosen for the imputation, giving the complete sequence of states for the patient as:

$$1 \quad 1 \quad 2 \quad 1 \quad \textit{2} \quad \textit{2} \quad 2 \quad 2 \quad 3 \quad 3 \quad 4.$$

There are several difficulties with this approach. One is its complexity compared with methods such as LVCF. A second difficulty is the assumption about the

Table 11.2 Probabilities of sequences for imputation (Based on Curran *et al.*, 1998a)

Possible sequence	All possible sequences with associated transition probabilities						Probability	Adjusted probability	Cumulative probability (%)
1 1	0.870*	**1**	0.870	**1**	0.130	**2**	0.098	0.329	32.9
1 2	0.870	**1**	0.130	**2**	0.871*	**2**	0.099	0.332	66.1
2 1	0.130	**2**	0.129*	**1**	0.130	**2**	0.002	0.007	66.8
2 1	0.130	**2**	0.871	**2**	0.871	**2**	0.099	0.332	100.0

* From Table 11.1: 76.0/(76.0 + 11.4) = 0.870 and 11.4/(76.0 + 11.3) = 0.130.

relative stability of transition probabilities over time. In our example, Table 11.1 was calculated using only information from QoL assessments four, five and six. It was judged that the transition probabilities would be stable over this period. However, perhaps probabilities are different for the first three assessments or from the seventh assessment onwards. It is difficult to make decisions about the stability of the transition probabilities over time. Another problem is that scales often have larger numbers of categories, leading to many cells in the corresponding table of transition probabilities. Consequently, these probabilities may be based upon relatively few observed patients and may be unreliable, making their use for imputation problematic.

However, an important advantage of this method over the deterministic LVCF or mean imputation methods is that the variability of the data is preserved in the augmented dataset, and hence the value of the *SD* is maintained.

HOT DECK IMPUTATION

Hot deck (a pack of playing cards) imputation selects at random, from patients with observed QoL data, the QoL score from one of these and substitutes this as the imputed value for the patient with the missing QoL assessment. The hot deck literally refers to the deck (here computer file) of responses of patients with observed data from which the missing QoL score is selected. The particular deck chosen may be restricted to those patients that, in some way, are "similar" to the patient with the missing QoL score.

Example

Curran *et al.* (1998a) indicate that in patients with prostate cancer the baseline WHO performance status (PS) affects the probability of being in a subsequent QoL state. Thus in Table 11.3, 73.3% of patients with PS = 0 at baseline were state 1 (Good PF), but this was so for only 20.0% for those with PS = 2.

To impute a missing value using information about the baseline PS, we first identify the corresponding "deck" of patients. Thus if a patient with a missing baseline QoL value has PS = 0, the deck consists of patients with this PS. Table 11.3 shows that, for this deck, state 1 (Good PF) would be imputed with probability 0.733 and state 2 (Bad PF) with probability 0.267. On the other hand if the deck is PS = 1, states 1 and 2 would be imputed with probabilities

0.476 and 0.524 respectively. Finally, if the deck is PS = 2, states 1 and 2 would be imputed with probabilities 0.200 and 0.800 respectively. Although the possible imputed values (states 1 or 2) remain the same for all patients with missing assessments, the probabilities attached to the (two) alternatives within the deck are varied according to baseline PS values. Thus the three PS decks considered here all consist of two types of "cards", Good or Bad PF, but these are present in the three decks in differing proportions.

Table 11.3 Probabilities for hot deck imputation (Based on Curran *et al.*, 1998a)

WHO performance status	1 = Good PF	2 = Bad PF
0	73.3	26.7
1	47.6	52.4
2	20.0	80.0

Curran *et al.* (1998a) describe how this method can be extended to more complex situations with differing imputation probabilities assigned taking into account WHO performance status, treatment group and initial pain levels.

COLD DECK IMPUTATION

Cold deck imputation refers to replacing a missing value of a QoL item or score by a constant value from an external source, such as a value from a previous study. This may be the value observed in a patient with very similar demographic and disease characteristics undergoing similar treatment in the same centre as the index case. Such a device is unlikely to be of practical utility in a clinical trial context.

EM ALGORITHM

When the missing values arise through a known censoring mechanism, the so-called *EM algorithm* can be used to impute missing values. (The E stands for expectation and M for maximum likelihood, but these details need not concern us.) The EM algorithm is particularly useful when many patients have missing forms at different assessment points, because then there may be few patients with complete data from whom we are able derive hot decks or transition probabilities.

To apply the EM algorithm, first, we need to decide upon an imputation method for estimating the missing items. This could be one of the methods described above, or could be multiple regression as described for missing items. If using regression models, we can of course include various factors that are expected to be predictive of the QoL outcomes; for example, age, gender, stage of disease. Let us assume we decide to use regression and have developed a regression model. The procedure of the EM algorithm is:

1. Replace all missing values with the estimates that are predicted from the regression.

2. With the new dataset, recalculate the parameters of the regression equation.
3. Now repeat from (1), using the revised regression equation as just calculated in (2).

This iterative procedure is continued until the values "put back" do not differ from those just "taken out". The process is then deemed to have converged.

When using regression methods, the EM algorithm will usually converge after only a few cycles. When there is much missing data, the resultant estimates will be far more reliable than if a simple (non-iterative) regression approach were used.

MULTIPLE IMPUTATION

It is clear that there are several options for the methods of imputation chosen. If deterministic methods such as LVCF are used then the augmented dataset will be unique. In contrast, if a random element is included in the choice of missing values, the resultant augmented dataset will be just a single random one out of many potential datasets. We can then use this dataset for analysis—for example, we might perhaps carry out a *t*-test or estimate *CI*s for a treatment comparison.

The idea of multiple imputation is that many alternative "complete" datasets can be created instead of just one. The analysis (*t*-tests, or whatever) can be repeated for each dataset. Common practice suggests that five repetitions should suffice. Rubin (1987) has given some rules for combining the separate analyses into a final summary analysis.

Multiple imputation is a powerful technique, and overcomes the disadvantages associated with both deterministic methods (such as underestimated *SD*s, *CI*s and correlations) and Markov or hot deck models (the randomly chosen values may be randomly atypical). It also allows "sensitivity" analyses, in which the stability of the imputation methods is examined against their impact upon the analyses.

11.8 COMMENTS

One possibility is not to impute any values at all and resort to either complete case or available case analysis. There are clearly difficulties associated with such an approach. For example, in the analysis of the breast cancer data of Figure 11.2, if we include only the 52 patients for whom up to five assessments are available we may be seriously misled. We might incorrectly conclude that the overall mean was 64.6 at baseline and that by the assessment at four months the mean QoL score has risen by 6.2 to 70.8. As can be seen from Figure 11.2, this method of analysis considerably overestimates the mean QoL score at all but the final assessment time points. Fairclough and Cella (1996) similarly conclude, from a comparison of alternative methods of imputing missing values, that case-wise deletion results in significant bias.

A major advantage of imputing missing values is that, once the values have been filled in, standard methods of analysis can be used (with some provisos). The dataset becomes an "augmented" dataset comprising the observed values and the imputed values. It can not be regarded as the same as if it consists only of complete real data.

Otherwise this can cause problems since, although summary statistics such as the mean and median may not be distorted, the corresponding *SD*s may be affected with knock-on consequences for the associated confidence intervals (*CI*). Even if the *SD* remains unaffected or is adjusted as we have described earlier, these *CI*s still have to take account of the corresponding degrees of freedom (*df*). A cautious approach to calculating the degree of freedom when there are missing data is to reduce the *df* by 1 for every patient with missing values for the variable under consideration. Thus suppose that there are *N* patients recruited to each of two treatment groups in a clinical trial and QoL information is available from all but *M* patients. Then if the *CI* of the difference in mean QoL between treatments is required, the degrees of freedom will be reduced from $2N - 1$ to $(2N - 1) - M$; that is, $2N - M - 1$ will be used to obtain the value of *t* from statistical tables, which will be then used in the calculation of the correct *CI*.

However, if this method is applied when there are single items missing within a scale and the scale score has been imputed, the final *df* may be too small as it is reduced by 1 for every such item. A possible compromise in this situation is to reduce the *df* by a fraction for every observation missing. For example, if an *L*-item scale is calculated for a particular patient but one item is missing, then *df* can be reduced by $1/L$. These fractions are then summed over all the *M* patients with missing data items to obtain

$$df = (2N - 1) - \frac{M}{L},$$

and this is rounded down to the nearest integer.

11.9   CONCLUSIONS

Many investigators are suspicious about using imputation techniques, because of the assumptions that are overtly involved. However, it should be remembered that *not* imputing missing data also involves making assumptions – namely, that the patients failing to respond are similar to those study patients for whom data have been recorded. One difference between imputing or not imputing is simply that the assumptions are explicit for the former and implicit for the latter. Thus, for example, if patients with poor baseline performance status tend to have follow-up QoL assessments missing, it is presumably better to make use of this baseline characteristic by imputing values than to (implicitly) assume that these patients are likely to be similar on average to the other patients in the study, many of whom are known to have a high performance status. Imputation tries to use the available information, so as to make better allowance for patients with missing data.

Of the imputation techniques described, the Markov chain imputation method and the hot deck imputation method seem the most efficient, as they take additional patient information into account in the imputation process, and they preserve the magnitude of the *SD*s, ensuring that the *CI*s can be correctly estimated. They also allow the user's prior knowledge and experience to be incorporated into the imputation process. In contrast, some approaches to non-response require new and specialised computer programs in order to handle the problem of missing data. One should caution against the use of very sophisticated mathematical techniques, as the processes utilised may not be readily understood.

An intrinsic difficulty, especially when there is a large amount of missing data, whether missing forms or items, is the final choice of imputation method. The best method may be specific to the individual missing items or scales concerned as well as the particular assessment sequence. In many QoL questionnaires there are so many items that to tailor the imputation for each component may not be practical. In any event it is probably important, at least in most circumstances, to decide the method of imputation in advance of examining the data. Previous experience with similar data will often guide the choice of method. Of particular concern are those few QoL items and scales that have been selected as the major endpoints for the study concerned. These should be the major focus for determining the imputation process. Secondary QoL endpoints may perhaps be imputed using the less sophisticated approaches. It is important to emphasise that estimating missing values is an extra burden on the analyst and therefore consumes resources, some of which may be better deployed by giving greater attention to patient compliance at an earlier stage in the study process. Sophisticated imputation methods are merely devices for facilitating the final analysis. They are no substitute for the real data.

12 Quality-adjusted Survival

Summary

The overall survival time following diagnosis in a patient with a life-threatening disease may be considered as partitioned into distinct periods during which the QoL levels of the patient may expect to differ. These states may include, for example, the active treatment period. Once the time in each of these states is determined, they can be used to calculate the *time without symptoms and toxicity* (TWiST); the time actually experiencing symptoms and/or toxicity (TOX): and the time in relapse following progression of the disease (PROG).

Utility coefficients (once defined) corresponding to each of these states can be used as multipliers of TOX, TWiST and PROG to obtain a weighted *quality-adjusted time without symptoms and toxicity* (Q-TWiST). These are then averaged over all patients receiving a particular treatment and so can be used to compare treatments.

Threshold analysis enables the investigation of how sensitive the difference in treatments so quantified is on the values of the utility coefficients of each state. The way in which Q-TWiST may be compared between different prognostic groups, and changes over successive time intervals from diagnosis, are described.

12.1 INTRODUCTION

The measures described so far in this book are sometimes called *profile* instruments because they provide a descriptive profile as to how each patient is feeling. This information may be used to describe groups of patients, as we have seen, or may be used for comparative purposes in a clinical trial. Thus it can be used by clinicians when deciding whether one treatment results in, on average, better or worse QoL and whether this should result in wider use of that treatment or even preclude its use altogether. Although the summary scores may seem at first sight difficult to interpret, Chapter 16 examines ways in which these scores may be interpreted clinically. The QoL profiles also provide a source of information about the possible consequences of therapy, and this information can be discussed with patients when deciding which treatment may be the most suitable. Thus, clinicians can contrast the potential therapeutic benefits against possible impact upon QoL, and this can be used as the basis for patient decisions when choosing between alternative treatments.

However, for some decision purposes it is desirable to weigh up the therapeutic benefits and contrast them more formally against the changes in QoL. Specifically, if the more efficacious therapy is associated with poorer QoL outcomes, is it worthwhile? Just as QoL can be assessed only by the patients themselves, so the value judgement of treatment preference should similarly be determined by asking the patients. Various methods are available for determining patient preference ratings, some of which aim to combine QoL and survival duration into a single summary score that may be broadly summarised as equating actual years of survival to the (smaller) number of equivalent healthy years. The aim of this is to enable overall benefits of various treatment or management policies to be contrasted.

12.2 PREFERENCES AND UTILITIES

When the outcomes are known in advance, patients can express a *preference* for one treatment or another. For example, if it can be stated that treatment will result in cure but at the cost of specified QoL disadvantages, patients can decide whether or not to accept the treatment. However, in most clinical situations there will be uncertainty regarding both the cure and the QoL outcomes. Usually we can state only that there is a certain probability of cure, and that this may be gained at possible QoL disadvantages. When preferences are assessed in the face of uncertainty they are called *utilities*, because a patient might make one selection under uncertainty but might express a different preference if it were known what outcome would ensue.

VISUAL ANALOGUE RATING SCALES (VAS)

The simplest form of establishing preference ratings is by means of a *visual analogue rating scale*, in which the extreme anchors are usually "best possible QoL" and "worst possible QoL", or some equivalent wording. The patient is then asked to indicate on the 10-cm line the position of their current state, and also to mark positions corresponding to various scenarios such as their likely condition during or following therapy. For the least favourable state, "death" is often avoided because some patients may declare particular states of health to be worse than death; thus for alternative wording one might consider "worst imaginable state of health".

This method has been found to be efficient and easy to use, and appears to provide meaningful values for relative preferences of various states of health and treatment. It can be extended to include the concept of uncertainty, thereby providing utilities, if the scenarios include suitably phrased descriptions that indicate a risk of side-effects or disease progression; in this case, extra care is needed in choosing appropriately worded endpoints for the scale.

TIME TRADE-OFF (TTO)

Time trade-off involves comparing QoL against length of survival. A typical strategy for evaluating TTO is to present a scenario under which health is impaired by specific disabilities or symptoms, and to ask the patient whether he or she would choose one year in perfect health or one year with impaired health; presumably, the healthy year would be selected. Then the duration of the healthy period is gradually reduced: "Would you choose 11 months in perfect health, or one year with impaired health?", and so on. At some stage equilibrium should be reached, and it may then be concluded that the value of impaired life is equivalent to a certain percentage of time relative to healthy life.

As we shall see, TTO is conceptually equivalent to the QALY approach (see Section 12.5), and might therefore seem attractive. Since it does not involve uncertainty, it is a method for eliciting patient *preferences*. However, many patients find the concepts difficult to apply.

STANDARD GAMBLE (SG)

The *standard gamble* method involves decisions in the face of uncertainty, where the uncertainty involves a risk of death or some other outcome. Thus SG attempts to estimate patient *utilities*.

For example, SG might be used to establish the value of anti-hypertensive therapy by offering the following alternatives to patients: "Suppose there is a $P\%$ chance of death within the following year if you do not take anti-hypertensive therapy, but on the other hand you would have to take therapy for the rest of your life and it has these side-effects. . . ." By varying the percentage, P, the point of indifference can be established. The value $(1 - P)$ then provides the utility value for impairment due to this form of therapy.

As for TTO, many patients find the concepts of SG unrealistic and have difficulty in making consistent responses. One particular problem is that it is frequently difficult to provide realistic scenarios for some of the medical conditions and therapies that are under consideration.

Example from the literature

De Haes and Stiggelbout (1996) compared VAS, TTO and SG methods in 30 testicular cancer patients. In line with other reports, the VAS method yielded the lowest scores, and TTO was slightly lower than SG. The authors noted that since many patients are reluctant to trade survival for QoL, and are willing to accept high levels of toxicity for a relatively modest increase in survival time, it is perhaps not unexpected that TTO results in higher scores than VAS. Similarly, SG patients are asked to consider the possibility of immediate death, which is even less acceptable to many. De Haes and Stiggelbout suggest that the choice between the three methods might be made according to the disease and the intended application of the ratings; for example, in a surgical trial that involves a risk of early death, the SG approach might be preferred.

WILLINGNESS TO PAY (WTP)

Whereas SG involves a gamble and the element of risk when comparing the value of different health states, and TTO uses varying time periods, *willingness to pay* introduces the concept of monetary value. The foundation for this is that people are accustomed to making decisions about how much they are willing to spend upon most things relating to life—from small items such as food and clothing, and medium-cost decisions such as annual holidays, through to major expenses including car and house. The amount that an individual is willing to pay is an indicator of the utility or satisfaction that they expect to gain from the particular commodity.

Various methods have been used to elicit WTP values, including basic questions such as "What is the most that you would be willing to pay for . . .". A variation on this is to present a list of options or a set of cards containing "bids" of increasing amounts, from which the respondent selects the amount they would be willing to pay.

WTP has rarely been used in QoL research.

CONJOINT ANALYSIS (CA)

A newer technique for assessing preferences of health states is *conjoint analysis*, which has been used extensively in market research and transport economics. CA involves constructing a number of realistic scenarios that represent combinations of different health states (item levels). Obviously there are too many possible states to be able to present them all (see Section 12.3), and so particular scenarios must be selected. The patient is then presented with two or more of the scenarios, and asked to rank them, rate them or indicate their preferred option. Since the majority of people are accustomed to making what are effectively pairwise comparisons and decisions on a daily basis, Ryan (1999) has argued that this may be the preferred approach for CA.

The resultant data consist of binary preferences, and must therefore be analysed using logistic (or the related probit) regression models; some of the models are complex, requiring specialised software for their fitting (Ryan, 1999).

12.3 MULTI-ATTRIBUTE UTILITY MEASURES

Having assessed patient preferences or utilities for individual items, for example by using rating scales, SG or TTO, there remains the issue of how to combine them. Some schemes use utilities as a form of item weighting for forming a summary index. However, there are few grounds for assuming that a patient with vomiting, pain and headaches should score the same as the sum of the three individual utility scores. *Multi-attribute theory* is a method for investigating the utilities associated with health states represented by a combination of item-scores.

If an instrument has, say, three 5-point scales, there are a total of $5^3 = 125$ possible combinations of scores. Each such combination is called a *state*, and for example a score of 4 on the first scale, 3 on the second, 4 on the third could be written as the state (4,3,4). Ideally, preferences or utilities should be established for each of these states, but for many instruments this would not be feasible—an instrument with as few as six 5-point dimensions would result in 15 625 states and the SF36, for example, has millions of possible combinations. This has led to some utility-based instruments being deliberately brief; the EuroQoL has five dimensions that result in a total of 243 states. Of course, it is also possible to base the assessment of patients upon a single global item, in which case all that is required are the utilities corresponding to each level of the global item. For longer instruments, there are a number of possible strategies. If it is thought reasonable to regard the dimensions as independent, only the "marginal" utilities are required and so each dimension can be studied separately when investigating the utilities. A multiplicative model is frequently used to combine "disutility" dimensions, where disutility is (1 – utility). The rationale for this is that symptoms or other deteriorations are likely to have the greatest impact if they are the first and only problem, and will reduce overall QoL to a lesser degree if they are but one of many problems. Equally, an improvement in a single area will not be sufficient to restore good QoL if there are many other problems. For example, with a three-dimension instrument, if a score of, say, 4 on the first dimension d_1 has utility $u_{d1}(4)$, a score 3 on dimension d_2 has utility $u_{d2}(3)$, and 4 on dimension d_3 has utility $u_{d3}(4)$, then

$$\text{Utility of } (d_1 = 4, d_2 = 3, d_3 = 4) = U(4,3,4)$$
$$= 1 - [1 - u_{d1}(4)] \times [1 - u_{d2}(3)] \times [1 - u_{d3}(4)].$$

More complex schemes are available for rendering manageable the task of assessing multi-state utilities, including for example those involving a combination of the marginal and "corner" state utilities such as (for scales from 1 to 4), $U(1,1,1)$, $U(1,1,1,4)$, $U(1,1,4,1)$ etc.

12.4   UTILITY-BASED INSTRUMENTS

Some QoL instruments have been designed explicitly with preference or utility methods in mind. The Quality of WellBeing scale (QWB) of Kaplan, Buck and Berry (1979) combines preference values with scale-scores for mobility, physical activity, social activity and symptoms. The preference values were obtained by using rating scales to assess each possible state on a VAS scale from 0 to 1, and were obtained from the general community. The resultant scores range from 0, death, to 1, full functioning without adverse symptoms. It has been suggested that, since this instrument is sometimes used for resource allocation, the preferences of the payers—the community—are more relevant than those of the patient. In any event, it is also often claimed that community-expressed preferences are usually not too dissimilar from patient opinions. The QWB was used extensively by the Oregon Health Services Commission in the USA, and in 1990 a priority list was produced based upon the rank-ordering of services according to cost-utility.

The Health Utilities Index (HUI) as described by Feeny *et al.* (1995), on the other hand, used patient-generated utilities, derived from TTO and SG methods. The HUI version III measures emotion, cognition, pain, dexterity, vision, speech, hearing and ambulation, each on five- or six-category scales.

Example from the literature

The HUI was used in the 1991 population health survey in Canada. Feeny *et al.* (1995) reported that 75% of the 11 567 participants were in the 12 most common states, with 30% reporting "perfect health".

Preference scores are available for the HUI, and it has been used to develop a population health index, comparing the health of different subgroups and monitoring changes over time.

The EuroQoL EQ-5D, with five dimensions each with three categorical levels, is a brief instrument intended for use in economic evaluation. However, this still results in a total of 243 health states, and so the designers decided to focus on 13 of the most commonly occurring states, covering a broad range of health conditions.

Example from the literature

Brooks *et al.* (1996) report the valuations for the 13 "common core" states of the EuroQoL EQ-5D, using VAS, TTO and SG. Although the three methods resulted in very different scores, the ranking of the health states was broadly similar.

12.5 QUALITY-ADJUSTED LIFE YEARS (QALYs)

Having established values for preference ratings or utilities, the next stage is to attempt to combine them with the patient's likely duration in each condition. *Quality-adjusted life years* (QALYs) allow for varying times spent in different states by calculating an overall score for each patient. In broad terms, if the state of health during disease or treatment has been assigned a utility of 60%, then one year spent in this state is considered equivalent to 0.6 of a year in perfect heath. Thus if a patient progresses through four states that have estimated utilities of U_1, U_2, U_3, U_4, spending time T in each state, we have:

$$\text{QALY} = U_1 T_1 + U_2 T_2 + U_3 T_3 + U_4 T_4. \tag{12.1}$$

This is analogous to the "area under the curve" (AUC) discussed in Chapter 9, but using utility values instead of scale scores. QALYs can be calculated for various medical conditions; and although the scores may be difficult to interpret in any absolute terms, they provide relative rankings for alternative states and treatments in different disease areas.

Since QALYs explicitly make use of patient-derived utilities when combining scales and when incorporating the survival, it is arguable that they are a more realistic method for deriving summary indexes of QoL than the more naïve summation across dimensions and AUC calculations. However, whether or not it is meaningful to combine such disparate dimensions as QoL and survival into a single number must remain debatable. Even more controversial is the use of QALYs in health-economic analysis, when the third dimension of cost is included, although this is clearly a convenient procedure for policy-making. Thus Fayers and Hand (1997b) point to the logical difficulties of declaring one treatment to be "better" than another when there are gains in some dimensions that are offset by losses in others; the comparison depends heavily upon the trade-off across dimensions, and different people will have different opinions about the relative values and these opinions will change over time, according to circumstances, contexts and experiences. Patients have different priorities from others, and community-averaged opinions may reflect only the views of a few central individuals. All the implicit assumptions regarding value judgements can too easily become obscured, or conveniently disguised, when only a single summary index such as cost per QALY is cited and presented in a league-table.

ASSUMPTIONS OF QALYs

The value of QALYs is that they provide a common unit that can be compared across different disease areas and treatment groups. However, this is at the expense of a number of assumptions.

Utility independence is the assumption that individuals value length of life in a health state independently of the value of that health state. For example, if one were indifferent to the choice between two years with severe pain and one-year survival that is pain-free, then one should also be indifferent to the choice between two weeks with severe pain and one-week pain-free survival.

Risk neutrality assumes a linear function for utility of life years, so that if one is willing to gamble on a 50–50 chance of dying in one year or living for four years versus the certainty of living for two years, then one should also be willing to gamble similarly in the future between a 50–50 chance of dying in 21 years or living to 24 years versus the certainty of living 22 years.

Constant proportional trade-off is the assumption that the proportion of remaining life that one is willing to give up for a specified improvement in quality of life is independent of the number of remaining years of life.

These are strong assumptions, and there is some evidence that none of them is realistic.

DISCOUNTING OF QALYs

Most people place a greater value upon benefits that are immediate rather than those that may arise many years later. Thus it may be relevant to "discount" distant gains by proportionally reducing that component of the QALYs that relate to distant benefits. This concept of discounting is widely applied in economic analyses, and appears equally important in the context of QALYs, especially when the utilities are derived from TTO evaluations.

COST-UTILITY RATIOS

One application for QALYs, albeit controversial, is to provide a single summary statistic for the economic evaluation of the cost-utility of interventions. This, coupled with the possibility of calculating QALYs in order to compare impact of treatment across different diseases, has led to their widespread use by economists.

The cost of each intervention is determined, and the cost-utility per expected number QALYs is estimated as

$$\text{Cost-utility per QALY} = \text{Cost}/\text{QALY}. \qquad (12.2)$$

When comparing a treatment T versus a control C, for example, we have

$$\text{Cost-utility per QALY gained} = (\text{Cost}_T - \text{Cost}_C)/(\text{QALY}_T - \text{QALY}_C). \qquad (12.3)$$

This can then arguably be used when assigning the most efficient use of healthcare funds.

Example from the literature

Hillner, Smith and Desch (1992) applied economic assessment to assess the efficacy and cost-effectiveness of autologous bone marrow transplantation (ABMT) for metastatic breast cancer. Physicians and nursing staff assigned preference values for 11 health states, from well (1) through stable disease (0.5) to death (0). Table 12.1 shows the differences between treatments that might be observed for a cohort of 45-year old women. The cost per gained QALY, from equation (12.3), was US$96 000. Costs and benefits were discounted at a 5% annual rate.

In the words of the authors: "To our surprise, the results of the analysis changed minimally when QALYs were used." It was concluded that if ABMT does not provide a chance of cure but simply increases survival by one or two years, "its attractiveness to women and its cost are both unacceptable".

Table 12.1 Cost per QALY of ABMT compared with standard chemotherapy (Based on Hillner *et al.*, 1992)

End point	ABMT	Standard chemotherapy	Difference
Median survival (months)	27.4	21.4	6.0
QALY	19.6	12.3	6.3
Cost (US$)	89 700	36 100	53 600
Cost per gained year of life (US$)	115 800		
Cost per gained QALY (US$)	96 000		

12.6 Q-TWiST

The Q-TWiST approach is similar in concept to QALYs, in that it uses utility scores to reduce the importance of years survived when health is impaired. Unlike QALYs, however, Q-TWiST can be applied to censored survival data and is therefore particularly appropriate for use in clinical trials. The principle is to partition the overall treatment-related survival curves into a few—typically three—regions that define the time spent in particular clinical states. The areas of the regions are then used to provide scores for these states, and the scores are weighted according to utilities that have been derived as for the QALY method.

CHOICE OF HEALTH STATES

The initial stage in calculating Q-TWiST is to define the health states. The overall survival time (OS) of each patient may include a time without symptoms or toxicity (TWiST). This will usually represent the optimal state, or the best possible QoL that is realistic and attainable for patients with chronic diseases such as cancer, and is therefore usually one of the health states included in a Q-TWiST analysis. This state has by definition a utility of 1. In contrast, death has a utility of 0. The other states are chosen according to clinical relevance, but two states might be, for example, the period with symptoms and toxicity (state 1 = TOX), and when in relapse (state 2 = REL). In this case, OS = TOX + TWiST + REL with disease-free survival (DFS) = TOX + TWiST; but other states might be more suitable for partitioning survival in other contexts.

Example

> Suppose a patient with operable lung cancer has the tumour surgically removed, so that in practical terms the patient is (almost) free of disease and hence symptom-free. However, post-operative chemotherapy of three cycles is given to sterilize any potential metastases. During the course of chemotherapy the patient experiences severe toxicity for 5, 3 and 7 days respectively following each cycle of chemotherapy. Thereafter the patient remains without either symptoms or toxicity until the disease recurs at 250 days after surgery when symptoms also reoccur and he dies 50 days later. Here TOX = 5 + 3 + 7 = 15, TWiST = 235, REL = 50 and OS = 15 + 250 + 650 = 300 days.

SURVIVAL CURVES

A standard survival analysis is based upon OS for each patient, and the treatment-specific groups can be compared using the Kaplan–Meier method as described by Parmar and Machin (1995). This form of analysis also takes into account survival times of patients who have not yet died at the time of analysis. In very broad terms the treatment that is most effective corresponds to the upper of these two survival curves, and the magnitude of the area between them represents the size of their difference.

To partition the survival curves, the time in each of the Q-TWiST states is quantified for each patient and summarised using the corresponding Kaplan–Meier estimates to graph the "survival" curves for the different states. The area beneath the corresponding Kaplan–Meier curve provides an estimate of the mean duration of time spent in each particular health state. The areas between the curves for TOX, DFS and OS are estimates of the respective mean health state durations. Thus the area between the DFS and TOX survival curves is an estimate of the mean duration of TWiST, while the area between the OS and TWiST survival curves is an estimate of the mean duration of REL.

Example from the literature

> Gelber *et al.* (1995) calculate the survival curves for OS, DFS and TOX for the individual treatments of the International Breast Cancer Study Group (IBCSG) Trial V. Their calculations for the Long (as opposed to Short) chemotherapy treatment are summarised in Figure 12.1. From these curves it can be seen that approximately 67% of patients lived to 84 months, and that of the other 33% about half lived to 38 months, giving an average OS = $0.67 \times 84 + 0.33 \times 38 = 69$ months. Similarly the average time in TOX and DFS can be estimated, and the averages for TWiST and REL obtained by subtraction. They estimated that mean times as TOX = 6, TWiST = 54 and REL = 9 months.

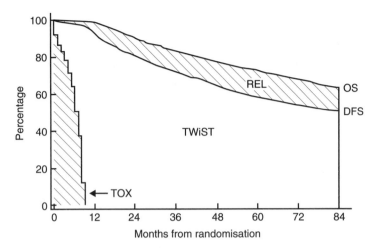

Figure 12.1 Partitioned survival curves for the Long duration chemotherapy treatment of the IBCSG Trial V (Based on Gelber *et al.*, 1995)

CALCULATING Q-TWiST

The period in TWiST is regarded as optimal, with a utility of 1, but we need utilities u_{TOX} for TOX, and u_{REL} for REL. These presumably have utilities between 0 and 1, and could be determined using the methods of VAS, SG or TTO, or could be chosen arbitrarily on the basis of experience of clinicians or other staff. The utilities might be specified as part of the protocol documentation, or could be collected during the trial itself. Q-TWiST is then calculated by summing the utility-weighted values for TOX, TWiST and REL. Thus:

$$Q\text{-}TWiST = (u_{TOX} \times TOX) + (u_{TWiST} \times TWiST) + (u_{REL} \times REL). \quad (12.3)$$

Since TOX, TWiST and REL are measured in units of time, such as months, Q-TWiST too is measured in the same time units.

Example from the literature

Gelber *et al.* (1995) gave the estimated mean times for their 3 states as TOX = 1, TWiST = 47 and REL = 16 months for the Short chemotherapy arm in the IBCSG Trial V. They also define $u_{TWiST} = 1.0$, $u_{TOX} = 0.5$ and $u_{REL} = 0.5$. Thus:

$$Q\text{-}TWiST = (0.5 \times 1) + (1.0 \times 47) + (0.5 \times 16) = 55.5 \text{ months}.$$

If the utilities used were different, then a different value of Q-TWiST would be obtained. For example, suppose relapse were followed by a period of much lower QoL than when TOX was being experienced. In such a case perhaps $u_{TWiST} = 1.0$ and $u_{TOX} = 0.5$ as previously, but $u_{REL} = 0.25$. Then:

$$\text{Q-TWiST} = (0.5 \times 1) + (1.0 \times 47) + (0.25 \times 16) = 51.5 \text{ months.}$$

Here the "value" of one month spent during the relapse period is one-quarter that spent with the better QoL of the TWiST interval, and one half of that during the period of symptoms and/or toxicity.

Example from the literature

Lenderking *et al.* (1994) describe a Q-TWiST approach to evaluate the role of zidovudine therapy for asymptomatic patients with HIV infection. In their situation, one health state corresponds to adverse events (AE) which are the symptomatic sequelæ associated with either treatment or disease. The second health state is progression (PROG). In their situation:

$$\text{Q-TWiST} = (u_{AE} \times \text{AE}) + \text{TWiST} + (u_{PROG} \times \text{PROG}).$$

The utility model of equation (12.4) makes the assumption that the quality-adjusted time spent in a health state is directly proportional to the actual time spent in the health state. It also assumes that the value of the utility coefficient for a health state is independent of the time the health state is entered. This implies, for example, that if toxicity is experienced on three separate occasions then the associated u_{TOX} will be the same for each occasion.

COMPARING TREATMENTS

In a randomised trial to compare treatments, Q-TWiST itself becomes the variable for analysis. In theory the value of Q-TWiST for each patient could be calculated, which would then enable the Mann–Whitney test described in Section 8.2 to be used for testing significance. However, the methods described above based upon partitioned survival curves are advocated for use with censored data or when there are missing values, and these result in a single summary statistic for each treatment group. One way of testing the statistical significance of this observed treatment difference is to use computer-based "bootstrap" methods to calculate confidence intervals and *p*-values, as described in Altman *et al.* (2000).

Example from the literature

Gelber *et al.* (1995) describe the steps taken in the calculation of Q-TWiST using data from the IBCSG Trial V. These calculations are summarised in Table 12.2. In broad terms they concluded that the advantages for long-term chemotherapy in terms of OS and DFS over the short-term chemotherapy are not offset by the disadvantages associated with the greater toxicity. Thus the Q-TWiST difference of 5 months favours the use of long-term therapy for these patients. Confidence intervals were calculated using bootstrap methods.

Table 12.2 Calculation of Q-TWiST from International Breast Cancer Study Group Trial V (Based on Gelber *et al.*, 1995)

Endpoint	Utility coefficient	Mean time (months)		Difference	Confidence interval
		Long	Short		
Survival (OS)	–	69	64	5	2–8
Disease-free survival (DFS)	–	59	48	11	8–15
Time with toxicity (TOX)	0.5	6	1	5	
TWiST	1.0	54	47	7	
Time in relapse (REL)	0.5	9	16	–7	
Q-TWiST	–	61.5	55.5	6	3–8

12.7 SENSITIVITY ANALYSIS

The final value of Q-TWiST depends critically on the values assigned to the utility coefficients. Thus in Table 12.2, had the utilities $u_{TWiST} = 1.0$, $u_{TOX} = 0.75$ and $u_{REL} = 0.25$ been used in place of 1.0, 0.5 and 0.5, then Q-TWiST$_{Long}$ = 60.75 and Q-TWiST$_{Short}$ = 51.75 months. Then the advantage of the Long regimen is extended to the equivalent of 60.75 – 51.75 = 9.00 disease-free months. Thus there is value in exploring how robust the conclusion is to changes from the utility coefficients specified. If this exploration concludes that whatever the values of the utilities provided there always remains an advantage to one particular treatment, then the message is clear. However, if there are conflicting suggestions depending on the choices made, then the situation may become unclear. Or at least, the choice of best treatment option should be based on individual (patient-specific) values.

Such a *sensitivity analysis*, or *threshold utility analysis*, begins by comparing equation (12.4) calculated for each of the two treatment options. For brevity we term these treatments A and B. For a particular clinical trial we will have calculated TOX$_A$, TWiST$_A$, REL$_A$ and TOX$_B$, TWiST$_B$, REL$_B$ and hence Q-TWiST$_A$ and Q-TWiST$_B$. The difference between these two values of Q-TWiST is termed the *Gain, G*:

$$G = \text{Q-TWiST}_A - \text{Q-TWiST}_B. \qquad (12.4)$$

Then:

$$G = u_{TOX} \times (\text{TOX}_A - \text{TOX}_B) + u_{TWiST} \times (\text{TWiST}_A - \text{TWiST}_B) + u_{REL} \times (\text{REL}_A - \text{REL}_B).$$

Further if we assume $u_{TWiST} = 1$, as will be the case in most applications, then G simplifies to

$$G = u_{TOX} \times (\text{TOX}_A - \text{TOX}_B) + (\text{TWiST}_A - \text{TWiST}_B) + u_{REL} \times (\text{REL}_A - \text{REL}_B). \qquad (12.5)$$

From equation (12.5) the gain will be zero, that is $G = 0$, if Q-TWiST for the two treatments is the same. To achieve this, one can search for values of the pair (u_{TOX}, u_{REL}) that once substituted in equation (12.6) make this true. The values of both u_{TOX} and u_{REL} are confined to the range between 0 and 1. We can also search for values of (u_{TOX}, u_{REL}) which have $G > 0$. In this case treatment A would be preferred to B. Similarly, we can search for values that have $G < 0$, in which case treatment B is preferred to A.

This sensitivity analysis can be presented as a two-dimensional plot of u_{TOX} against u_{REL} (Figure 12.2). The straight line in Figure 12.2 is called the *threshold line*, and indicates all pairs of utility coefficients (u_{TOX}, u_{REL}) for which the two treatments have equal Q-TWiST. The threshold line is determined by setting $G = 0$ in equation (12.7). In effect we rewrite equation in the following way:

$$u_{TOX} = -\frac{(TWiST_A - TWiST_B)}{(TOX_A - TOX_B)} - u_{REL}\frac{(REL_A - REL_B)}{(TOX_A - TOX_B)}. \tag{12.6}$$

This is in the form of the equation of a straight line $y = \alpha + \beta x$, where

$$y = u_{TOX}, \quad x = u_{REL}, \quad \alpha = -\frac{(TWiST_A - TWiST_B)}{(TOX_A - TOX_B)} \quad \text{and} \quad \beta = -\frac{(REL_A - REL_B)}{(TOX_A - TOX_B)}.$$

Example from the literature

For the IBCSG Trial V comparing Long and Short chemotherapy, Gelber *et al.* (1995) use the data of Table 12.2 to specify equation (12.7). This gives

$$G = u_{TOX} \times (6 - 1) + (54 - 47) + u_{REL} \times (9 - 16)$$
$$= 5u_{TOX} + 7 - 7u_{REL}.$$

Setting $G = 0$ we have, from equation (12.7):

$$u_{TOX} = -\frac{7}{5} + \frac{7u_{REL}}{5} = -1.4 + 1.4u_{REL}$$

This implies that the threshold line has intercept $\alpha = -1.4$ and slope $\beta = 1.4$. In fact the authors quote $u_{TOX} = -1.2 + 1.4u_{REL}$ but the difference between the two expressions is due to rounding to whole numbers when presenting the summary calculations.

To fix this line in a graph we choose two convenient values of u_{REL} and determine the corresponding u_{TOX}. If we choose $u_{REL} = 0$ in their equation, $u_{TOX} = -1.2 + 1.4 \times 0 = -1.2$ (ignore for a moment that a negative value has no interpretation), and if we choose $u_{REL} = 1$ then $u_{TOX} = -1.2 + 1.4 \times 1 = 0.2$. These two pairs of values, that is (0, -1.2) and (1, 0.2), can be plotted and fix the straight line (the threshold) which is drawn between them. This line divides the region (the square box) of possible and realistic values of u_{TOX} and u_{REL} into two parts.

The area above the line in the box of Figure 12.2 has $G > 0$ and gives all combinations of values of u_{TOX} and u_{REL} for which Long will be preferable to Short, whereas the area below the line has $G < 0$ and give values of u_{TOX} and u_{REL} for which Short will be preferable to Long. It is clear that the Short option will be preferable only in circumstances when u_{REL} is very close to unity; that is, when survival after relapse is given the same quality as survival before relapse.

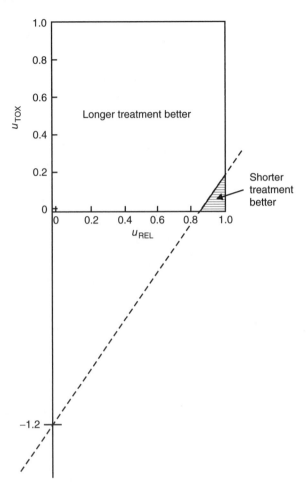

Figure 12.2 Threshold utility analysis (Based on Gelber *et al.*, 1995)

There is no meaning to the "hatched" part of this line (below and to the side of the box of possible values of u_{TOX} and u_{REL}) but it is included here to aid exposition. This was used only to help establish the position of the straight line, and would not be presented when reporting the results of the study.

12.8 PROGNOSIS AND VARIATION WITH TIME

PROGNOSTIC FACTORS

In many clinical situations the appropriate treatments and the patients' final choice of therapeutic option may differ depending on circumstances. Nevertheless there may be groups of patients, perhaps pre-menopausal women with breast cancer, who might choose a different approach from that chosen by post-menopausal women with the same disease. The Q-TWiST methodology extends to this situation and can also be used for comparing patient groups receiving the same treatment. From such studies one may conclude, for example, that pre-menopausal women gain additional disease-free equivalent days by use of a particular therapy when compared with the post-menopausal women receiving the same treatment. More generally one can make comparisons between treatments within each of these patient groups.

Example from the literature

In describing a Q-TWiST analysis, Cole *et al.* (1994) present the mean times spent in TOX, TWiST and REL for four groups of women according to treatment (Short or Long chemotherapy) received. The prognostic groups comprised women who were pre-menopausal with small tumours and few nodes; pre-menopausal with large tumours and numerous nodes; post-menopausal with small tumours and few nodes; and post-menopausal with large tumours and numerous nodes. Their results are summarised in Table 12.3.

In Table 12.3 there are differences between treatments with respect to the time spent in each of the states TOX, TWiST and REL. In addition there are some major differences between patient groups. For example, for the pre-menopausal women with small tumours receiving short-duration chemotherapy, Q-TWiST = $0.8u_{TOX} + 74.5 + 19.0\,u_{REL}$, whereas for those who are pre-menopausal but have large tumours it is $0.8u_{TOX} + 38.1 + 23.5\,u_{REL}$. Thus whatever the values given to

Table 12.3 Average number of months in each of three health states for four groups of patients with breast cancer receiving one of two chemotherapy regimens (Based on Cole *et al.*, 1994)

	Chemotherapy	
	Short	Long
Tumours <2 cm and <4 nodes		
Pre-menopausal		
TOX	0.8	5.8
TWiST	74.5	83.5
REL	19.0	7.7
Post-menopausal		
TOX	0.8	5.8
TwiST	80.1	87.9
REL	16.8	6.7
Tumours ≥2 cm and ≥4 nodes		
Pre-menopausal		
TOX	0.8	5.8
TWiST	38.1	50.1
REL	23.5	9.9
Post-menopausal		
TOX	0.8	5.8
TWiST	43.9	55.8
REL	22.1	9.4

u_{TOX} and u_{REL} by these two groups of women, those with the smaller tumours will have the greater Q-TWiST with short-duration therapy. The TWiST values of 74.5 and 38.1 months, respectively, dominate the corresponding Q-TWiST values.

VARIATION OF Q-TWiST WITH TIME

The preceding sections have summarised Q-TWiST in a single figure, essentially encapsulating the period from diagnosis to subsequent death of the patient. This may be relevant to patients with relatively poor prognosis, but not for those whose prognosis is good. However, the principles involved in calculating Q-TWiST are not changed if the time from diagnosis is divided into segments—perhaps into yearly or even shorter intervals.

Thus in some situations patients diagnosed with a certain disease receive an aggressive treatment for a relatively short period (say less than one year) during which they experience both treatment-related toxicity and symptoms of their disease. Thereafter they may have an extensive period in which they are disease-free, followed by the remote possibility of relapse and the emergence of long-term side-effects of treatment. In this example, for all patients on therapy, the first post-diagnosis year may be dominated by TOX, and the remaining parts with TWiST and REL within this year may be of relatively short duration. Whereas in the second post-diagnosis year a few patients may be still experiencing toxicity, the majority are disease-free, while a few may relapse. Thus the balance between TOX, TWiST and REL may change. This implies that the Gain, G, of equation (12.6) may well vary from period to period following diagnosis.

Example from the literature

Gelber *et al.* (1995) show, with their example of Short and Long chemotherapy regimens of the IBSCG Trial V, how the Gain changes with time during the first seven years post-diagnosis. In Figure 12.3, the bold central line shows the relative Gain when $u_{TOX} = 0.5$ and $u_{REL} = 0.5$, and the shaded region denotes the range of Q-TWiST Gains as the utility coefficients vary between zero and one.

Thus Figure 12.3 illustrates how the balance in the first year after diagnosis favours the Short regimen. This is clearly because all the active treatment occurs in this period and the TOX component of Short is much less than that of Long. As a consequence Q-TWiST, when confined to this period, will be dominated by TOX unless the associated utility coefficient, $u_{TOX} \approx 0$. However, in later years the contribution of TOX to Q-TWiST is reduced in any event, so that the balance between the two options shifts in favour of the Long regimen.

Thus with Q-TWiST potentially varying with time following diagnosis, the attending physician may discuss with the patient with breast cancer the pattern of possible Gain over the coming years. This in turn may then influence the patient's choice for treatment.

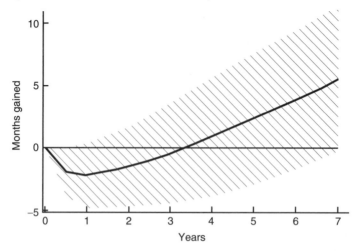

Figure 12.3 Change in Q-TWiST Gain (months) over time for women with breast cancer receiving Short or Long term chemotherapy (Based on Gelber *et al.*, 1995)

12.9   HEALTHY-YEARS EQUIVALENT (HYE)

Various alternatives to QALYs and Q-TWiST have been proposed, but few have gained matching popularity. *Healthy-years equivalent* (HYE) is one of the principal alternatives, and is claimed by its advocates to be superior to QALYs because it avoids some of the assumptions.

The principle of HYE is to avoid the need for expressing the preferences of patients in terms of utilities, which are an abstract concept, but instead to obtain an estimate of the equivalent number of years in full health that the patients would trade for their health state profile.

The original procedure involved a two-stage estimation to obtain patients' HYE values, but it has been shown that HYE is very closely related to QALYs calculated using TTO. The difference is as follows. For QALYs, we need to know the utility of each health state, and the overall QALY score is calculated by assuming that this utility then applies uniformly to the time in that particular health state, as in equation (12.1). In the HYE formulation, the number of HYEs has to be measured for every possible duration of time in each possible health state. Thus HYEs avoid the "risk-neutrality over time" assumption of QALYs, but at the major expense of having to evaluate HYEs for every possible state-duration.

Whether or not HYEs have benefits over QALYs and Q-TWiST remains controversial. In any event, in a clinical trials setting HYEs will rarely be feasible.

12.10   CONCLUSIONS

Utility approaches attempt to combine QoL with survival, enabling a comparison of different policies of management when both QoL and survival vary simultaneously. They do this by equating a year of survival with good QoL as being equivalent to a longer period with poor QoL. However, there are clearly some difficulties with assessing this quality-adjusted survival. These include the determination of the utilities themselves, and the rather simplified concept of health states during which QoL remains essentially constant. Although cost utility may remain constant, a patient's attitude and hence QoL with respect to successive cycles of chemotherapy may well be very variable and far from even approximately constant. Thus although the threshold analysis examines the robustness of this approach to some extent it does not challenge some basic assumptions.

Another problem is that different patients may have very different sets of utilities. The concept of asking patients to assess their utilities for themselves is likely to be feasible only in a relatively small groups of patients. Furthermore, an individual patients' utilities need not remain constant, but may change over time or according to experience and circumstances. Thus unless a threshold analysis confirms that conclusions regarding treatment superiority hold for a very wide range of utilities, it would be difficult to maintain that the results have general applicability.

In summary, in many situations it would seem preferable to report the observed QoL and the overall survival differences, and let the individual—whether he or she be a patient, clinician, or healthcare planner—decide what relative importance to attach to the separate dimensions. In other words, one possibility is to aim to present sufficient information to let the individual apply their own set of utilities.

D Practical Aspects and Clinical Interpretation

13   Clinical Trials

Summary

Inclusion of QoL in clinical trials, and especially multi-centre clinical trials, presents a number of difficult organisational issues. These include standardisation of the procedures for assessment and data collection, specification of measurement details to ensure consistent QoL assessment, methods for minimising missing data, and the collection of reasons for any missing responses. In particular, many trials report serious problems in compliance. As emphasised in Chapter 11, there are problems for interpretation of results when data are missing. Hence it is important to seek methods of optimising the level of compliance, both of the participating institution and of the patient. In this chapter we describe a number of methods for addressing these issues, which should be considered when writing clinical trial protocols involving QoL assessment. A checklist is provided for points that should be covered in protocols.

13.1   INTRODUCTION

The success or failure of the trial will depend on how well the protocol was written, since a poorly designed, ambiguous or incompletely documented protocol will result in a trial which will not be able to answer the questions of interest. The protocol must be concise, yet detailed and precisely worded with all the requirements clearly indicated so that the trial is carried out uniformly by all participants. Protocols should contain a statement about the rationale for assessing QoL, justifying its importance to the participating clinician. Sometimes this may be brief, although a more detailed discussion might be appropriate when QoL is a major endpoint of the study.

Poor compliance with completion of QoL forms bedevils randomised clinical trials, leading to serious problems of analysis and interpretation. In some instances the potential for bias in the analyses could even render the results uninterpretable. Compliance can be greatly enhanced by ensuring that all those involved in the trial, from medical staff to patients, are aware of, and agree with, the relevance of QoL as a study endpoint.

Equally, it is important to recognise that QoL assessment should be incorporated in a clinical trial only when it really is relevant to do so. This may depend on the aims of the trial, and the precise objective in including a QoL assessment. QoL is not necessarily relevant to all clinical trials. It is usually unnecessary to measure QoL in small early phase I or phase II trials, although it can be useful to do so on an exploratory basis or as a pilot study when developing instruments for subsequent studies. QoL is mainly of importance in phase III clinical trials. Chapter 1 described and gave examples of situations in which it is particularly relevant. The following situations can be identified:

1. Trials in which the new treatment is expected to have only a small impact on such clinical endpoints as long-term survival, cure or response, and any small improvement in the primary clinical endpoint may have to be weighed against the negative aspects upon QoL of an intensive therapy. This appears to cover the majority of long-term chronic diseases, including cancer.
2. Equivalence trials, where the disease course in both arms is expected to be similar but there are expected to be QoL benefits or differences in morbidity. In these trials, QoL may be a primary endpoint.
3. Trials of treatments which are specifically intended to improve QoL. This includes trials in palliative care, for example palliative radiotherapy for cancer, and bisphosphonates for metastatic bone pain. In these studies QoL is most often the primary endpoint.
4. Studies involving health economic cost-effectiveness review contrasted against QoL.

13.2 CHOICE OF INSTRUMENT

In Chapter 1 we illustrated the wide diversity of QoL instruments. The choice of instrument may be crucial to the success of a study, and although many question-naires exist, not all have been extensively validated. The selection must be made with care, and expert advice is important. Generic instruments focus on broad aspects of QoL and health status, and are intended for use in general populations or across a wide range of disease conditions. If it is considered important to compare the results of the clinical trial with data from other groups of patients, including patients with other diseases, a generic instrument may be most appropriate. For example, a generic instrument could be used when applying health economics to a range of disease areas, to compare treatment costs versus treatment effects upon health status.

In contrast, disease-specific instruments are usually developed so as to detect subtle disease and treatment-related effects. They will contain items reflecting issues of importance to the patients. When considering a single clinical trial, a disease-specific instrument will frequently be chosen because it is expected to have better sensitivity to the health states that may be experienced by patients in the study. Disease-specific instruments may also provide detailed information that is of clinical relevance to the management of patients.

Although it may occasionally be possible to use a combination of both a generic and a disease-specific instrument, the result may be a questionnaire package that takes unacceptably long to complete and which contains questions that are more-or-less repeated in different formats. Extensive reviews of general and disease-specific questionnaires exist; for example Bowling (1995, 1997), Anderson, Aaronson and Wilkin (1993) and Salek (1998).

The separation of instruments into generic and specific can function at different levels. For example, the EORTC QLQ-C30 and the FACT-G are examples of instruments that are generic for a class of disease states. These instruments are core modules that are intended for use with supplementary modules focusing on particular diseases and treatments. Since they were designed to be modular, both the core and a supplementary module can be used together on each patient. Other instruments assess specific dimensions of QoL, such as pain, fatigue, anxiety and depression, and if these dimensions are of particular interest in the trial the questionnaires may be used alongside disease-related or generic instruments.

General considerations when selecting an instrument include the following.

- There should be documentation concerning the development and psychometric properties of the instrument, and in particular concerning its validation, reliability, sensitivity and responsiveness.
- There should be evidence that the instrument has been developed for and tested in a wide range of patients with the target disease states or receiving the intended treatment modalities.
- There should be evidence that the instrument has been tested and found valid for use with patients from the relevant educational, cultural and ethnic backgrounds.
- If additional language versions are required, they should be developed using formal procedures of forward and backward translation and tested on a number of patients who also complete a debriefing questionnaire.
- If a generic instrument is used, it must be checked whether disease- or treatment-specific questionnaires, as may be required for the trial, are compatible with the main instrument.
- Consider the feasibility of the instrument: How lengthy is the questionnaire; how long does it take to complete; how easily understood are the questions; and are there any difficult or embarrassing items?
- Is there a global question or a global measure of overall QoL? Is there, or is it necessary to provide, an open-ended question about "other factors affecting your QoL, not covered above"? Are treatment side-effects covered adequately?
- Are there any reference data or interpretation guidelines? These are required both for estimating sample size when designing a trial, and for interpretation and reporting of the results.

The study protocol should document the reasons for selecting a particular instrument.

13.3 COMPLIANCE

When QoL is assessed in a clinical trial, it is important to ensure that the information collected is representative of the study patients. However, when data are missing for some patients, a question arises as to whether the patients with missing data differ from those who returned completed forms. As a consequence, missing data present severe problems in analysis and interpretation of results. Therefore the amount of missing data in a trial should be minimised. Data may be unavailable for two principal reasons:

- unavoidable reasons, of which the most common in some disease areas is patient attrition due to early deaths
- low compliance, in which forms that should have been completed by patients and returned to the trials office may be missing; this has frequently been a serious problem in clinical trials.

Example from the literature

The MRC Lung Cancer Working Party (Fayers *et al.*, 1997b) assessed aspects of QoL with a five-item daily diary card that patients completed at home. Only 47% of the expected patient Daily Diary Cards were returned, and a third of the patients provided no data at all. It was noted that there were major differences in compliance rates according to the centre responsible for the patient, providing strong support for the belief that much of the problem is institution-compliance rather than patient-compliance.

Compliance has continued to be a problem in later MRC trials, when other instruments have also been used, and when assessments have been made while patients attended the clinic.

MEASURING COMPLIANCE

Compliance is defined as the number of QoL questionnaires actually completed as a proportion of those expected. The number of patients alive at each protocol assessment point represents the maximum number of QoL forms, as patients must be excluded upon death.

It is important to verify that the forms received have indeed been completed at the scheduled times. For example, if the scheduled QoL assessment is on day 42 and the corresponding QoL form is not completed until (say) day 72, then the responses recorded may not reflect the patient QoL at the time point of interest. However, it is necessary to recognise the variation in individual patient's treatment and follow-up, and so a time frame or *window* may be allowed around each scheduled protocol assessment time. The exact definitions will depend upon the nature of the trial, but the initial assessment will usually be given a tight window such as no more than three days before randomisation, to ensure that it represents a true pre-treatment baseline. During the active treatment period, the window may still have to be narrow, but it should allow for treatment delay. Similarly, if an assessment is targeted at, say, two months after surgery, a window of acceptability must be specified. Later, during follow-up assessments, the window may widen, particularly in diseases for which there is a reasonable expectation of long survival and follow-up. Finally, since it is unlikely that QoL forms will be completed until the day of death, it may be appropriate to impose a cut-off point at some "reasonable" time prior to death.

Example from the literature

In a trial comparing two chemotherapy regimens for palliative treatment of patients with small-cell lung cancer, the number of questionnaires received (and completed on schedule) was 764 (53%) of the 1445 anticipated (Medical Research Council Lung Cancer Working Party, 1996). Table 13.1 indicates the windows used for the seven QoL assessments that were scheduled during the first six months. Compliance within these windows was initially good but declined markedly after chemotherapy stopped.

Table 13.1   MRC Lung Cancer Working Party trial of four-drug vs. two-drug chemotherapy in the palliative treatment of patients with small-cell lung cancer (from Medical Research Council Lung Cancer Working Party, 1996)

Assessment	Time due (day)	Window (days)	Dead	Alive (forms expected)	(No.)	(%)
			Patients		Forms received	
Baseline	0	−7 to +1	0	310	232	75
Week-3 chemotherapy	21	14 to 28	58	252	165	66
Week-6 chemotherapy	42	35 to 49	72	238	137	58
Month 3	91	77 to 105	116	194	78	40
Month 4	122	108 to 136	137	173	66	38
Month 5	152	138 to 166	159	151	49	33
Month 6	183	169 to 197	183	127	37	29
Overall				1445	764	53

Various trials groups use different definitions of windows, making it difficult to compare reported compliance rates. Clearly a group using a window of plus or minus a week from the time of surgery might expect to report worse values for compliance than if they used a window of plus or minus two weeks. Given this variation in defining compliance, it is slightly surprising to find that the reported experience of other groups has been similar. Serious problems in compliance with QoL assessments have been reported in many multi-centre clinical trials, especially in palliative trials involving poor-prognosis patients. In some trials only about half the expected post-baseline QoL questionnaires were returned. However, poor compliance is not necessarily attributable to lack of patient compliance. Compliance rates have repeatedly been found to vary widely according to institution, which has often led, perhaps unfairly, to poor compliance being attributed to the lack of commitment by clinicians; in busy clinics, lack of resources for assisting patients, for example, can be an equally important institution-related component. Thus single-centre trials can frequently achieve better compliance, especially if a research nurse is assigned solely for the purpose of QoL collection.

When patients become increasingly ill with progressive disease, they can find it difficult to continue completing questionnaires. This poses a methodological problem for investigators who wish to assess effects in settings such as palliative care during terminal stages of disease. In some studies it may be necessary to use home-care staff or home-visit nurses to assist the patients in completing questionnaires.

Example from the literature

> Sadura *et al.* (1992) developed and implemented a comprehensive programme specifically aimed at encouraging compliance. They reported overall compliance of above 95% in three Canadian trials, which they attributed to their programme.
>
> However, they acknowledged that it remained unclear whether similar success could be obtained with different questionnaires, in different types of trials, in different institutions, and during long-term follow-up. Also, the Canadian group used a level of resources, which may not be available to other groups conducting international multi-centre randomised trials: in one study, "nurses called the patients at home on the appropriate day to remind them to complete the questionnaire". Given careful planning, and provided adequate resources are made available, it *is* possible to achieve high compliance.

Unfortunately, it is well recognised that if questionnaires are missing there may be serious bias in the results of analyses, and the estimates of treatment differences and the overall level of QoL may be inaccurate and misleading. For example, patients with poor performance status may provide less data than those with good performance, and this could distort the assessment of treatment effects.

Example from the literature

> Hopwood *et al.* (1994) describe an MRC trial in which information was provided by 92% of patients whom the clinician assessed as having good performance status (normal activity, no restrictions), through to only 31% of those assessed as very poor (confined to bed or chair).
>
> It was concluded: "At present, given the rapid attrition in lung cancer trials and the rather low levels of compliance in completing questionnaires, there is no entirely reliable way of analysing data longitudinally."

Example from the literature

> However, other patients may respond differently, and Cox *et al.* (1992), illustrating the problems with data for heart transplant patients using the Nottingham Health Profile (NHP), found the reverse effect: those about to die or to be lost to follow-up tended to have poorer QoL scores than those who missed their next follow-up.
>
> Cox *et al.* suggested another reason for poor compliance is that: "those experiencing fewer problems may not be so diligent in returning questionnaires".

At best, low compliance raises questions about whether the results are representative, and at worst it may jeopardise interpretation of the treatment comparisons. This is especially so when compliance rates differ according to treatment group and patients' performance status. In addition, poor compliance means that there are

Has the patient filled in the scheduled quality of life questionnaire?
0 = no, 1 = yes |__|

If **no**, please state the main reason:

|__| 1 = patient felt too ill

|__| 2 = clinician or nurse felt the patient was too ill

|__| 3 = patient felt it was inconvenient, takes too much time

|__| 4 = patient felt it was a violation of privacy

|__| 5 = administrative failure to distribute the questionnaire to the patient

|__| 6 = (at baseline) patient didn't speak the language or was illiterate

|__| 7 = other, please specify ....

Figure 13.1 Questionnaire to ascertain the reason why a patient has not completed the current QoL assessment

fewer data items available for analyses, and thus there may be questions about the adequacy of the sample size. However, if this were the only issue one solution would be to recruit extra patients so as to compensate for the losses due to non-compliance. Unfortunately, this does not address the more serious issue of potential bias in the results; if compliance rates stay the same then, no matter how much patient numbers are increased, the bias will remain.

REASONS FOR NON-COMPLIANCE

Missing data, and hence low compliance, may arise from many causes, including clinicians or nurses forgetting to ask patients to complete QoL questionnaires, and patients refusing, feeling too ill or forgetting. Low "compliance" does not necessarily imply fault on the part of the patient or their medical staff.

One advantage of studying QoL as an integral part of a clinical trial is that additional clinical information about treatment or disease problems can be collected at each visit of the patient, and this information can indicate why QoL data has not been collected. The reasons for not completing the questionnaire should be collected systematically, for example as in Figure 13.1. This information should be summarised and reported, and may also be used as an indication of whether particular missing data is likely to have occurred at random, in which case the imputation of the corresponding missing values may be improved.

13.4 ADMINISTRATION OF QoL ASSESSMENT

For QoL to be successfully incorporated into a clinical trial, practical steps have to be taken to ensure good standards of data collection and to seek as many methods as possible for improving compliance.

Because of heavy workloads, many clinicians are unable to give the necessary attention to data collection in a QoL study. Responsibility for explaining about

QoL assessment and distributing questionnaires is often allocated to research nurses or other staff associated with the clinical trial. As pivotal members of the research team, nurses and data managers need a clear view of their job-specific tasks to improve efficiency and quality of data. Research nurses play a major role in the education of patients and therefore may be influential for generating interest in the QoL part of the study. Suitably trained personnel can ensure better compliance of QoL data through standardisation and continuity of working procedures, and comprehensive programmes of training are important. These should be supplemented by written operating procedures and guidelines for administration of QoL assessment in clinical trials. One example of detailed guidelines for improving data quality and compliance in clinical trials is the manual written by Young *et al.* (1999).

THE PATIENT

Most patients are willing to complete QoL questionnaires, especially if they are assured that the data will be useful for medical research and will benefit future patients. Therefore patients should be given full information about the procedures, and any of their concerns answered.

- Patients should be given a clear explanation of the reason for collecting QoL data.
- Information sheets should supplement the verbal information given to patients, detailing the rationale for collecting QoL data and explaining aspects of the procedure. The information sheet should include the frequency and timing of assessments, the need to answer all questions, and the importance of completing the questions without being influenced by the opinions of others.
- Patients should be told how their questionnaires will be used. In particular, they should be told whether the information will be seen by the clinician or other staff involved with their management, or whether it will remain confidential and used solely for scientific research purposes.
- The questionnaire should not be too lengthy, and should contain clear written instructions.
- Patients should be thanked for completing the questionnaire, and given the opportunity to discuss any problems. They should be encouraged to help with future assessments; for example, patients could be asked to remind staff if later questionnaires are not given out.

THE MEDICAL TEAM

Similarly, the medical team deserves to receive explanation of the value of QoL assessment in the particular study. Sceptical staff make less effort, and will experience greater difficulty in persuading patients to complete questionnaires.

- The role of QoL assessment should be emphasised. If it is a primary endpoint for the study, patients should be randomised only on condition that relevant QoL assessments have been or will be completed.

- It is useful to assign a research assistant or a research nurse to QoL studies. Clinicians may be engaged in other tasks when patients come for their treatment.
- Named individuals at participating institutions should be identified for specific roles, especially if the clinical trial is multi-centre. At some institutions this might involve several individuals for the different tasks. Responsibilities include:
  - explaining to the patient the rationale for QoL assessment and the implications
  - giving QoL questionnaires to patients (one possibility is that questionnaires should be completed whilst awaiting to be seen by the clinician)
  - providing a quiet, private and comfortable place for the patient to complete them
  - ensuring that help is readily available for patients who require it
  - collecting and checking questionnaires for completeness
  - sending reminders and collecting overdue or missing questionnaires
  - forwarding completed questionnaires to the clinical trial office and responding to queries arising.
- It is important to consider the provision of systematic training to accompany the written instructions for staff responsible for administering the questionnaires.
- Regular feedback should be given, to maintain motivation. This might include reports of data quality (numbers of completed forms, compliance rates, details of missing items) and tabulation of baseline, pre-randomisation data.
- Finally, the medical team should be reminded that experience shows that most patients are willing to complete QoL questionnaires.

Example from the literature

Hürny *et al.* (1992) reported that compliance in a trial of small-cell lung cancer varied between 21% and 68%, with larger institutions having highest rates of compliance. Institution was the only significant factor for predicting compliance. Patient age, sex, education and biological prognostic factors at randomisation were not found to be predictors.

It was suggested that smaller institutions might be at a disadvantage, as they usually do not have the resources to dedicate a full-time staff member to data management and quality assurance. However, with an organised effort at the local institutional level, high-quality data collection could be achieved. It was also recommended that to achieve good-quality QoL data there is a need for systematic training and commitment of staff at all institutions.

13.5 RECOMMENDATIONS FOR WRITING PROTOCOLS

Protocols should aim to be concise, practical documents for participating clinicians, covering all aspects of the day-to-day running of the clinical trials. It is to be hoped that brevity encourages reading and observance of the content of the protocols. There is no consensus as to the optimal way of presenting all the relevant background information and justification of QoL study design. Different approaches are used by different trials organisations, according to their needs and preferences and according to the nature of individual trials. Thus whilst it is important to consider the study objectives and details of the design, it is unclear how much of this should be incorporated in the working protocol or whether it should be recorded separately. One possibility is to mention these issues briefly in the main study protocol, and to address them in greater detail in written accompanying supplementary documents. These additional documents should comprise part of the package that is also sent to the Protocol Review Committee and to the Local Ethics Committees (Institutional Review Boards). The following examples are taken from a range of protocols, with specific illustrations of text that has been used in MRC protocols (Fayers *et al.*, 1997b).

RATIONALE FOR INCLUDING QoL ASSESSMENT

A section in the protocol should explain the reasons why QoL is being assessed. Some clinicians are less committed to QoL evaluation than others, and so it is important to justify the need for the extra work that the participants are being asked to carry out.

> **Quality of life follow-up**
>
> Quality of life is an important endpoint in this study. The timing of treatment may have a considerable impact on patients. The long-term palliation and prevention of symptoms are important factors in the treatment of relapsed disease. **It is important therefore that all centres participate in this study**.

EMPHASISING GOOD COMPLIANCE

The need for good compliance should be stressed to participants, telling them that a serious effort is being made to ensure completeness of QoL data collection. In trials where QoL is a major endpoint or the principal outcome measure, optimal compliance is clearly essential; patients who fail to return QoL data do not contribute information for analysis. In extreme cases a trial Data Monitoring Committee (DMC) could recommend early closure of the trial if the level of QoL compliance is unacceptable. Thus protocols should emphasise the importance of QoL assessment, and should also encourage doctors to emphasise this to patients.

> Such data will be an **essential** source of information for comparison between the two arms in this study.
>
> Emphasise to the patient that completion of these forms helps doctors find out more about the effects of treatment on well-being.

IDENTIFY CONTACT-PERSONS

We have described the need to identify personnel within the medical team, to take responsibility for the various tasks associated with administering QoL questionnaires. It is recommended that one named person be identified to serve as the contact at each centre. This person is responsible for collecting the QoL data and ensuring that the forms are checked and returned to the trials office. This might or might not be the clinician responsible for the patients, although in general it is recommended that a person other than the responsible clinician should administer the questionnaire to the patient, so that the form may be completed prior to consultation with the doctor. In addition, it has been suggested that patients try to please their doctor or nurse, and thus the responses may be distorted if the person responsible for managing their treatment is present whilst they complete the forms.

> A named person in each centre must be nominated to take responsibility for the administration, collection and checking of the QoL forms. This may or may not be the clinician responsible for the patients.

WRITTEN GUIDELINES FOR ADMINISTERING QoL QUESTIONNAIRES

There should be written guidelines aimed at those administering the questionnaires in the clinical setting. These address the issues of poor compliance at the level of the participating institute. The topics covered should range from suggestions about adopting a sympathetic approach towards patients who may be feeling particularly ill or may have just been informed about progression of their disease for example, through to instructions about the need to ensure backup staff for times when the normal QoL personnel are on leave or absent.

There should be instructions about checking of forms, including procedures for patients who fail to complete answers for all questions—for example, how to handle patients who have not understood what is required, or who do not wish to respond to particular questions ("Explain the relevance and importance of those particular questions, and the confidentiality of the information"). The guidelines should indicate any questions that are anticipated to present particular problems. For example, staff might be warned: "Some patients omit to answer the question about sexual interest, because they find it embarrassing and consider it irrelevant. However, it is included as an indicator of the general health and well-being of the patient." Similarly, for a question about loss of appetite: "Patients may be confused between inability to eat due to symptoms such as dysphagia or inability to eat because of lack of appetite; it is the latter meaning which is intended."

> An information pack is sent to all participating centres detailing the procedures for quality of life assessment and providing guidelines for ensuring optimal compliance.

CHECKING FORMS BEFORE THE PATIENT LEAVES

When clinical data are missing from a form it is frequently possible to retrieve the information from hospital notes. QoL is different; once the patient has left the hospital it will be too late to retrieve missing or unclear information, except by contacting the patient by telephone or post. Therefore there should be statements about the need for the QoL forms to be checked before the patient has left the clinic, and any action to be taken in the event of missing data. There should also be instructions regarding procedures to follow when questionnaires are missing: should the patient be contacted, possibly by a post with a reply-paid envelope or by telephone, or should the data be accepted as missing and only the reason recorded?

The questionnaire must be collected before the patient leaves and **checked to ensure that all questions have been answered**. If necessary, go back to the patient immediately and asking him or her to fill in any missing items.

If a questionnaire assessment is missed because of administrative failure, the patient should be contacted by telephone or letter and asked to complete and return a mailed questionnaire as soon as possible.

BASELINE ASSESSMENT

There will usually be a "baseline" assessment, taken before randomisation. In addition to providing a pre-treatment baseline against which the patients' subsequent changes can be compared, this also enables a baseline comparison between the randomised study groups. If differences are present, it may be necessary to make compensatory statistical adjustments to later QoL measurements. When follow-up data are missing, the baseline information can also allow examination of the patterns of missingness, and can often be used to minimize the systematic biases that may arise from data that are not missing at random.

The baseline assessment should be made before the patient has been informed of the randomised treatment allocation; otherwise, knowledge of the treatment assignment may cause different levels of, for example, anxiety within the two treatment groups. Furthermore, by ensuring that QoL is assessed before randomisation and made a randomisation eligibility criterion, we can try to ensure that form completion is 100%.

Randomisation

Patients should be randomised by telephoning the Trials Office. The person telephoning will be asked to confirm that the eligibility criteria have been met, and that the patient have completed their initial quality of life questionnaires.

ASSESSMENT DURING THERAPY

Some trials have used a daily diary card, obtaining a complete picture of the changing symptomatology and QoL before, during and after therapy. More commonly, and especially in large multi-centre clinical trials, it is necessary to identify specific time points when a QoL questionnaire should be used. Since administering and completing questionnaires imposes burdens on the patient, it is desirable to limit the number and frequency of questionnaires.

Frequently, for administrative convenience, assessment times during treatment will be chosen to coincide with patient visits to the clinic. For diseases such as long-term treatment for hypertension, patients' condition may be expected to be relatively stable and so the precise time point may not be critical. In this situation, timing of QoL assessment becomes relatively easy. For other diseases, such as cancer, patients commonly attend at the start of each course or cycle of chemo-therapy treatment, with the patient completing the QoL questionnaire whilst waiting to be reassessed by the clinician. However, some QoL instruments specify a time frame of "during the last week . . .", and will therefore collect information about how the patient recalls feeling only during the week preceding the next course of therapy. If treatment courses are for example pulsed at intervals of three to four weeks, this may or may not be what is ideally wanted, as the impact of transient toxicity might remain undetected. That is, the investigators will have to decide whether temporary toxicity-related reductions in QoL are of importance, or whether the longer-term effects as seen later during each cycle are more important. Some-times it may be appropriate to assess QoL at, say, one week after therapy.

Another point to be considered is that sometimes treatment may be delayed, possibly because of toxicity, in which case if assessments are made immediately preceding the next (delayed) course of treatment, the impact of the toxicity upon QoL may not be noticed.

In principle, it is desirable to use the same timing schedule in all treatment arms, with QoL assessments being made at times relative to the date of randomisation. In practice, this may be difficult in trials that compare treatments of different modality or where the timing of therapy and follow-up differs between the randomised groups. In these settings, patients may attend the clinic at different times and therapy in the treatment arms may also be completed at different times. This leads to differences in the timing of assessments within the arms of the study, which can make interpreta-tion of results difficult if patients are deteriorating as a consequence of their disease progressing from the time of randomisation.

In summary, there are compromises to be made in those studies that investigate QoL in the context of treatment events such as surgery and intermittent courses of chemotherapy and radiotherapy. Assessments may be made relative to the treatment events, or relative to the randomisation date. They may also be timed to occur after but relative to the date of the previous course of treatment, or immedi-ately preceding the following course. Sometimes a combination of strategies can be used.

Clearly the general timing of the assessments must be specified—for example, two weeks after surgery. However, a more precise specification might specify a window within which assessments are valid—for example, at least two, but not more than three, weeks after surgery.

> The quality of life questionnaire should be completed by the patient **before** randomisation, at 6 weeks, 12 weeks, 6 months and 1 year.
>
> Most patients are expected to keep to their protocol treatment time schedule, but to allow for occasional delays a window of one week around each 6-week time-point will be accepted.

FOLLOW-UP (POST-TREATMENT) ASSESSMENT

There may also be follow-up assessments after completion of treatment. Sometimes the primary scientific question concerns QoL during therapy, and if post-treatment assessment is thought necessary perhaps one suffices. In other studies, it may be important to continue collecting data in order to explore treatment-related differences in the long-term impact of therapy and control of disease progression. Sometimes it is relevant to continue assessment until and after any relapses may have occurred, and in some studies, such as studies of palliative care, assessments may continue until death. In all these situations, to eliminate bias, long-term assessments in both treatment groups should normally be at similar times relative to the date of randomisation. If the questionnaires are mailed to patients any appropriate schedule can be used, but if they are to be handed out at clinics the choice of times may be restricted for logistic reasons.

SPECIFYING WHEN TO COMPLETE QUESTIONNAIRES

Generally it is advisable for QoL to be assessed before the patient is seen by the clinician. Usually this is a convenient time for the clinic (whilst the patient is in the waiting room); it means that the patient will not have been affected by anything occurring during their consultation, and it enables the clinical follow-up form to include the questions: "Has QoL been assessed? If not, why not?"

> **Follow-up**
>
> The patient should complete the questionnaires whilst waiting to be seen in the clinic—this should be done in a quiet area.

Patients should also be encouraged to request their QoL forms upon arrival at the clinic, since this will help to prevent QoL assessments being forgotten and there is usually suitable time to complete the forms whilst waiting to be seen by the clinician.

> If you are not given a questionnaire to complete when you think it is due, please remind your doctor. You can, of course, decline to fill in a questionnaire at any time.

Some instruments relate to "the past week". In many trials, the patient attends hospital three or four weeks after the previous cycle of chemotherapy or radiotherapy, and thus assessments at these times may not always include the period during which therapy was received. It is important that patients be aware of the time frame of the questions.

> It is important to explain to the patient that the questionnaire refers to how they have been feeling **during the past week**.

HELP AND PROXY ASSESSMENT

Nurses, doctors and family members often underestimate the impact of those items which most distress the patient. Therefore it is important that the patients should complete the QoL questionnaire themselves. Patients may be influenced by the opinions of others when completing questionnaires.

Example from the literature

Cook *et al.* (1993) compared the same questionnaire when interviewer- or self-administered, on a sample of 150 asthma patients. When using the self-administered version, patients recorded more symptoms, more emotional problems, greater limitation of activities, more disease-related problems and greater need to avoid environmental stimuli. On average, 47% of items were endorsed when self-administered, but only 36% when interviewed.

Thus it is advisable that patients should receive help only when it is absolutely necessary, and doctors, nurses and spouses should all be discouraged from offering help unless it is really needed.

However, some patients may be unable to complete the questionnaire by themselves or have difficulty understanding the questions. Examples range from vision problems and forgotten glasses, to cognitive impairment. In these cases help should be provided, as assisted completion is better than either total absence of data or incorrect information through misapprehension. Similarly, if a few patients are too ill or too distressed to complete the forms, someone familiar with their feelings may act as a proxy. Proxies are typically a "significant other" such as a partner, spouse or close family member, but may include staff such as a nurse who knows the patient well. For some trials, such as those in psychiatry or advanced brain malignancies, it might be anticipated that the majority of patients will be unable to complete questionnaires and it may be appropriate to make extensive—or even exclusive—use of proxy assessment. Proxy assessment may also be needed for young children who are unable to complete questionnaires, even though parents and other adults usually have a very different set of priorities from children, and value emotional and physical states differently. Sometimes it can be anticipated that a large proportion of the patients will become unable to complete questionnaires as the trial progresses, for example in trials of palliative care that involve rapidly deteriorating patients. In these cases the use of proxy respondents could be considered as an integral part of the trial. In general, however, proxy assessment is acceptable only as the last resort, and remains controversial.

The instructions to the patients should normally ask them to complete the forms on their own, that is, without conferring with others. The study forms should collect details of assistance or use of proxies.

> The patient should complete the questionnaire without conferring with friends or relatives, and all questions should be answered even if the patient feels them to be irrelevant. Assistance should be offered only if the patient is unable to complete the questions personally.

WILL QoL FORMS INFLUENCE THERAPY?

There are differing opinions as to the value of having QoL forms available for use by the treating clinician, or whether they should be confidential. For example, those patients who are keen for their therapy to be continued may be reticent about revealing deterioration in QoL or side-effects of treatment if they believe that their responses might cause treatment reduction. Also, some patients try to "please" their clinician and nursing staff, and may respond over-positively. Although evidence for this remains scanty, there is support from studies showing differences between QoL assessments completed by self-administered questionnaire versus interview-administered questionnaire, in which interview-assisted completion resulted in reduced reporting of impairments. A tendency for "yea-saying" or response acquiescence when filling in QoL questionnaires has also been noted (Moum, 1988). Thus it can be an advantage to assure patients that the QoL information is confidential and will not be seen by the clinician, and some trials supply pre-stamped envelopes that are addressed to the Trials Office.

On the other hand, in some hospitals the clinicians and nurses use the QoL forms to assist with patient management—which is of advantage to the trial organisation in that it may increase compliance with form completion. In addition, there are considerations of individual and collective ethics. From the point of view of guaranteeing bias-free interpretation, there are arguably grounds to maintain—and assure the patient of—confidentiality. Thus there are both advantages and disadvantages to keeping the forms confidential and not using them to influence therapy, but in either case the procedures should be standardised and specified.

> You will be given a folder of questionnaires and some reply-paid envelopes in which to return them. We would like you to complete one of these questionnaires just before you go to hospital at the start of each course of chemotherapy, for other treatment or at a routine check-up.
>
> [Reply-paid envelopes are addressed to the Trials Office]

PATIENT INFORMATION LEAFLETS

An initial leaflet may be provided prior to requesting informed consent from the patient. This can be combined with the general information leaflet that the patient receives when completing QoL questionnaires, or may be a separate brief document that is specifically given out during the consent process. In addition to describing the nature of randomised trials and discussing issues of relevance to consent, it should explain the reasons for evaluating QoL, and indicate what this involves. It should mention the frequency and timing of assessments.

If QoL is the primary endpoint in a trial it may be included as a condition on the patient consent form. Patients who are unwilling to contribute towards the primary endpoint of a trial should be ineligible for randomisation.

> We will also ask you to fill in a form, which assesses your quality of life, before you receive treatment and at 3, 6, 12 and 24 months after your treatment starts. The quality of life questionnaire is a standard form that is used for other patients and allows us to compare quality of life across various diseases. Because of this, there are some questions that may not seem relevant to your disease and its treatment. **However, please try to answer them all**.

The Patient QoL Information Leaflet is a detailed document that the patient may take away for reference. It should introduce the reasons for using questionnaires, explain aspects of the QoL assessment, and attempt to answer queries that patients commonly ask. Figure 13.2 shows an example.

RANDOMISATION CHECKLIST

Completion of the initial QoL assessment is often made a pre-requisite for randomisation. Not only does this provide baseline QoL data for all patients, but it also ensures that patients understand the procedure and, by implication, agree to participate in the study of QoL.

> **RANDOMISATION CHECKLIST**
>
> ELIGIBILITY (please tick to confirm)
>
> ⊔   Patient consents to participate in the trial, and patient is willing and able to complete QoL questionnaires.
> ⊔   Patient has completed the first QoL questionnaire.
>
> . . . . . .
>
> TO RANDOMISE, TELEPHONE THE TRIALS OFFICE.

QUALITY OF LIFE QUESTIONNAIRE

About your questionnaires

We are concerned to find out more about how patients feel, both physically and emotionally, during and after different treatments. In order to collect this information, brief questionnaires have been designed that can be completed by patients themselves. We would like you to complete questionnaires before, during and after your treatment at this hospital.

The questionnaires refer to how you have been feeling **during the past week** and are designed to assess your day-to-day well-being, as well as to monitor any side-effects you may be experiencing. Your questionnaires will be sent to the Medical Research Council where they will be treated in confidence and analysed together with those from patients in other hospitals to help plan future treatments.

We enquire about a wide range of symptoms as the questionnaires are designed for use in many different areas of research, but please feel free to discuss any symptoms or concerns with your doctor.

Completing the questionnaires

If possible, complete the questionnaires on your own. Please try to answer all the questions but do not spend too much time thinking about each answer as your first response is likely to be most accurate. If a question is not applicable to you, please write alongside 'not applicable' or 'N/A', but do not leave any question blank.

When you attend hospital for the first time, you will be asked to complete a questionnaire. We would like you to complete further questionnaires each time you come into hospital for an assessment. If you are not given a questionnaire to complete, please remind your doctor. You can, of course, decline to complete a questionnaire at any time without affecting your relationship with your doctor; however, the questionnaire will help us to acquire the knowledge to improve the treatment of patients with your condition.

Thank you for your help

Figure 13.2   Patient QoL Information Leaflet

CLINICAL FOLLOW-UP FORMS

The question "Has patient completed QoL forms?" serves as a reminder to the clinician and should protect against patients leaving the hospital before completing the questionnaire. Furthermore, in the event of refusal or other non-compliance—for example, if the patient feels too ill to complete the questionnaire—it is important to obtain details regarding the reasons. There should be a question "If no, give reasons . . . .". This information helps decide how to report and interpret results from patients for whom QoL data are missing.

The follow-up forms should also document whether significant help was required in order to complete the questions, or whether a proxy completed them.

FOLLOW-UP FORM

Has patient completed Quality of Life form?   ☐ Yes ☐ No
If **NO**, please state reason:

_____

If **YES**, indicate whether the patient required help completing the
form, and if so please give details:

_____

13.6 STANDARD OPERATING PROCEDURES

Although not usually part of the main clinical trial protocol sent to participating
clinicians, there is also a need for documentation of the standard operating procedures (SOPs) at the trials office, and an outline of the intended analysis plan. This
should be specified at the inception of the trial, and covers all aspects of the clinical
trial. In particular, for QoL it should detail the statistical analysis and interpretation
of the clinical trial results when there are missing data. Nowadays, the SOP is a
standard part of Good Clinical Practice (GCP).

13.7 SUMMARY AND CHECKLIST

There are many considerations when incorporating QoL assessment into clinical
trials. The most readily apparent of these is *compliance*. However, compliance is but
one of the issues that need to be addressed in a protocol, and it remains far too easy
to omit other necessary details. Hence the use of checklists is important. By ensuring
that all the details are covered, and provided there is adequate resources and
training, it should be possible to optimise the quality of the information collected
and the level of compliance achieved.

1. During the design stage of a study, sufficient financial resources should be
   available to provide an adequate infrastructure to manage the study and to
   integrate the QoL assessment into the normal daily practices of a clinic.
2. Objectives of the study should be presented clearly in the protocol, including
   the rationale for QoL, particularly if it is a main study endpoint.
3. It is preferred that QoL not be an optional evaluation.
4. Based on the objectives of the study, an appropriate valid instrument should
   be selected and if necessary additional treatment-specific questions should be
   developed, tested and added as appropriate. However, the number of items
   should be kept to a minimum.
5. The QoL questionnaire should be available in the appropriate languages in
   relation to potential participants in the clinical trial. If additional translations
   are required, they should be developed using tried and tested translation procedures.

6. The schedule of assessments should not be too much of a burden for the patient, yet at the same time it should be frequent enough and at appropriate time points to provide a relevant picture of the patients' QoL over the study period. For practical reasons, the schedule of QoL assessments should coincide with the routine clinical follow-up visits for the trial.

7. Statistical considerations in the protocol, including anticipated effect size, sample size and analysis plan, should be clear and precise.

8. Protocols should include guidelines on QoL data collection procedures for clinicians, research nurses and data managers.

9. There should be a policy of education for all those involved, from training for staff through to information documents for patients.

10. A cover form should be attached to the questionnaire. This should be completed if the patient did not complete the questionnaire, providing reasons for non-completion.

Figure 13.3 summarises the issues discussed in this chapter, and a protocol for a clinical trial should normally address all of the points enumerated here.

Are the following points addressed in the protocol?

1. ☐ Is rationale given for inclusion of QoL assessment?
2. ☐ Is importance of good compliance emphasised?
3. ☐ Is a named contact-person identified as responsible in each participating centre?
4. ☐ Are there written guidelines for the person administering the questionnaires?
5. ☐ Are all forms checked for completion whilst patient still present?
6. Timing of assessments:
   a. ☐ Are baseline assessments specified to be pre-randomisation?
   b. ☐ Is timing of follow-up assessments specified (valid window)?
   c. ☐ Is timing of follow-up assessments specified (before/whilst/after seeing clinician)?
7. ☐ Is it specified whether help and/or proxy assessment are permitted?
8. ☐ Will QoL forms be used to influence therapy or patient management?

Are the following forms and leaflets available?

9. PATIENT CONSENT INFORMATION LEAFLET (Pre-Consent Form):
   ☐ Is QoL assessment explained?
10. PATIENT QoL INFORMATION LEAFLET:
   ☐ Is there a leaflet for the patient to take home? [See specimen in Figure 13.2]
11. RANDOMISATION CHECKLIST:
   ☐ Is QoL completion a pre-randomisation eligibility condition?
12. CLINICAL FOLLOW-UP FORMS:
   a. ☐ Do follow-up forms ask whether QoL assessment has been completed?
   b. ☐ Do follow-up forms ask about reasons for any missing QoL data?
   c. ☐ Do follow-up forms ask whether help was needed?

Figure 13.3   Checklist for writing clinical trials protocols

14 Sample Sizes

Summary

This chapter describes how sample sizes may be estimated for QoL studies. To obtain such sample sizes it is necessary to specify, at the planning stage of the study, the size of effect that is expected. The type of statistical test to be used with the subsequent data needs to be stipulated, as do the significance level and power. Situations in which means, proportions, ordered categorical, and time-to-event outcomes are relevant are described. Sample size considerations are included for the difference between groups, comparison with a reference population and equivalence studies, as well as unpaired and paired situations. The consequences of comparing more than two groups or simultaneously investigating several endpoints are discussed.

14.1 INTRODUCTION

In principle, there are no major differences in planning studies using QoL assessment as compared with using, for example, a comparison of blood pressure levels between different groups. The determination of an appropriate design and study size remains as fundamentally important in this context as in others. A number of medical journals, including those specialising in QoL, stipulate in their statistical guidelines that a justification of sample size is required (Staquet *et al.*, 1996). A formal calculation of the sample size is an essential prerequisite for any clinical trial, and, for example, guidelines from the Committee for Proprietary Medicinal Products (CPMP, 1995) make it mandatory for all studies in the European Union. However, it must be recognised that one is usually designing a study in the presence of considerable uncertainty—the greater this uncertainty the less precise will be our estimate of the appropriate study size. Machin *et al.* (1997) provide detailed consideration of sample size issues in the context of clinical studies and also provide a PC-based program for the calculations.

14.2 SIGNIFICANCE TESTS, *P*-VALUES AND POWER

Previous chapters have referred extensively to statistical significance tests and *p*-values, for example when comparing two or more forms of therapy. Since patients vary both in their baseline characteristics and in their response to therapy, an apparent difference in treatments might be observed due to chance alone, and this need not necessarily indicate a true difference due to a treatment effect. Therefore it is customary to use a significance test to assess the *weight of evidence* and to estimate the probability that the observed data could in fact have arisen purely by chance. The results of the significance test will be expressed as a "p-value". For example, $p < 0.05$ indicates that so extreme an observed difference could only be expected to have arisen by chance alone less than 5% of the time, and so it is quite likely that a treatment difference really is present.

If few patients were entered into the trial then, even if there really is a true treatment difference, the results are likely to be less convincing than if a much larger number of patients had been assessed. Thus the weight of evidence in favour of concluding that there is a treatment effect will be less in a small trial than in a large one. In particular, if a clinical trial is too small it will be unlikely that one will obtain sufficiently convincing evidence of a treatment difference, even when there really is a difference in efficacy of the treatments. Small trials frequently conclude "there was no significant difference", irrespective of whether there really is a treatment effect or not. In statistical terms, we would say that the sample size is too small, and that the "power of the test" is very low. The *power*, $1 - \beta$, of a significance test is a measure of how likely a test is to produce a statistically significant result, on the assumption that there really is a true difference of a certain magnitude. The larger the study, the more likely it is to detect treatment effects that may exist, and so the higher its power.

Suppose the results of a treatment difference in a clinical trial are declared "not statistically significant". Such a statement indicates only that there was insufficient weight of evidence to be able to declare that the observed data are unlikely to have arisen by chance. It does not mean that there is no clinically important difference between the treatments. If the sample size was too small, the study might be very unlikely to obtain a significant p-value even when a clinically relevant difference is present. Hence it is of crucial importance to consider sample size and power both when planning studies and when interpreting statements about "non-significance".

14.3   ESTIMATING SAMPLE SIZE

To estimate the required sample size it is necessary to specify the test size α (significance level), the power $1 - \beta$, and the anticipated difference (effect size) in QoL that may be expected between alternative groups. Precedence often dictates that test size is two-sided at 5% and power is set as a minimum of 80%. However, in contrast to other endpoints in clinical studies, such as survival time in patients with cancer, there is seldom a large body of prior experience to quantify the anticipated differences with much precision. In addition, QoL is seldom summarised in terms of a single outcome variable; for example, the EORTC QLQ-C30 has 30 questions that are combined to produce essentially 15 different outcomes. Not only are there 15 different outcomes but they will often all be assessed on different occasions throughout the study thereby generating a longitudinal profile for each patient. Typically, in a clinical trial setting, assessments start immediately before randomisation, are at relatively frequent intervals during active therapy, and perhaps extend less frequently thereafter until death.

As we have already indicated, the anticipated effect size must be determined for each study based on experience, published data or pilot studies in order to estimate the appropriate sample size. However, it is first essential to identify and rank the QoL variables (scales or items) in order of importance for the specific study under consideration. For example, the investigators may know, from previous observation of patients with the specific disease and receiving standard therapy for the condition, that patients experience considerable fatigue. If one objective of the new therapy is to alleviate symptoms then fatigue could be regarded as the most important aspect of QoL and, in the context of a clinical trial, would be used for sample size determination purposes. The remaining QoL items then play a secondary role.

Once the principal endpoint variable has been established it is then necessary to identify how this is to be utilised to assess the outcome on a patient-by-patient basis. This may not be easy. As we have indicated in Chapter 8, this QoL variable is likely to be assessed several (perhaps many) times in each patient so that a summary is first required of each patient's profile. Thus Matthews et al. (1990) recommend that a series of observations be analysed through a series of summary measures obtained from each patient; for example the change from baseline QoL assessment to that at the end of active therapy, the time above a certain level, or the area under the curve (AUC).

Once this summary is determined, an average of this for each of the study therapies needs to be estimated. In the context of planning a randomised trial of two alternative therapies, these might be a standard or control treatment (C) and a test treatment (T). The control average can be obtained from previous experience of other or similar patients; for some instruments, such as the EORTC QLQ-C30, published reference data are available (Fayers et al., 1998b). It is then necessary to specify the benefit in QoL that is anticipated by use of the test therapy in place of the control. This too may be obtained from previous experience or may have to be elicited in some way using clinical opinion.

This benefit or effect size, Δ, has been variously defined as the "minimum value worth detecting" or a "clinically important effect" or "quantitatively significant" (see Chapter 16). Sometimes there may be neither the experience nor agreement of what constitutes a meaningful benefit to the patient (Hopwood et al., 1994). Cohen (1988) has suggested that, when there is an absence of other information about relevant sizes for effects, a small effect usually corresponds to $\Delta = 0.2$, a moderate effect to $\Delta = 0.5$ and a large effect to $\Delta = 0.8$ (see also Chapter 16). In general, the smaller the effect the larger the study.

Example

Chapter 1 introduced the Hospital Anxiety and Depression Scale (HADS) which is one method of assessing the psychological aspects of QoL in studies of cancer patients. Julious et al. (1997) provide a detailed summary of some HADS anxiety and depression data generated from 154 patients with small-cell lung cancer in a randomised trial conducted by Medical Research Council Lung Cancer Working Party (1996). The data for the anxiety scores are given in Table 14.1.

A practical advantage of the HADS instrument is that an estimate of clinically important levels of distress can be made using recommended cut-off scores for each subscale. Thus a score of 15 or more is regarded as a potential clinical case, perhaps signalling more detailed clinical examination and possibly treatment; a score between 8 and 10 is regarded as borderline, and one of ≤ 7 is regarded as normal. As a consequence, sometimes the actual score may be ignored and analysis based upon comparison of the proportions in these three categories for the different treatment groups.

Suppose we assume that the HADS domain for anxiety is the most important of the two domains and that the summary measure of most relevance is the HADS assessment two months post-randomisation. Then the endpoint of interest is one of the simplest possible.

Table 14.1 Frequency of responses on the HADS for anxiety for patients with small-cell lung cancer two months post-randomisation (Based on MRC Lung Cancer Working Party, 1996)

Category	Anxiety score	No. of patients
Normal	0	7
(0–7)	1	5
	2	20
	3	11
	4	11
	5	11
	6	11
	7	17
Borderline	8	13
(8–10)	9	7
	10	13
Case	11	7
(11–21)	12	2
	13	6
	14	4
	15	5
	16	2
	17	1
	18	0
	19	1
	20	0
	21	0
Total		154
Normal	0–7	93 (60.39%)
Borderline	8–10	33 (21.43%)
Case	11–21	28 (18.18%)
Median anxiety score	6	
Mean anxiety score	6.73	
SD	4.28	

There are several possible approaches to calculating the sample size required for data such as those of Table 14.1. One is to assume the data have (at least approximately) a Normal distribution. The second is to categorise the data into binary form; for example, "case" or "not case". A third is to categorise into more than two categories—for example, "case", "borderline" or "normal"—or to consider the full form of the data as an ordered categorical variable with, in our example, $\kappa = 22$ levels. Nevertheless, each approach requires specification of an anticipated effect size.

In the formulae given below, we give the total number of subjects required for a clinical study for a two-sided test size (or significance level) α and power $1 - \beta$. In these formulae, $z_{1-\alpha/2}$ and $z_{1-\beta}$ are the appropriate values from the standard Normal distribution for the $100(1 - \alpha/2)$ and $100(1 - \beta)$ percentiles respectively, obtained from Table T1.

Example calculations

The illustrative calculations in the examples use a two-sided significance level of 5% and a power of 80%. Thus, from Table T1, $z_{1-\alpha/2} = 1.96$ and $z_{1-\beta} = 0.8416$. The term $(z_{1-\alpha/2} + z_{1-\beta})^2$ occurs in many of the sample size equations, and for these values of power and significance level it equals 7.849.

14.4 COMPARING TWO GROUPS

MEANS—UNPAIRED

In a two-group comparative study where the outcome measure has a Normal distribution form, a two-sample t-test would be used in the final analysis (see Campbell and Machin, 1999). In this case the (standardised) anticipated effect size is $\Delta_{Normal} = (\mu_T - \mu_C)/\sigma$, where μ_T and μ_C are the anticipated means of the two treatments and σ is the SD of the QoL measurements and which is assumed the same for both treatment groups. On this basis, the number of patients to be recruited to the clinical trial is:

$$N_{Normal} = \frac{4(z_{1-\alpha/2} + z_{1-\beta})^2}{\Delta_{Normal}^2} + \frac{z_{1-\alpha/2}^2}{2}. \tag{14.1}$$

Example

The mean HADS anxiety score is $\bar{x} = 6.73$ with a large $SD = 4.28$, indicating a rather skew distribution far from the Normal form, as does the full anxiety distribution in Table 14.1. Consequently, it may not be advisable to use equation (14.1) directly to calculate sample size.

However, if the data are transformed using a logarithmic transformation then the transformed variable may have a distribution that approximates better to the Normal form. To avoid the difficulty of a logarithm of a zero score, each item on the scale can be coded 1 to 4 rather than of 0 to 3—with corresponding changes in boundaries, so that $y = \log_e(x + 7)$, where x is the HADS anxiety score on the original scale. In this case, the data of Table 14.1 lead to $\bar{y} = 2.5712$ and $SD(y) = 0.3157$. The distribution has a more Normal form on this transformed scale, and equation (14.1) could be applied once the effect size Δ_{Normal} is specified. Unfortunately there is no simple clinical interpretation for the y-scale, and so the inverse transformation is used to obtain scores corresponding to the HADS scale. Thus, for example, the value corresponding to $\bar{y}$ is $x = \exp(\bar{y}) - 7 = 6.0815$, and this is closer to the median than the original $\bar{x}$.

The object of therapy is to reduce problems of anxiety in the patients—that is, to increase the proportion classified as "normal"—and this corresponds to a desired reduction in HADS. We may postulate that the minimum clinically important difference to detect is a decrease in this equivalent to one unit on the HADS; that is, from 6.0815 to 5.0815. This is then expressed as an anticipated effect on the y scale as $\Delta_{Normal} = (\mu_T - \mu_C)/\sigma = [\log_e(5.0815 + 7) - \log_e(6.0815 + 7)]/0.3157 = (2.4917 - 2.5712)/0.3157 = -0.25$. This would be regarded as a small effect size, using the guidelines proposed by Cohen (1988). Using equation (14.1) with $\Delta_{Normal} = -0.25$ gives $N_{Normal} = 504$ patients or approximately 250 patients in each group.

The sample size obtained depends only on the absolute value of the anticipated difference between treatments and is independent of the direction of this difference. Thus the same sample size would be obtained if $\Delta_{Normal} = +0.25$ corresponding to, for example, a new more toxic therapy being investigated when an increase in HADS (corresponding to an increase in anxiety) was likely.

MEANS—PAIRED

Some QoL studies may be designed in a matched case–control format. In this situation, patients with a particular condition may be of interest and we may wish to compare their QoL with a comparative (non-diseased) group. This could be a comparison of elderly females with rheumatism against those without the disease. Thus for every patient identified, a control subject (female of the same age) is chosen and their QoL determined. The paired or matched difference between these two measures then gives an indication of their relative difference in QoL. These differences are then averaged over all N_{Pairs} of the case–control pairs, to provide the estimate of group differences.

On this basis, the number of patient–control pairs to be recruited to the clinical trial is

$$N_{Pairs} = \frac{(z_{1-\alpha/2} + z_{1-\beta})^2}{\Delta^2} + \frac{z_{1-\alpha/2}^2}{2}. \tag{14.2}$$

This expression is of a similar form to equation (14.1) but here there is a major difference in how $\Delta = \delta/\sigma_{Difference}$ is specified. Thus $\sigma_{Difference}$ here is the anticipated SD of the N differences between the case–control pairs. It is neither the SD of the case values themselves nor the SD of the corresponding control values, which is often of similar magnitude.

Machin et al. (1997, page 73) point out that there is a relationship between the SD for each subject group σ and the SD of the difference $\sigma_{Difference}$. Thus:

$$\sigma_{Difference} = \sigma\sqrt{2(1 - \rho)} \tag{14.3}$$

where ρ is the correlation coefficient between the values for the cases and their controls. An exploratory approach is to try out various values of ρ to see what influence this may have on the proposed sample size.

Example

Regidor *et al.* (1999, Table 3) give the mean physical functioning (PF) measured by the SF-36 Health Questionnaire in a reference group of 1063 women aged 65 years and older as 55.8 with $SD \approx 30$. The large SD here suggests that the distribution of the PF score may be rather skewed.

Suppose we are planning a case–control study in women 65 years or older who have rheumatism. It is anticipated that these women will have a lower PF by as much as 5 points. How many case–control pairs should the investigators recruit?

It is first worth noting that even if the distribution of PF scores is not itself of the Normal distribution form, the differences observed between cases and controls may approximate to this pattern. This is what is assumed.

In this example $\delta = 5$, and in order to determine the anticipated effect size $\Delta = \delta / \sigma_{Difference}$ we need a value for $\sigma_{Difference}$ itself, although we can assume $\sigma = 30$. Table 14.2 shows the different values for $\sigma_{Difference}$ depending on the value of ρ. For each of these values there is an effect size Δ, and finally the number of case–control pairs required is calculated from equation (14.2). Various options for the eventual study size are summarised in Table 14.2.

We can see from Table 14.2 that there is a wide range of potential study size which depends rather critically on how ρ effects $\sigma_{Difference}$ and hence Δ and ultimately N_{Pairs}. The numbers in this table have been rounded upwards to the nearest 10 subjects to acknowledge the inherent imprecision in the sample estimation process.

Table 14.2 Variation in size of a case–control study (two-sided $\alpha = 0.05$ and power $1 - \beta = 0.8$), assuming $\alpha = 5$ and $\sigma = 30$

ρ	0.0	0.2	0.4	0.6	0.8	0.9	0.95
$\sigma_{Difference}$	42.4	37.9	32.9	26.8	19.0	13.4	9.5
Δ	0.12	0.13	0.15	0.19	0.26	0.37	0.53
N_{Pairs}	550	470	360	220	120	60	30

PROPORTIONS—UNPAIRED

The statistical test used to compare two groups when the outcome is a binary variable is the Pearson χ^2 test for a 2×2 contingency table (see Campbell and Machin, 1999). In this situation the anticipated effect size is $\delta_{Binary} = (\pi_T - \pi_C)$, where π_T and π_C are the proportions of "normals" (however defined) with respect to depression in the two treatment groups. On this basis, the number of patients to be recruited to the clinical trial is

$$N_{Binary} = \frac{2(z_{1-\alpha/2} + z_{1-\beta})^2[\pi_T(1 - \pi_T) + \pi_C(1 - \pi_C)]}{\delta_{Binary}^2}. \tag{14.4}$$

Alternatively, the same difference between treatments may be expressed through the odds ratio (*OR*) which is defined as

$$OR_{Binary} = \frac{\pi_T(1 - \pi_C)}{\pi_C(1 - \pi_T)} \qquad (14.5)$$

This formulation leads to an alternative to equation (14.4) for the sample size. Thus:

$$N_{Odds\text{-}Ratio} = \frac{4(z_{1-\alpha/2} + z_{1-\beta})^2 / (\log OR_{Binary})^2}{\bar{\pi}(1 - \bar{\pi})}. \qquad (14.6)$$

where $\bar{\pi} = (\pi_C + \pi_T)/2$. Equations (14.4) and (14.6) are quite dissimilar in form, but Julious and Campbell (1996) show that they give, for all practical purposes, very similar sample sizes, with divergent results occurring for relatively large (or small) OR_{Binary}.

Example

Table 14.1 indicates that there are approximately 60% of patients classified as "normal" with respect to anxiety. Suppose it is anticipated that this may improve to 70% in the "normal" category with an alternative treatment. The anticipated treatment effect is thus $\delta_{Binary} = (\pi_T - \pi_C) = (70 - 60)\% = 10\%$. This equates to a total sample size of $N_{Binary} = 706$ from equation (14.4).

Alternatively, this anticipated treatment effect can be expressed as $OR_{Binary} = (70/30)/(60/40) = 1.5556$. Using this in equation (14.6), with $\bar{\pi} = (0.70 + 0.60)/2 = 0.65$, also gives a total sample size of $N_{Odds\text{-}Ratio} = 706$ patients. As noted, the difference between the calculations from the alternative formulae is usually small and inconsequential.

PROPORTIONS—PAIRED

In the matched case–control format discussed above, the comparison of elderly females with rheumatism to those without the disease may be summarised as "Good" or "Poor" QoL. Thus the possible pairs of responses are (Good, Good); (Good, Poor); (Poor, Good) and (Poor, Poor). The McNemar test for such paired data (see Campbell and Machin, 1999) counts the number of the N_{Pairs} which are either (Good, Poor) or (Poor, Good). If these are s and t respectively, the odds ratio for comparing cases and controls is estimated by $\psi = s/t$, and the proportion of discordant pairs by $\pi_{Discordant} = (s + t)/N_{Pairs}$. To estimate the corresponding study size, anticipated values for ψ and $\pi_{Discordant}$ need to be specified. Then:

$$N_{Pairs} = \frac{\left\{ z_{1-\alpha/2}(\psi + 1) + z_{1-\beta}\sqrt{(\psi + 1)^2 - (\psi - 1)^2 \pi_{Discordant}} \right\}^2}{(\psi - 1)^2 \pi_{Discordant}} \qquad (14.7)$$

Example

Suppose in the case–control study discussed previously in women 65 years or older who have rheumatism, their overall QoL is to be summarised as Good or Poor and so is that of their controls. It is anticipated that a major difference in the odds ratio will be observed, so a value of $\psi = 4$ is specified. It is further anticipated that the discordance rate will probably be somewhere between 0.5 and 0.8. How many case–control pairs should be recruited?

In this example $\psi = 4$, which is itself the anticipated effect size, we also need to specify $\pi_{Discordant}$. Table 14.3 shows some options for the study size differing for values of $\pi_{Discordant}$ calculated using equation (14.7).

The numbers in this table have been rounded upwards to the nearest 10 subjects in recognition of the inherent imprecision in the sample estimation process.

Table 14.3 Variation in size of a matched case–control study, assuming $\psi = 4$ (two sided $\alpha = 0.05$ and power $1 - \beta = 0.8$)

$\pi_{Discordant}$	0.5	0.6	0.7	0.8
N_{Pairs}	90	60	50	40

Just as we saw for paired means, it is often difficult to anticipate the impact of pairing upon sample size estimates because the calculations require more information than for unpaired designs. Usually, the purpose of pairing or matching is to obtain a more sensitive comparison—that is, to reduce sample size requirements. Thus the sample size needed for a paired design should usually be less than for an unpaired one, and may often be appreciably less.

ORDERED CATEGORICAL DATA

Transformation of the data when dealing with a variable that does not have a Normal distribution leads to difficulties in interpretation on the transformed scale and, in particular, the provision of an anticipated effect size. It would be easier if the original scale could be preserved for this purpose. In fact the data of Table 14.1 are from an ordered categorical variable and the statistical test used when the outcome is ordered categorical is the Mann–Whitney U-test with allowance for ties (see Conover, 1998). Thus it would be more natural to extend from the comparison of two proportions, which is a special case of an ordered categorical variable of $\kappa = 2$ levels, to $\kappa = 22$ levels for the HADS data. Formulating the effect size in terms of OR_{Binary} rather than δ_{Binary}, enables this extension to be made. The estimated sample size is given by Whitehead (1993) as

$$N_{Categorical} = \frac{12(z_{1-\alpha/2} + z_{1-\beta})^2 / (\log OR_{Categorical})^2}{\left[1 - \sum_{i=0}^{\kappa-1} \bar{\pi}_i^3\right]}, \tag{14.8}$$

where the mean proportion expected in category i ($i = 0$ to $\kappa - 1$) is $\bar{\pi} = (\pi_{Ci} + \pi_{Ti})/2$, and π_{Ci} and π_{Ti} are the proportions expected in category i for the treatment groups C and T.

The categories are labelled as 0 to $\kappa - 1$, rather than 1 to κ, so that they correspond directly to the actual HADS category scores of Table 14.1. Here, the $OR_{Categorical}$ is an extension of the definition of OR_{Binary} given in equation (14.8) and is now the odds of a subject being in category i or below in one treatment group compared with the other. It is calculated from the cumulative proportion of subjects for each category 0, 1, 2, . . . , $(\kappa - 1)$ and is assumed to be constant through the scale.

The effect size in equation (14.8), as summarised through $OR_{Categorical}$, implies an assumption of proportional odds. This means, that each adjacent pair of categories for which an OR can be calculated, that is OR_1, OR_2, . . ., OR_{21} for the HADS, all have the same true or underlying value $OR_{Categorical}$. Thus the odds of falling into a given category or below is the same irrespective of where the HADS scale is dichotomised. This appears to be a very restrictive assumption but, for planning purposes, what is of greatest practical importance is that although the ORs may vary along the scale, the underlying treatment effect should be in the same direction throughout the scale. Thus all ORs are anticipated to be greater than 1 or all are anticipated to be less than 1.

When using an ordered categorical scale the ORs are a measure of the chance of a subject being in each given category or less in one group compared with the other. For the HADS data there are 21 distinct ORs. However, the problem is simplified because the OR anticipated for the binary case, that is the proportions either side the "caseness" cut-off, can be used as an average estimate of the OR in the ordered categorical situation (Campbell, Julious and Altman, 1995). Thus, if the trial size is to be determined with a Mann–Whitney U-test in mind rather than the χ^2 test for a 2×2 table, then the anticipated treatment effect is still taken to be OR_{Binary}.

Julious *et al.* (1997) illustrate the evaluation of equation (14.8). First Q_{Ci}, the cumulative proportions in category i for treatment C, are calculated using, for example, tables of reference values. Then, for a given (constant) $OR_{Categorical}$ the anticipated cumulative proportions for each category of treatment T are given by

$$Q_{Ti} = \frac{OR_{Category} Q_{Ci}}{OR_{Category} Q_{Ci} + (1 - Q_{Ci})} \qquad (14.9)$$

After calculating the cumulative proportions, the anticipated proportions falling in each treatment category, $\bar{\pi}_{Ti}$, can be determined from the difference of successive Q_{Ti}. Finally, the combined mean of the proportions of treatments C and T for each category is calculated.

We have assumed here that the alternative to the binary case ($\kappa = 2$) is the full categorical scale ($\kappa = 22$). In practice, however, it may be more appropriate to group some of the categories but not others to give κ categories, where $3 \leq \kappa < 22$. For example, merging the HADS scores into the "caseness" groups defined earlier would give $\kappa = 3$, while $\kappa = 5$ if the "caseness" categories are extended in the manner described below.

Although there are 22 possible categories for the full HADS scales, it is reasonable to ask whether the full distribution needs to be specified for planning purposes. In many situations, it may not be possible to specify the whole distribution precisely, whereas to anticipate the proportions in a somewhat fewer number of categories may be plausible. The HADS scale is often divided into three categories for clinical use: "normal" (≤ 7), "borderline" (8 to 10) and "clinical case" (≥ 11). For illustration purposes only, we define two additional categories: "very normal" (≤ 3) and "severe case" (≥ 16). Thus HADS scores 0 to 3 are "very normal", 4 to 7 "normal", 8 to 10 "borderline", 11 to 15 "case", and finally 16 to 22 "severe case".

Example

Table 14.4 gives, for the data of Table 14.1, the number of cases and cumulative proportions anticipated in each category for the anxiety dimension if we re-categorised the HADS anxiety scale into five categories as above.

Assuming $OR_{Categorical} = OR_{Binary} = 1.5556$ as we calculated above, then, for example, the anticipated proportion for category 2 of treatment T is from equation (14.6):

$$Q_{T2} = OR_{Category} \, Q_{C2}/[OR_{Category} \, Q_{C2} + (1 - Q_{C2})]$$
$$= 1.5556 \times 0.6039/[1.5556 \times 0.6039 + (1 - 0.6039)] = 0.7034.$$

The remaining values are summarised in Table 14.2. Values of π_{Ti} are calculated from the difference of successive Q_{Ti}; for example, $\pi_{T2} = 0.7034 - 0.3760 = 0.3274$. The final column of the table gives the corresponding values of $\bar{\pi}_i = (\pi_{Ci} + \pi_{Ti})$. The denominator of equation (14.5) is therefore

$$1 - [0.3276^3 + 0.3260^3 + 0.1929^3 + 0.1320^3 + 0.0214^3] = 1 - 0.0793 = 0.9207,$$

and finally from equation (14.8), $N_{Categorical} = 524$.

Repeating the calculations with the three categories for HADS (normal, borderline, case), the corresponding sample size is $N_{Categorical} = 680$. Finally, reducing the categories to "normal" versus the remainder ("borderline" and "cases"), $N_{Binary} = 712$. The increasing sample size suggests that the more we can assume about the form of the data then, provided the appropriate analysis is also made, the smaller the study need be.

Table 14.4 Number of patients with small-cell lung cancer two months post-randomisation categorised into "caseness" groups following assessment using HADS for anxiety. Cumulative proportions observed on standard therapy C and anticipated with test therapy T (Data from MRC Lung Cancer Working Party, 1996)

| Category | Anxiety score | Number of C patients | π_{Ci} | Cumulative proportions | | π_{Ti} | $\bar{\pi}_i$ |
				Q_C	Q_T		
Very normal	0–3	43	0.2792	0.2792	0.3760	0.3760	0.3276
Normal	4–7	50	0.3246	0.6039	0.7034	0.3274	0.3260
Borderline	8–10	33	0.2143	0.8182	0.8750	0.1716	0.1929
Case	11–15	24	0.1558	0.9740	0.9831	0.1081	0.1320
Severe case	16–22	4	0.0260	1	1	0.0169	0.0214
Total		154					

TIME-TO-EVENT DATA

Sometimes the endpoint of interest can be the time from randomisation until a patient achieves a particular value of their QoL. For example, suppose patients with a HADS of 10 or less (normal and borderline) will be recruited into a trial, and that it is also known that many of these patients will experience deterioration (increasing HADS) whilst receiving active therapy, but may then achieve improvement over their admission values. If a clinically important improvement is regarded as a HADS decrease of 2 points, then, with repeat assessments, one can observe if and when this first occurs. For those patients who experience the defined improvement, the time in days from baseline assessment to this outcome can be determined. For those who do not improve sufficiently, perhaps deteriorating rather than improving, their time to improvement will be censored at their most recent QoL assessment. The eventual analysis will involve Kaplan–Meier estimates of the corresponding cumulative survival curves, where here "survival" is "time to improvement", and comparisons between treatments can be made using the logrank test (Parmar and Machin, 1995).

To estimate the size of a trial, one can utilise the anticipated proportion of patients who have improved at, say, 12 weeks in the C and T groups respectively. However, in the actual study we will be determining as precisely as possible the exact time that the patient shows the QoL improvement specified.

In this situation the size of the anticipated effect is determined by the *hazard ratio*, Δ, the value of which can be obtained from

$$\Delta = \frac{\log_e \pi_C}{\log_e \pi_T} \tag{14.10}$$

where, in this case, π_C and π_T are the anticipated proportions improving (here by 12 weeks) with C and T therapy respectively. Once Δ is obtained, the number of patients that are required for the study is given by

$$N_{Survival} = \frac{2\left[\frac{(z_{1-\alpha/2} + z_{1-\beta})(1 + \Delta)}{(1 - \Delta)}\right]^2}{(2 - \pi_T - \pi_C)}. \tag{14.11}$$

Example

Suppose, $\pi_C = 0.65$ but it is anticipated that the test treatment will be effective in improving this to $\pi_T = 0.75$ at 12 weeks. In this case, $\Delta = \log_e 0.75/\log_e 0.65 \approx 1.50$. Substituting these values in equation (14.10) gives $N_{Survival} = 660$.

One aspect of a trial, which can effect the number of patients recruited, is the proportion of patients who are lost to follow-up during the trial. Such patients have censored observations determined by the date last observed, as do those for whom the event of interest (here decreasing HADS anxiety score of 2 points) has not occurred at the end of the trial. If the anticipated proportion of censored patients is w, then the sample sizes given in equation (14.11) should be increased to compensate by dividing by $1 - w$.

14.5 COMPARISON WITH A REFERENCE POPULATION

If a study is comparing a group of patients with a reference-population value for the corresponding QoL measure, then effectively one is assuming that the reference-population value is known. As a consequence, this is not estimated from within the study and so subjects are not needed for this component. Hence fewer subjects will be required overall.

MEANS

In this case, when the population or reference mean QoL is known the sample size necessary is given by equation (14.1), but with the 4 removed from the numerator in the first term. This effectively reduces the sample size required, compared with a two-group comparison, by one quarter. The final term of equation (14.1) is important only in small samples and usually may be omitted. For example, in the case of $z_{1-\alpha/2} = 1.96$ the final term is $1.96^2/2 \approx 2$.

PROPORTIONS

If a study is comparing the proportion of patients with (say) good QoL with a reference-population value for the same QoL measure, then effectively one is assuming that the reference-population proportion is known and is not estimated from within the study. In this case, provided the proportions are close, the sample size necessary is given as approximately one-quarter that given by either equations (14.4) or (14.6).

TIME-TO-EVENT DATA

In time-to-event studies the hazard ratio Δ is the measure of the effect size. Suppose a pilot study is planned to compare the time taken for patients to return (post-operatively) to good QoL in a hospital just introducing a new procedure. The reference population value, $\pi_{Reference}$, may be obtained as the proportion reported in a review of the literature. In this case the sample size necessary is given by

$$n = \frac{\Delta^2 (z_{1-\alpha/2} + z_{1-\beta})^2}{(1 - \Delta)^2 (1 - \pi_{Reference})}. \tag{14.12}$$

Example

Suppose in the above pilot study the proportion who return (post-operatively) to good QoL in the reference-population value is 0.7 at 3 weeks. The hospital has made some changes to the techniques and hopes to do better than that, possibly to achieve 0.8 by the same point in time. In this case, equation (14.10) gives an anticipated $\Delta = \log 0.7/\log 0.8 = 1.598$ and equation (14.12) gives $n = 187$ patients.

However, if it is anticipated that for various reasons up to 10% of patients may not be assessable for one reason or another, then $w = 0.1$, and the sample size may be increased to 187/0.9, which is approximately 210 patients.

14.6 EQUIVALENCE STUDIES

Sometimes, in a clinical trial of a new treatment for patients with (say) a life-threatening disease such as cancer, it may be anticipated that the treatment will at best bring only modest survival advantage. In such circumstances, any gain might be offset by a loss of QoL. Or, perhaps a new treatment is more convenient or cheaper. From the QoL perspective, we may wish to know that the new treatment is *equivalent* to the standard treatment with respect to QoL outcomes. However, it is important to realise that failure to find a "statistically significant" difference between treatments after completing a trial does not mean the two treatments are equivalent. It frequently means the trial was too small to detect the (small) actual difference between treatments. Indeed, with a finite number of subjects one can never prove that two groups are exactly equivalent. However, having conducted a study to compare groups, one can calculate the summary QoL at a key stage for each group, and a $100(1 - \alpha)\%$ confidence interval (*CI*) for the true difference, δ, between them. This *CI* covers the true difference with a given probability, $1 - \alpha$. At the design stage of an equivalence study, we need to specify α and also a limit, ε (> 0), which is termed the *range of equivalence* or the maximum allowable difference between the QoL measure in the two groups. We set this so that if we ultimately observe an actual difference no greater then ε, then we would accept that the two groups are essentially equivalent. We also need to specify the power, $1 - \beta$, that the upper confidence limit (*UL*) for δ, calculated once the study is completed, will not exceed this pre-specified value ε.

Earlier, when comparing two means or two proportions, we implied a null hypothesis of $\theta_1 = \theta_2$, where θ_1 and θ_2 are the parameters we wish to estimate with our study. Thus in the conventional test of significance we seek to test $\delta = \theta_1 - \theta_2 = 0$. In testing for equivalence this is modified to testing $\theta_1 = \theta_2 + \varepsilon$ against the alternative one-sided hypothesis $\theta_1 < \theta_2 + \varepsilon$. These considerations lead to a $100(1 - \alpha)\%$ confidence interval for $\delta = \theta_1 - \theta_2$ of

$$LL \text{ to } [Difference + z_{1-\alpha}SE(Difference)]. \tag{14.13}$$

Here the value of *LL* (the lower confidence limit) depends on the context but not on the data (see below). Note that since this is a so-called one-sided *CI* it uses $z_{1-\alpha}$ not $z_{1-\alpha/2}$.

The earlier formulae give the total number of subjects required for a clinical study for a two-sided test size (or significance level) α and power $1 - \beta$. In this section the calculations use a one-sided significance level of 5% and a power of 80%; thus from Table T1, $z_{1-\alpha} = 1.6449$ and $z_{1-\beta} = 0.8416$.

MEANS

When two means are compared, the lower limit for the *CI* of equation (14.13) is $LL = -\infty$; that is, negative infinity. The total sample size, $N_{Equivalence}$, required for a comparison of means from two groups of equal size and anticipated to have the same population mean and *SD*, σ, is

$$N_{Equivalence} = \frac{4(z_{1-\alpha} + z_{1-\beta})^2}{\Delta^2},$$ (14.14)

where $\Delta = \varepsilon/\sigma$ can be thought of as the effect size.

Example

Suppose that, following a period in hospital, elderly patients with no potential family support may either be discharged to their own home, with additional home-help provided, or to institutional care. Although home-care is considered the best option, there is concern that QoL may be compromised in those referred for institutional care.

Regidor *et al.* (1999, Table 3) give the mean social functioning (SF), measured by the SF-36 health questionnaire in a reference group of women aged 65 years and older, as 78.1 with *SD* approximately 25. In the group to be studied, SF will be less and may be closer to 65. The clinical team will regard the two approaches to be essentially equivalent if SF in the institutional care group is no more than 5 points below this figure.

Thus setting $\varepsilon = 5$ and $\sigma = 25$ gives $\Delta = 5/25 = 0.2$ and, from equation (14.14), $N_{Equivalence} = 620$ subjects, with half to be discharged home and the others to institutional care.

PROPORTIONS

We assume that the outcome of the trial can be expressed as the proportion of patients with good or poor QoL. After testing for equivalence of the treatments, we would wish to assume the probabilities of Good QoL are for all practicable purposes equal, although we might have evidence that they do in fact differ by a small amount. For this comparison $LL = -1$ in equation (14.13), as that is the maximum difference in the proportion of responses in the two groups.

The total sample size, $N_{Equivalence}$, required for a comparison of proportions from two groups of equal size and anticipated to have the same population proportion π is

$$N_{Equivalence} = \frac{4\pi(1 - \pi)(z_{1-\alpha} + z_{1-\beta})^2}{\varepsilon^2},$$ (14.15)

14.7   CHOICE OF SAMPLE SIZE METHOD

It is important when designing any study to obtain a relevant sample size. In so doing it is important to make maximal use of any background information available. Such information may come from other related studies and may be quite detailed and precise, or it may come from a reasonable extrapolation of observations from unrelated studies, in which case it may be regarded as very imprecise. It is clear that the more we know, or realistically assume, of the final outcome of our trial at the planning stage the better we can design the trial. In our example, we have detailed knowledge of HADS outcome at 2 months, based on more than 150 patients. We may be fairly confident, therefore, that provided the treatment C in a planned new trial remains unaltered and the patient mix remains the same, we can use this distribution for planning purposes. If the trial is to test a new therapy T, then possibly apart from some very preliminary data, we may have little information about the effect of T on QoL. In this case, we suggest that the investigator has to decide if he or she wishes to detect, say, a 1-, 2- or 3-point change in the average HADS score. This change has then to be expressed as an anticipated effect size before the sample size equations given here can be applied. The smaller the anticipated benefit, the larger the subsequent trial. If an investigator is uncomfortable about the assumptions then it is good practice to calculate sample size under a variety of scenarios so that the sensitivity to assumptions can be assessed.

In general, when designing a clinical trial there will often be other variables (covariates), apart from allocated treatment itself, such as gender, age, centre or stage of disease. These may or may not affect the clinical outcome. Such variables may be utilised to create different strata for treatment allocation purposes, and can also be used in the final analysis. If the QoL variable itself can be assumed to have a Normal distribution, then the final analysis may adjust for these variables using a multiple regression approach. If a binary type of measure of QoL has been used, then the covariates can be assessed by means of a logistic regression model (Campbell and Machin, 1999). Similarly, if a "time-to-event" measure of QoL is being used then the covariates can be assessed by means of a Cox proportional hazards model as described by Parmar and Machin (1995).

We have used a transformation approach for non-Normal data, illustrated by the logarithmic transformation, and made sample size calculations accordingly. Other common transformations for this purpose are the *reciprocal* or *square-root*. A difficulty with the use of transformations is that they distort the scales and makes interpretation of treatment effects difficult. In fact, only the logarithmic transformation (with, in order to remove zeros, each item on the HADS coded 1 to 4 instead of 0 to 3 and corresponding changes in boundaries) gives results interpretable on the original scale (Bland and Altman, 1996). The logarithmic transformation expresses the effect as a ratio of geometric means. A geometric mean of n positive observations is the nth root of the product of all these observations. However, this ratio will vary in a way which depends on the geometric mean value of treatment C. For example, if the geometric mean for treatment C is 6 and treatment T induces a change in HADS of -1 compared with this level, then this implies an effect size of log $(5/6) = -0.18$. On the other hand, for a geometric mean of 14 for treatment C but the same numerical change of -1 induced by T implies an effect size of log $(13/14) = -0.07$. Thus although in this example the effect size is -1 in both cases when expressed on the HADS scale, the logarithmic transformation results in one effect size which is less than half $(-0.07/-0.18 = 0.39)$ the former. This makes interpretation difficult.

As we have indicated, it is not uncommon that, when designing a trial where a QoL measure is the primary measure of interest, there is little prior knowledge of the full distribution of the scores. Thus the very detailed information provided by Table 14.1 might not be available. However, this need not necessarily present a major problem for the full ordered categorical approach to sample size calculation.

Whitehead (1993) indicates that knowledge of the anticipated distribution within four or five broad categories is often sufficient. This information, which may be solicited from experience gained by the clinical team, can then be used to aid the design of studies using HADS and other QoL instruments.

For sample size purposes when repeated measures of the same QoL item are involved, a recommended approach to design and analysis is to choose either a key observation time as the endpoint observation; or to use a summary statistic such as the *AUC*. A summary of these basic observations will then provide the values for the groups being compared and the basis for the sample size determination.

In circumstances where three or more groups are being compared, then we recommend calculating the sample size appropriate for each possible comparison. This will provide a range of possible sample sizes per treatment group. It is then a matter of judgement as to which should be used for the final study—the largest of these will be the safest option but may result in too large a study for the resources available. If the number of groups is large, then some note may have to be taken of the resulting numbers of significance tests. One possibility is to use a Bonferroni adjustment (see the next section) for the sample size. In some circumstances, the different groups may themselves form an ordered categorical variable; for example, no intervention, limited intervention and intensive intervention. In this case, there is a structure across the intervention groups, and a test for trend may be appropriate. Then no Bonferroni adjustment need be considered.

14.8 MULTIPLE ENDPOINTS

Earlier in this chapter we indicated that it is very important to decide on a principal QoL endpoint. If there are additional endpoints, then it is advisable to rank these in order of importance. We recognise that in many situations there may be a very long list of QoL variables but would urge that those that are to be included in a formal analysis should be confined to at most four or five. The remainder should be consigned to exploratory hypothesis-generating analyses or descriptive purposes only. However, if analyses of the four or five endpoint variables are to be made, then some recognition of the multiple statistical testing that will occur should be taken into account during the planning process.

In practice, it is very unlikely that the anticipated effect sizes would be of the same magnitude or direction. Thus, for example, $k = 4$ endpoints denoted (in rank order of importance) by $\Omega_{(1)}$, $\Omega_{(2)}$, $\Omega_{(3)}$ and $\Omega_{(4)}$ might be used separately in four sample size calculations and four different estimates are likely to result. The final study size is then likely to be a compromise between the sizes so obtained. Whatever the final size, it should be large enough to satisfy the requirements for the endpoint corresponding to $\Omega_{(1)}$ as this is the most important endpoint and hence the primary objective of the trial.

To guard against false statistical significance as a consequence of multiple testing, it is a sensible precaution to consider replacing the test size α in the various equations by an adjusted size using the *Bonferroni correction*, which is

$$\alpha_{Bonferroni} = \alpha/k. \qquad (14.16)$$

Thus $\alpha_{Bonferroni}$ is substituted instead of α in the sample size equations given above. For $k = 4$ and $\alpha = 0.05$, $\alpha_{Bonferroni} = 0.05/4 = 0.0125$. Such a change will clearly lead to larger sample sizes since, for $\alpha = 0.05$, $z = 1.96$ from Table T1; whereas for $\alpha = 0.0125$, z is approximately 2.50 and the numerators of, for example, equation (14.1) will both be larger.

14.9 CONCLUSION

When designing any study there is usually a whole range of possible options to discuss at the early design stage. We would therefore recommend that various anticipated benefits be considered, ranging from the optimistic to the more realistic, with sample sizes being calculated for several scenarios within that range. It is a matter of judgement, rather than an exact science, as to which of the options is chosen for the final study size.

In QoL studies there are many potential endpoints. As we have stressed, it is important that a clear focus be directed to identifying the major ones (at most five). This is clearly important for sample size purposes, but it is also necessary to state these endpoints clearly in the associated study protocol and to ensure that they are indeed the main focus of the subsequent report of the completed study.

We would recommend, when an ordered categorical variable such as HADS is the QoL outcome measure, that equation (14.5) is utilised directly. This is preferable to seeking a transformation that enables the formula for a Normal variable (equation (14.1)) to be used. The major reason is that this retains the "benefit" on the original QoL scale and therefore will be more readily interpreted. Although the associated methods of analysis are less familiar, statistical software is now available for these calculations.

Finally, it should be noted that if time-to-event endpoints are to be determined with any precision, there must be careful choice of the timing of QoL assessments. This is to ensure that for each patient the date when the event occurs can be determined reasonably precisely. Time-to-event techniques are unlikely to be useful if the assessment intervals are lengthy.

15   Practical and Reporting Issues

Summary

At various stages in the book we have indicated issues on which decisions have to be made when analysing, presenting and reporting QoL studies. With the wealth of data that are usually generated, it is clear that compromises have to be made and these mean that the major focus will need to be placed on a relatively few aspects. Choices made will have implications ranging from the way compliance is summarised to which particular comparisons will be presented with the associated confidence intervals. Although QoL data pose unique difficulties, there are general aspects of presenting and reporting the results of clinical studies that should always be adhered to. We assume that good reporting standards are indeed followed, and our focus will be on those aspects that relate to QoL studies in particular.

15.1   INTRODUCTION

Guidelines to assist investigators on reporting QoL studies have been suggested by Staquet *et al.* (1996). These have, by their very nature, addressed aspects of QoL but also contain more general recommendations for all types of clinical studies. Thus these guidelines contain elements of the *BMJ* checklists (*British Medical Journal*, 1996) for evaluating the statistical aspects of medical studies, and the later CONSORT statement (Begg *et al.*, 1996) on reporting clinical trials. The checklists were developed following experience in statistical assessment of papers submitted to medical journals, whilst CONSORT arose as a direct consequence of poor reporting standards for randomised clinical trials in particular.

Nevertheless, and perhaps owing to the unfamiliarity of clinical researchers, editors of medical journals and regulatory agencies with the field of QoL studies, the reporting of such studies calls for improvement. Weaknesses of the published reports of QoL in clinical trials have ranged from lack of information on specific items such as the psychometric properties of the instruments, and the handling of missing data caused especially through patient attrition.

15.2   DESIGN ISSUES

INSTRUMENTS

The justification for the selection of a health profile (descriptive) and/or a patient preference (utility) approach for the QoL assessment as well as of a particular questionnaire should be given. If a QoL instrument is not well known or is new, it must be described in detail and the psychometric properties should be summarized. The rationale for creating a new instrument and the method by which the items were created is indispensable. For disease-specific instruments an indication as to whether or not the psychometric properties were established in the same type of population as the study subjects is essential.

Of particular importance are the time frame over which the subject has to assess their responses to the items of the questionnaire (for example, the past week), and the method by which the instrument was administered (for example, by face-to-face interview). If appropriate, information on the process by which the measure was adapted for cross-cultural administration must be detailed.

Sources relevant to the development and format of the chosen QoL instruments should be referenced. When an instrument, item or scale is being used in a new population or disease from that in which it was originally developed, the psychometric properties of the instrument in the new context must be reported.

The choice of instrument will often be specific to the type of patients involved— for example, oral health (Slade, 1998) or vision-related QoL (Frost et al., 1998).

TYPE OF STUDY

The choice of study design is always crucial. However, in most situations the QoL assessment will be repeated with each subject on two or more occasions, and hence the study will be both prospective and longitudinal in nature. The design options are therefore limited in number. It could either be a follow-up study of a single cohort of subjects with any comparisons made between subject types within the cohort, or a two (or more) group comparison of which the randomised parallel group trial is a specific example. Rarely, if ever, will a crossover design be appropriate in QoL studies.

SIZE

In a comparative study, and particularly a randomised trial, the anticipated effect size that it is planned to detect should be specified. As indicated in Chapter 14, an estimate of the required sample size calculated on the basis of the endpoints of the study should be provided. The test size (α) and power ($1 - \beta$) must be specified. If a one-sided test is used it needs to be justified.

ORGANISATIONAL ISSUES

There are often choices within a QoL study as to when and by whom the instrument is to be completed. Even in the context of self-completed QoL instruments there will be occasions when help is needed, perhaps for an elderly person who can comprehend but not easily complete a questionnaire, or for someone with vision difficulties. It is often important to specify if the instrument is to be completed before or after a clinic appointment with the responsible physician, and whether or not the physician has knowledge of the patient responses when conducting the medical examination. Some of these options may influence the responses.

PROTOCOL

As with any clinical study, it is important to describe the details of the study in a protocol. This may also be a requirement of the investigators' local Ethical Committee. The protocol should not only describe the main purpose of the study and the target subjects or patient group, but also address specific issues. These issues include the principal hypotheses and the QoL outcomes to which they relate; the definition of "clinically important QoL differences" used for sample size estimation; and strategies for minimising the number of missing QoL forms.

15.3 DATA ANALYSIS

When describing the choice of instrument, it is important to give details of how the responses are scored, preferably by reference to a published scoring manual or other available source document. Any departure from such procedures should be detailed and justified. Information on how to interpret the scores is necessary; for example, do higher scores indicate better or worse functioning or symptoms?

Ideally, only those QoL endpoints that were defined before the trial commenced should be used for the formal analysis. For these endpoints, confidence intervals and *p*-values should be quoted. Other variables will be used only for descriptive purposes and to generate hypotheses for testing in later studies.

The statistical methods of analysis must be described in sufficient detail for other researchers to be able to repeat the analysis if the full data were made available. When appropriate, assumptions about the distribution of the data should be indicated. It should be indicated whether the analysis is by "intention to treat" or otherwise. In case of multiple comparisons, attention must be paid to the total number of comparisons, to the adjustment, if any, of the significance level, and to the interpretation of the results. If applicable, the definition of a clinically important difference should be given.

MISSING ITEMS

It is imperative to document the causes of all missing data. Several types of missing data are possible and should be identified and documented separately in the publication. If patients or subjects fail to compete all items on a QoL instrument, possibly accidentally, then the corresponding Scoring Manual for the instrument will usually describe methods of calculating scale-scores when there are a few missing values for some items. Particular note should be taken if missing data tend to concern particular items on the QoL instrument or occur with a certain type of patient.

In the study report, the percentages of missing data for each item in the questionnaire should be compared, always focusing on the pre-specified major endpoints. Any difference in the percentages by patient group should be commented upon.

MISSING FORMS

It should be specified whether missing data are due to informative (non-random) censoring—that is, due to the patient's health state or particular treatment—or to non-informative (essentially random) censoring mechanisms. The methods by which missing data were defined and analysed, including any imputation methods, must be clearly stated. In appropriate contexts, it is important to specify how data from patients who die before attaining the study endpoints are dealt with in the analysis.

As described in Chapter 11, missing the whole of a QoL form, and not just some items, poses a particular problem as their absence may lead to serious bias and hence incorrect conclusions. When forms are missing, there is no easy solution for eliminating this potential bias. Therefore, emphasis must always be placed upon avoiding the problem by ensuring optimal compliance with assessment. Any form of correction to the analysis is second best and the study results will be convincing only if compliance is high and missing data are kept to a minimum. Data forms may be missing for a variety of reasons, ranging from death of the patient to refusal to comply for no given reason.

Compliance with completion of the questionnaires can be defined as the percentage of completed forms received by the investigator from the number anticipated by the study design, taking due account of factors which would make completion impossible, such as the death of the patient. Thus the number of expected forms is based on the number of people alive. A special issue of the journal *Statistics in Medicine* is devoted to this topic alone (Bernhard and Gelber, 1998).

CHOICE OF SUMMARY STATISTICS

In certain cases—for example, if a QoL variable follows an approximately Normal distribution shape (it need not be continuous for this)—the mean and *SD* encapsulate the essential features of the data. As we have discussed, the Normal distribution form may require a transformation from the original scale of measurement. If the underlying QoL variable is of an ordered categorical form we would not recommend such an approach; rather we would use the median as the measure of location and the range as the measure of spread as are used in the box-whisker plot of Figure 8.4. In some situations, especially if the number of categories is small, there may be a tendency for the observations to cluster towards one or other end of the scale; that is, to take the minimum or maximum values sometimes termed the floor and ceiling values. In this situation, the median and minimum (or maximum) may coincide. In such cases, there is no entirely satisfactory summary that can be used. We suggest that for these variables the simple proportion falling in the first (or last) category be quoted, thus converting the ordered categorical variable to a binary one.

CHOICE OF ANALYSIS

QoL data are mostly either continuous or of an ordered categorical form (a binary variable is a special case of the latter), and standard statistical methods as described in Chapter 8 can be used for between-(two)-group comparisons. These methods can be extended to the comparison of three or more groups and can be adjusted to take account of patient characteristics (for example, age), which might also be influencing QoL apart from group membership itself. This lead us, in the case of a variable that has a Normal distribution, from the comparison of two means via the z- or t-tests, to ANOVA for three or more groups and the F-test, to multiple regression to adjust for patient characteristics. Similarly, we are led from the comparison of two proportions using the z- or χ^2-tests, to logistic regression with between-group differences expressed in terms of the odds ratio (OR), to the extension to an ordered categorical variable and finally to multiple logistic regression.

All the methods described are interconnected and are examples of multiple regression analysis with either continuous or categorical variables. As a consequence, it is usually best to approach analysis in this way. It should be noted, however, that the computer programs for multiple regression and multiple logistic regression are not the same.

SIMPLE COMPARISONS

Many of the complications in analysis arise because studies that assess QoL usually assess each patient at multiple time points. When cross-sectional analyses are carried out many of the problems disappear. Sometimes straightforward comparison of two means is required so that t-tests may be appropriate with associated confidence intervals. Some of these comparisons may need to be adjusted by multiple regression techniques to examine the effect of prognostic variables upon QoL outcomes. Non-parametric tests, such as the Wilcoxon or Mann–Whitney, may often be better because many of the QoL single items and some of the functioning scales can have asymmetric (non-Normal) distributions. Where single items are, for example, four-point scales, ordered logistic regression might be appropriate if one wants to examine the effect of prognostic variables.

For single items, a percentage rather than a mean may be a better summary of the corresponding variable. When percentages are used, the analyses often reduce to comparisons of binomial proportions by use of simple logistic regression.

MULTIPLICITY OF OUTCOMES

A typical QoL instrument contains many questions often with supplementary modules containing additional items and scales. Thus there are potentially many pairwise statistical comparisons that might be made in any two-group (or more) clinical study. Even if no treatment effect is truly present, some of these comparisons would be "statistically significant", and hence be false positives.

One way of avoiding this problem is to identify in the protocol itself one or two QoL outcomes as being the ones of principal interest. These few outcomes will then be the main focus of the analysis, and therefore there will be no problem of multiple testing. We recommend (with caution) that the p-values for these should not be corrected but perhaps a comment made to the problem of multiple testing in the discussion of the results. This approach is recommended by Pernegger (1998) who concludes that: "Simply describing what tests of significance have been performed, and why, is generally the best way of dealing with multiple comparisons." For these comparisons we suggest a corresponding confidence interval be reported. A precautionary recommendation here may be to have in mind a 99% confidence interval as an aid to interpretation. For the remaining QoL variables we would recommend less exhaustive analysis. All these analyses may then be regarded as primarily hypothesis generating and the associated p-values merely indicative of possible differences to be explored at a later stage in further study. Even here it may be sensible to adopt "conservative p-values" when the more stringent $p < 0.01$ or $p < 0.001$ could be used or the related Bonferroni correction using k times the calculated p value as the final p-value for the individual tests.

The guidelines by Staquet *et al.* (1996) state: "In the case of multiple comparisons, attention must be paid to the total number of comparisons, to the adjustment, if any, of the significance level, and to the interpretation of the results." Seldom will a global multivariate test producing a single (or composite) p-value be of use.

REPEATED MEASUREMENTS

This raises similar issues to those just preceding but here, rather than the numerous items on a QoL instrument leading to many comparisons, it is the longitudinal nature of the patient follow-up which can lead to repeat statistical testing of the difference between treatments at successive time points. Thus, of the various methods available, one of the simplest and yet most informative approaches is to use graphical displays (Chapter 9) and accompany these by cross-sectional analyses (Chapter 8) at a few specific time points. Ideally, the study protocol will have pre-specified that the analysis will focus both upon the aspect of QoL concerned and the particular time points. Nevertheless, the difficulty remains—there are still repeated tests and the problems associated with false positives remains.

A more satisfactory alternative is to encapsulate these repeated measurements into a single summary for each patient. Examples are: the overall mean QoL, the worst QoL experienced during therapy, or the *AUC* (Chapter 9). The choice of which to use will depend on the study objectives. The analyses can then compare and test using these summaries as the basic data for each patient in an appropriate cross-sectional manner.

MODELLING

For the truly primary endpoints, more sophisticated methods are available and these allow for the auto-correlation between QoL values at successive time points. The main methods include the hierarchical or multilevel models of Chapter 10 and the use of generalized estimating equations (GEE) to cope with missing values (Chapter 11). Some of these methods do ideally require specialist statistical software to implement, such as MLwiN (Goldstein *et al.*, 1998) or HLM (Bryk, Raudenbush and Congdon, 1996) for multilevel models, and BUGS (Spiegelhalter *et al.*, 1996) for Bayesian modelling. However, many of the methods are also becoming more widely available in standard statistical packages; for example, GEE is available in SAS and STATA.

In general, we would not recommend use of multivariate analysis of variance (MANOVA) for repeated measures, because the conclusions to be drawn from, for example, a statistically significant result are in many instances far from clear.

A sensible precaution before embarking on the modelling process (or for that matter using repeated measures ANOVA and related techniques) is first to plot the data. This will give a general idea of models that may or may not be appropriate. For example, there is unlikely to be a linear trend in values of (say) nausea and vomiting when assessed before active treatment commences, several times during chemotherapy and then several times during post-treatment follow-up in cancer patients. However, indiscriminate use of statistical packages leads some analysts to simply read off the significant p-values giving little thought to the appropriateness or otherwise of the underlying statistical procedure.

CLINICAL SIGNIFICANCE

Although it is not possible to give a clear definition of clinical significance, nevertheless specific examples are given in Chapter 16. It is clear that statistical and clinical significance should not be confused. Statistical significance tells us whether the observed differences can be explained by chance fluctuations alone, but says nothing about clinical significance. Despite the difficulty of determining what is "clinically significant", an idea of its magnitude has to be elicited for trial planning purposes.

15.4 ELEMENTS OF GOOD GRAPHICS

Exploratory and descriptive data analyses, explore, clarify, describe and help to interpret the QoL data. These less formal analyses may reveal unexpected patterns in the data. Because these analyses are less concerned with significance testing, graphical methods are especially suitable. Judicious use of graphics can succinctly summarise complex data that would otherwise require extensive tabulations, and can clarify and display the complex interrelationships of QoL data. At the same time, graphics help to emphasise the high degree of variability in QoL data. Current computing facilities offer unrivalled facilities for the production of extensive and high-quality graphics.

SIMPLE GRAPHICAL SUMMARIES

Perhaps the simplest summaries of all are histogram and bar charts, which show the frequency distribution of the data. These are often used for the initial inspection of data, and to establish basic characteristics of the data. For example, prior to using a t-test one ought to check whether the data are distributed symmetrically and whether they appear to follow a Normal distribution. Thus Figure 8.1 illustrates a histogram of baseline emotional functioning (EF) in patients with multiple myeloma. This is a common method of displaying information.

Although this is a simple graphical display, there are a number of variations that may improve the presentation. Thus Figure 15.1 shows the same information, adding blank "lines" to make it visually easier to assess the height of the histogram bars, and using light shading of the blocks.

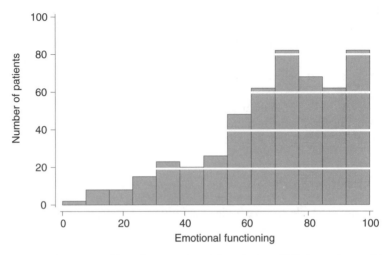

Figure 15.1 Histogram of baseline emotional functioning (EF) in patients with multiple myeloma (Data from Wisløff *et al.*, 1996)

COMPARISON OF TWO GROUPS

One common way of displaying the differences between two treatments or two groups of patients is a bar chart. An example is shown in Figure 15.2a, which displays the mean fatigue levels for males and females at various times over the duration of the study.

However, the format of Figure 15.2b is preferable since it more readily conveys the shape of the relationship with time and helps quantify more readily the gender differences. Also, in contrast to Figure 15.2a, the unequal time intervals between assessments are correctly represented along the horizontal axis. This figure could be further enhanced to provide confidence intervals.

ASSOCIATION OF VARIABLES

When showing the association between two variables the simplest graphic is perhaps the scatter plot, as shown for age versus anxiety in Figure 15.3a. In this example, a so-called rangefinder box plot is superimposed. The central cross marks the point of intersection of the two medians, and the lines all extend to cover the 25% to 75% interquartile range. The outer lines show boundaries after excluding the extreme outliers.

One of the difficulties with the plot of Figure 15.3a, and in many other situations, is that two or more patients may supply the same pair of values and the plotting symbols are overprinted and their true impact lost. One device to expose this overlap is to "jitter" these multiple observation points about the true plotting position. Thus Figure 15.3b represents exactly the same data as Figure 15.3a but there now "appears" to be more data. The second figure gives a more complete picture of the true situation. In the latter figure the marginal box-and-whisker plots for EF and age are added above and to the right hand side of the main panel to assist interpretation further.

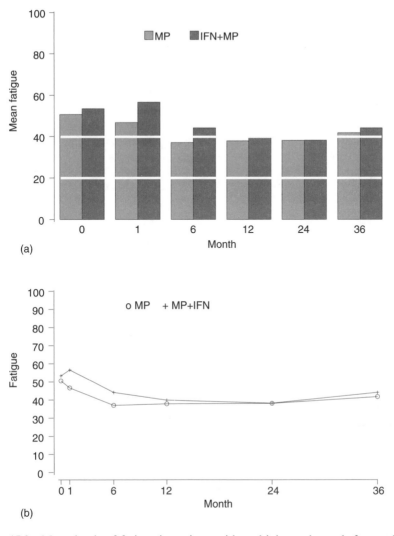

Figure 15.2 Mean levels of fatigue in patients with multiple myeloma, before and during treatment with MP or IFN+MP: (a) Bar chart; (b) line plot (Data from Wisløff *et al.*, 1996)

15.5 SOME ERRORS

BASELINE VARIABLES

In the reporting of any study, presentation of, for example, basic demographic and other baseline data in tabular format by patient group is always valuable. In this respect QoL studies are no different. However, these tables are usually for descriptive purposes only and so would usually contain, for example, means and *SD*s or means, minimum and maximum values, rather than means and confidence intervals. In most situations, statistical tests of significance between groups are also

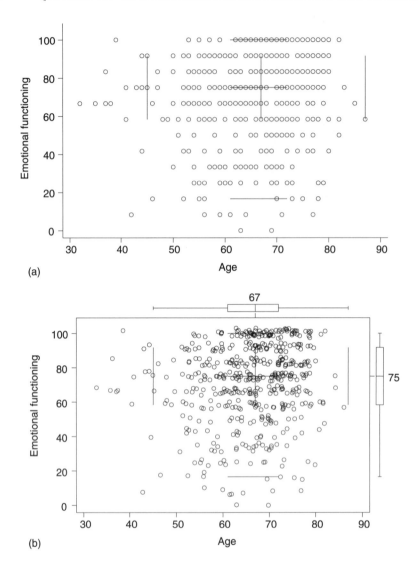

Figure 15.3 Baseline EF by age, in patients with multiple myeloma: scatter plots with (a) rangefinder box plot; (b) "jitter" rangefinder box plot, and marginal box plots (Data from Wisløff *et al.*, 1996)

not pertinent. This is particularly the case if the group membership was determined "at random", as would be the case of allocation to treatment groups in a randomised trial. Statistical tests and confidence intervals should be confined to the endpoint variables alone, although these comparisons may be adjusted for baseline variables which were included in the tabulation just referred to. A common mistake is to calculate and quote confidence intervals of (say) the mean of each group separately, whereas in any comparative study it is the confidence interval of the difference between groups that is relevant. As already indicated, these problems are not confined to QoL studies alone, but they are compounded in such studies as the number of baseline and endpoint measures may be very large.

CONFIDENCE INTERVALS

In published QoL research, some investigators summarise differences between subject groups for each of the QoL items or scales under study by merely reporting in a tabular format the corresponding p-value. Often they do not quote the precise p-value unless it is less than 0.05, instead using the notation NS (not statistically significant). This is very bad practice and is now actively discouraged by the leading medical journals since NS covers a range of p-values from a little over 0.05 to 1. The conclusions drawn from a result with p-value = 0.06 are quite different from one for which it is 0.6. It is important, even when there is no statistically significant difference, to provide not just the p-values but also an estimate of the magnitude of the difference between groups together with the associated confidence interval. This is emphasised by Altman et al. (2000), with clear recommendations.

GRAPHICAL

One disadvantage to profile plots is that there may be a tendency for naïve readers of such plots to assume that the different dimensions may be compared—for example, in Figure 8.5 to think that overall quality of life (ql), is slightly greater than or "better" than role functioning (rf), and social functioning (sf) is much "better" than both ql and rf. However, responses to items on QoL questionnaires are rarely scaled uniformly, and it is meaningless to describe whether one item or scale takes higher (or lower) values than other items and scales.

A common and, at first sight, apparently reasonable form of analysis is to compare change in QoL scores for patients against their baseline values. Thus one might seek to determine whether patients who start with a poor QoL are likely to have an even poorer QoL after treatment, or whether they tend to improve. Hence one might plot the baseline score (QoL_0) against the change between baseline and (say) month-one (QoL_1) values. Thus Figure 15.4a, for emotional functioning, shows a moderate degree of correlation between the change ($QoL_1 - QoL_0$) and the baseline measurement.

However, this plot cannot be interpreted. This is because a similar plot can be obtained by replacing the initial EF observations by random numbers over the same range of possible values and using these in the calculation of the change from baseline! Such a "random numbers" plot against initial EF is shown in Figure 15.4b. The reason for the association in Figure 15.4a is that the vertical axis measure $y = (QoL_1 - QoL_0)$ and the horizontal axis measure $x = QoL_0$ both contain the same quantity QoL_0. Thus, in part, one is correlating $-QoL_0$ with $+ QoL_0$ itself, and this correlation is perfect but negative. This correlation then dominates both panels of Figure 15.4, creating the illusion of an association.

A comparison of change against initial value may be of clinical importance, and more rigorous methods of analysis are available. These issues are discussed by Bland and Altman (1986) who suggest plots corresponding to change in score ($QoL_1 - QoL_0$) against the average score ($QoL_1 + QoL_0$)/2.

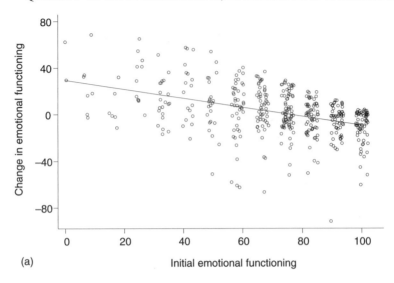

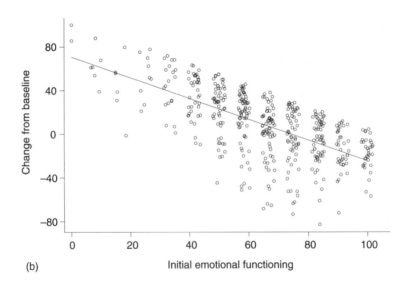

Figure 15.4 Change in EF from baseline plotted against the baseline EF, in patients with multiple myeloma: (a) plotting ($EF_1 - EF_0$) against EF_0; (b) substituting random numbers for the initial measurements, EF_0 (Data from Wisløff *et al.*, 1996)

15.6 GUIDELINES FOR REPORTING

In recent years, the number of clinical trials incorporating measurement of health-related QoL has substantially increased. We introduce here general guidelines for the reporting of clinical trials that include a QoL measurement. These proposals are intended for researchers reporting a new study as well as for those who are asked to evaluate critically the published reports.

CHECKLIST

Some of the headings in this section repeat those already mentioned above, but the topics are collected here as a reminder or checklist. The associated comments add some detail not included previously. This list is based on the checklist of Staquet *et al.* (1996).

- **Abstract**. Describe the purpose of the study, the methods, the key results, and the principal conclusions.
- **Introduction**. (a) Describe the objective of the study in detail. Its rationale must be supported with a comprehensive review of the literature relevant to the disease or the treatment of interest. (b) The natural history of the disease and its treatment should be described succinctly so that it is clear why QoL is being assessed. (c) The pre-study hypotheses for QoL assessment must be stated clearly, including which domains or scales were expected to show a difference between treatment arms. The definition of QoL should be presented.
- **Materials and methods**.
- **Population and sample**. (a) A description of the patient population, including the study inclusion and exclusion criteria, is mandatory. The population sample must be described with appropriate demographic data, for example age, gender, and ethnicity depending on the context. Other variables, such as the clinical and mental status, if they were likely to alter the ability of the patient to answer a questionnaire, should also be included. (b) It is important to indicate how and from where the patients were recruited to the study. For instance, indicate whether the sample was random or one of convenience, and the number of centres involved. If a subset of the total sample size is deemed to be sufficient for the QoL part of the trial, the method used to select the patients in the subset must be explained.
- **QoL instrument selection**.
- **Trial size**.
- **Endpoints**. The dimension(s) or the item(s) of the instrument that were selected as endpoint(s) before subject accrual need to be stated. Endpoints not chosen before the start of the trial are to be avoided. When QoL is not the primary endpoint, the major endpoints of the trial should be provided.
- **Timing of study assessment**. The scheduled times of instrument completion must be given (for example, every four weeks), as should the timing of the follow-up assessment—for instance at the completion of treatment or discontinuation of treatment, every three months, or at the end of the study, and so on.
- **Data**. The means by which the data were collected and the procedure for evaluating their quality should be described. The criteria for what is to be considered adequate/inadequate must be specified.
- **Method of analysis**.
- **Results**.
- **Presentation of data**. The results of planned primary and secondary analyses should be presented along with the results of appropriate tests of statistical significance, such as *p*-value, effect size, and confidence intervals. The report should include reference to all the other items or scales from each instrument used in the study. In particular, it is important not to pick and choose which

scales to report from an instrument without indicating very clearly why this has been done.

- **Patient data**. (a) All patients entered in the study must be accounted for and their characteristics presented; for example, how many centres were involved, how many eligible patients were approached, how many were accrued, how many refused to participate, how many were unable to complete the questionnaires, and so on. (b) In the context of a clinical trial or comparative study, numbers of patients should be given for each group. Thus details are required on the numbers: eligible and entered; excluded from the analysis (with inadequate data, with missing data); losses to follow-up and death; adequately treated according to protocol; failed to complete the treatment according to protocol and received treatments not specified in the protocol.
- **Scheduling of instrument administration**. Descriptive information is required that contributes to an understanding of treatment schedules, patient compliance, time windows, median follow-up times, and other practical aspects of QoL data collection and follow-up.
- **Missing data and compliance**.
- **Statistical analysis**. The main analysis should address the hypothesis identified in the introduction. Although it is recognised that there are often large numbers of items on a QoL questionnaire, the particular and few dimensions which were selected as design endpoint(s) should be the most relevant part of the report. Analysis of other variables as well as any subgroup analysis not pre-specified should be reported only as "exploratory" or tentative. If appropriate, the reasons for not adhering to the pre-trial sample size should be discussed. In the case of a graphical presentation, it is important to specify the number at risk by treatment group beneath the time axis in the plot.
- **Discussion and conclusions**. The findings should be discussed in the context of results of previous studies and research. Some particular issues in the interpretation of QoL data should be addressed here, including (as appropriate) the clinical interpretation of score change. A summary of the therapeutic results should be reported alongside the QoL results so that a balanced interpretation of the trial results can be made.
- **Appendices**. For instruments or battery of instruments or measure(s) selected for the trial which are not well known or which have been modified from the original version, it is appropriate to provide a copy. For a copyright instrument, it is appropriate to give information about where the instrument can be obtained.

CONSORT

The CONSORT statement includes a list of 21 items that should be reported in the paper. There is also a flow chart describing patient progress through the trial, which should be included in the trial report. In addition, a few specific subheadings are suggested within the Methods and Results sections of the paper. In the spirit of the times, the recommendations are evidence-based where possible, with common sense dictating the remainder.

In essence the requirement is that authors should provide enough information for readers to know how the trial was performed, and thus so that they can judge whether the findings are likely to be reliable. The CONSORT suggestions mean that authors will no longer be able to hide study inadequacies by omission of important information.

The full details are provided by Begg *et al.* (1996).

16 Clinical Interpretation

Summary

Interpretation of QoL scores raises many issues. The scales and instruments used may be unfamiliar to many clinicians and patients, who may be uncertain of the meaning of the scale values and summary scores. We describe various methods aimed at providing familiarity of scale scores and understanding the meaning of changes in scores. We describe the use of *population-based* reference values from healthy individuals and from groups of patients with known health status and various illnesses. We also discuss *patient-orientated* methods. These include identification of the minimal changes in QoL that are discernible by patients, or are important to patients; the impact of QoL states upon behaviour; and the changes in QoL that are caused by major life events. *Data-derived* "effect sizes", which consider the random variability of the observed data, provide yet another method and can be particularly useful when reference values and patient-orientated information are not available.

16.1 INTRODUCTION

Previous chapters have described methods of collecting, analysing and summarising QoL data. What do the results mean? What is the clinical relevance of a particular score for QoL, and how important are the observed changes in patients' QoL?

Sometimes results for single items are reported. For example, when a seven-point global question about overall QoL has been used, the results might indicate that treatment improves overall QoL by, say, on average 0.8 points. A clinician (or a patient) might quite reasonably demand to know how to interpret such a change. If QoL for an individual patient changes by that amount, would it be a noticeable change? Would it be an important change? Similarly, when scores are calculated for multi-item scales, what do they mean? What are the clinically important differences between groups of patients?

Although some clinicians may hope to identify a single value that will serve as a clinically significant difference in QoL, it can be argued that this is a demand that is unfairly imposed more frequently upon QoL scales than other clinical scales. Suppose we consider blood pressure (BP) measurement. Systolic and diastolic BP are two of the most widely used medical measurements, and the association between elevated BP and increased mortality is well recognised. The epidemiology of BP and its relationship with age and gender are also well established. Yet there is little consensus as to what critical levels should be taken as indication of hypertension demanding treatment. Most clinicians would probably consider initiating therapy if repeated diastolic BP measurements exceed 100 mmHg in men or 105 mmHg in women, but some might start at 95 and 100 respectively. Some would use diastolic BP in conjunction with systolic BP. Some would make allowance for age when setting the threshold for commencing therapy. Given this poor degree of agreement about thresholds, it is not surprising to find that there is even less agreement as to what *differences* are clinically worthwhile. If beta-blockers lower diastolic BP by 20 mm, from 120 mmHg to 100 mmHg, is it worth continuing long-term therapy? Many might agree, yes. But suppose the change is 10 mm? Or even as little as 5 mm?

One could level similar arguments against other, simple measurements. If a course of cytotoxic drugs prolongs survival by an average of 50% in small-cell lung cancer patients, is it worth giving routinely? Most might agree that it is worthwhile for good-prognosis patients, but how about those with advanced disease who are expected to have very short survival and for whom a 50% increase results in a gain of only a few weeks? Would therapy still be worthwhile if it prolongs average survival by less than 10%? Clearly there is little consensus about survival, either. It appears to be recognised and accepted that clinically important survival benefits are very much a matter of personal value judgement, on the part of both the patient and the treating clinician.

One obvious distinction is familiarity with the scales. Most people can understand the concept of survival, and thus many patients justly demand to be involved in decisions about their survival. Patients have less feeling for the meaning of BP measurement, but realise that their clinicians have a better understanding of it than they do. Therefore they expect the clinician to help assess the value of treatment. Unfortunately, with QoL scales, both patients and clinicians rarely have a feel for what a change of, say, 10% means. Hence the need for information about the levels of QoL that are to be expected for ill patients, and guidelines to help decide what magnitude change in QoL is worthwhile.

No single approach is likely to provide a complete feel for the meaning of QoL measurements, and thus it is important to use a variety of methods for obtaining familiarity with QoL scores.

16.2 STATISTICAL SIGNIFICANCE

The meaning of statistical significance and the power of tests was covered in Chapters 4 and 14. Here, we merely emphasise that statistical significance does not imply clinical significance. Statistical significance tests are concerned solely with examining the observed data values, to determine whether differences or changes can be attributed to chance and patient variability, or whether there is sufficient weight of evidence to claim that there is almost certainly a pattern in the data. Highly statistically significant p-values indicate little about the magnitude of the differences, and tell us only that the differences are probably real as opposed to chance events. They tell us even less about the *clinical significance* of the observed changes.

It is particularly important to bear this in mind when reading reports of survival studies. Many of these enrol large numbers of patients, in order to be certain of detecting small, yet clinically important, differences in survival. Sample sizes of several hundred are not uncommon in multi-centre randomised trials, and some recruit thousands of patients. QoL is often a secondary endpoint in those clinical trials that aim to compare two treatments for survival differences. This large sample size means that if there is even a very small difference in QoL it will be detected and found to be statistically highly significant. A p-value of, say, under 0.01 tells us that, because of the large sample size, it is unlikely (a chance of less than 1 in 100) that we would have observed such extreme data purely by chance. Therefore we are reasonably confident that there is likely to be a difference in QoL. However, despite being "highly significant" in statistical terms, the observed difference in QoL (which is our best estimate of the true difference between patients taking these treatments) might in fact be very small. It might be clinically unimportant.

Conversely, in a small study of QoL a difference might be found to be barely significant at the 5% level ($p < 0.05$). Yet the observed difference in QoL could be substantial and, if confirmed to be true, might be exceedingly important in clinical terms.

In summary, statistical significance does not necessarily indicate clinical relevance of the findings. Statistical "significance tests" are concerned solely with evaluating the probability that the observed patterns in the data could have arisen purely by chance.

16.3 ABSOLUTE LEVELS AND CHANGES OVER TIME

Interpretation of QoL scores will take different forms according to the application for which QoL is being assessed.

- *Cross-sectional studies* may collect data representing the levels of QoL in a group of patients, and often it will be appropriate to contrast the observed average values against reference data from other groups, such as the general population.
- *Follow-up studies* that collect repeated QoL measurements for each patient may be interested in the same issues as cross-sectional studies, but in addition they are likely to place greater emphasis upon changes over time rather than absolute levels. Large follow-up studies have the power to detect small variations in the mean level of QoL, and some of these changes may be so small that they are of little consequence to individual patients.
- *Clinical trials* place the focus upon differences between the randomised groups. Usually the investigators will carry out a significance test to determine whether there is evidence that the observed differences are larger than can be attributed to chance alone. If statistical significance is established, they will next want to know whether the between-group differences are large enough to be clinically important. They may also want to know whether one or both groups of patients in the trial have lower or higher QoL scores than reference groups such as the general population. Also, assessments of QoL in clinical trials are usually made at baseline, during treatment, and during follow-up.

In these situations, investigators are interested in either differences between groups of people, or within-person changes in QoL over time.

1. If one group has a worse (or better) QoL than another group, are the differences large enough to be important?
2. If QoL changes over time, how large do the changes need to be before they are noticed?
3. What magnitude of change in QoL is big enough to be important?
4. Do differences between the groups diminish over time, and if so, when do they cease to become clinically important?
5. Do some individuals have such a large reduction in QoL that psychosocial intervention is necessary?

Many forms of information are necessary to answer the above questions. The interpretation of QoL data may often be based upon consideration of absolute levels relative to a reference population, combined with a judgement concerning the magnitude and clinical importance of observed differences between groups of patients and changes over time. We need to define a reference population. Often this will consist of healthy people or the general population. We need to know what levels of QoL are present in the reference population, and how much variability there is in the data. This variability is often summarised by the *SD* calculated from the reference population. We need to know what magnitude of differences or changes are perceived by patients or others as being noticeable, important and worthwhile.

16.4 THRESHOLD VALUES, PERCENTAGES

One of the simplest forms of presentation—and therefore one of the simplest for interpretation—is to show the percentage of patients above some specific value. For example, when comparing treatment groups one might tabulate the percentage of patients that report "good" QoL. For a few instruments, such as the HADS, there are guidelines for values that denote "cases" and "doubtful cases" requiring treatment. Even without such guideline levels, many readers seem to find it intuitively easier to visualise a comparison based upon the percentage of patients above and below some arbitrary cut-point rather than a difference in group means.

In some situations, such as when many of patients rate themselves at the maximum (ceiling) value, it may be helpful to compare the proportion of patients at this maximum.

Similarly, when using odds ratios (*OR*) it is also in principle possible to choose a critical value and compare the proportion of patients lying above and below that threshold. This approach has not been widely used and so for most instruments it is less clear what critical values might be appropriate.

16.5 POPULATION NORMS

Interpretation of QoL scores may use population-based reference values, which provide expected or typical scores that are called "norms." Tables of normative data, taken from surveys of randomly selected subjects from the general population, provide a useful guide for interpretation. Norms can consist of values for the general population as a whole, or for various subgroups such as healthy people or those with particular disease conditions. Norm-based interpretation of QoL scores consists of defining one (or more) reference groups for whom norms are available, and treating these scores as target values against which the scores observed in an individual patient, or the average for a group of patients, can be compared. For comparative purposes, the average patient values and the norms can be listed side-by-side. A possibly better method is to regard the norms as anticipated values, and subtract them from the patient averages to give the difference of observed from expected values. These differences can be standardised, to allow for differences in variability of the measurements and scales. Usually, if a measurement scale has a small *SD* in the general population (indicating that most people have very similar values to each other), even a small difference from the norm will be noticeable and important. Conversely, if the population *SD* is large, there will be a large amount of variation from one person to another and only large differences between the observed patient values and the norms will be clinically important. Therefore the standardised differences, in which the differences are divided by the *SD*, may be easier to interpret than plain observed-minus-expected differences. Standardisation is also related to the concept of effect sizes, as described in Section 16.8.

What reference population should be chosen? The two obvious choices are the general population, which includes both the healthy and those with chronic or acute illness, or the healthy population after excluding those with illnesses. Random samples from the general population may find that more than half of the subjects report chronic illnesses of varying severity, although the proportions will vary according to the composition of the sample (for example, age range and distribution) and the definition of chronic illness. Often the optimal choice of reference population will be debatable. In some studies, patients who are recruited into the study will be as likely as the general population to have concomitant diseases. For example, a study of QoL in patients with cardiovascular diseases may find that many patients have chronic lung disease, too. In such cases the general population would seem the most suitable choice. This is the reference population that is most frequently used. However, the healthy population could be used to provide an indication of the "ideal" target value. Sometimes the healthy population may be more appropriate as the reference group. For example, some clinical trials may have eligibility criteria that exclude patients with serious comorbid conditions. In such trials contrast with values from the healthy population is preferable. In other circumstances neither reference population is ideal. For example, when considering the meaning of QoL states in patients who are receiving active therapy or recovering from side-effects, sometimes the target and potentially achievable QoL might be defined as that obtained by long-term survivors or cured patients. These data are less frequently available for QoL instruments, and most investigators make use of the general population or, less commonly, the healthy population.

Normative data, also called *reference values*, are available for many QoL instruments. Mostly, these are based upon cross-sectional surveys of the general population and are presented as values tabulated by age and gender. Norms are also sometimes available for different disease groups. Less common, although important, are norms from longitudinal studies, showing the changes over time that may be expected for healthy or ill subjects. For example, it could be important for interpretation of results to know the anticipated rate of change in palliative care patients, or in those responding to therapy.

Example from the literature

Hjermstad *et al.* (1998a) report normative data for the EORTC QLQ-C30 in a randomly selected sample of 3000 people from the Norwegian population, aged between 18 and 93. Data were available for 1965 individuals. Table 16.1 summarises their results, by age and gender, for the functioning and global health/QoL scales of the QLQ-C30 (version 2.0).

Apart from emotional functioning, all functioning scales and the global score showed a decline with age. The fall was particularly marked for physical functioning above the age of 50. Men tended to have markedly higher levels than women. These patterns are clearly shown in Figure 16.1. The authors also presented bar charts of the data, showing that there is a large amount of variability in the data; the distributions are inevitably asymmetric since the mean values are close to the ceiling of 100.

Table 16.1 Mean scores for EORTC QLQ-C30 (version 2.0) functioning scales and global health/QoL, by age and sex, in a Norwegian population (Based on Hjermstad *et al.*, 1998a)

	Male							Female							Totals
	All	18–29	30–39	40–49	50–59	60–69	≥70	All	18–29	30–39	40–49	50–59	60–69	≥70	
Number:	(1016)	(205)	(228)	(182)	(153)	(114)	(134)	(949)	(185)	(159)	(147)	(145)	(142)	(171)	(1965)
Functioning scales															
Cognitive	87.1	91.6	88.9	89.5	86.5	82.7	77.6	85.8	89.5	87.3	86.9	86.1	86.4	77.9	86.5
Emotional	85.4	87.8	83.7	84.6	83.9	84.8	87.7	79.9	78.7	77.2	76.8	83.2	79.4	84.4	82.8
Physical	93.2	98.0	97.3	91.1	92.9	89.1	77.7	86.4	97.6	93.6	89.9	87.6	78.2	67.7	89.9
Role	85.7	92.4	91.0	85.5	84.4	79.0	73.3	80.6	88.4	85.9	82.6	81.3	75.5	68.1	83.3
Social	87.7	94.5	89.4	89.0	84.4	80.9	81.6	83.6	88.9	84.0	80.0	83.9	83.4	80.1	85.8
Global health/QOL	77.3	80.1	78.8	79.0	75.9	75.2	71.4	73.2	77.9	75.7	72.7	74.1	70.2	67.6	75.3

One way of using normative data for interpreting values observed in individual patients is to note the decrease in levels with increasing age. Physical functioning declines by nearly 5 units per decade of life, both for men and for women. This may help give a feeling for what an average change of 5 units might mean to patients. Similarly, Global health/QoL declines by approximately 2 units per decade, role functioning by 3.5, cognitive functioning and social functioning by 2, and emotional functioning by 0.5.

ADJUSTING FOR AGE AND GENDER

The patterns in Figure 16.1 emphasise the need to allow for age and gender when contrasting normative data against groups of patients who may have very different age–gender profiles. People with chronic health problems may tend to be older than those who are healthy, and for many disease areas the patients in clinical trials may be older than people in normative samples. Thus an adjustment should be made for differing age and gender distributions.

There are two principal approaches to this problem. Firstly, it is possible to regard the age distribution of the reference population as being the standard to which all other datasets should be adjusted. The age-specific scores for the patients

328

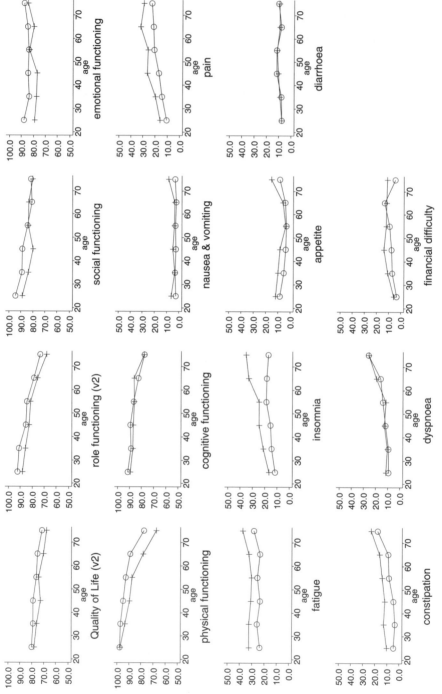

Figure 16.1 Age-distribution of the mean scores for the subscales of the EORTC QLQ-C30 (+3), for males (0) and females (+) from the general Norwegian population (Based on Hjermstad *et al.*, 1998a)

Table 16.2 Age and gender distribution of a group of cancer patients (Based on Hjermstad *et al.*, 1998b)

Age group	Female	Male
18–29	0	0
30–39	4	4
40–49	3	1
50–59	7	7
60–69	14	9
≥70	29	13
Totals	57	34

are calculated, and the age distribution of the reference population is used with these scores so as to estimate the mean level of QoL that would be expected for the reference age-structure. This leads to adjusted, or standardised, mean scores for each of the disease groups. This procedure is equivalent to *direct standardisation* as used in epidemiology. This method is not often used because, if the disease group is small, age-specific mean scores cannot be estimated very accurately.

The second approach, illustrated in Table 16.2, is based upon the concept of calculating "expected" mean scores for the disease group. The population reference values are used to calculate the expected scores that would be observed for subjects of the same age and gender distribution as in the disease group. Since each disease group will have a different age–gender distribution, separate expected values are calculated for each group. The calculations use basic reference data, such as those in Table 16.1. Similar *indirect standardisation* is used in epidemiology when comparing incidence or prevalence rates amongst different subgroups.

Although we illustrate the calculations using the age-grouped data presented in Table 16.1, a variation on this approach is to use the individual patient raw-data and apply regression modelling to fit an equation that includes age and gender. This can be used to generate expected (predicted) values for each individual. In principle this should be a more accurate method, since it makes full use of the individual values and involves fitting a smooth curve. In practice, however, it usually makes negligible difference to the estimates and has two disadvantages: it requires access to the individual patient data, and the regression models will often involve different nonlinear functions of age for each gender.

Example

The study of Hjermstad *et al.* (1998a,b) included 91 cancer patients, with an age–gender distribution as given in Table 16.2 and a mean global health/QoL score of 59.9. There are four females aged 30–39, and if we examine the comparable age–gender group in the normative data of Table 16.1, we see that the expected value of their global health/QoL is 75.7. Therefore the expected total score for these four females is $4 \times 75.7 = 302.8$. Similarly, we can estimate the expected total score for the remaining female groups. Combining these gives an expected total score of

$(0 \times 77.9) + (4 \times 75.7) + (3 \times 72.7) + (7 \times 74.1) + (14 \times 70.2) + (29 \times 67.6) = 3982.8.$

Similarly, for the 34 males:

$(0 \times 80.1) + (4 \times 78.8) + (1 \times 79.0) + (7 \times 75.9) + (9 \times 75.2) + (13 \times 71.4) = 2530.5.$

The expected total score for all 91 cancer patients is therefore 3982.8 + 2530.5 = 6513.3, giving an expected mean score 6513.3/91 = 71.6. Hence the cancer patients have a global health/QoL mean score of 59.9 that, even after allowing for age and gender, is lower than that of the general population by 71.6 − 59.9 = 11.7.

Note that if we had not allowed for age and gender, but used the mean score for the total normative sample directly, then the difference (75.3 − 59.9 = 15.4) between cancer patients and the general population appears almost 4 points larger.

Example

Bjordal *et al.* (1999) used the EORTC QLQ-C30 to assess QoL of head and neck cancer patients. A subgroup of 287 patients from this study completed QoL questionnaires on three occasions during treatment. The Norwegian reference data of Table 16.1 were used to obtain typical values for the general population. A summary of the results is shown in Figure 16.2. The mean values from the reference data, adjusted for an age and gender distribution equivalent to that of the cancer patients, are shown in bold. It is apparent that the cancer patients have, on average, lower functioning scores than the general population. Role functioning is particularly affected. Whereas high scores for functioning indicate better functioning, high symptom scores indicate worse symptomatology. Hence, patients have higher levels of symptomatology, and appetite is particularly affected. The scores for the three repeated assessments were broadly similar.

Although the format of Figure 16.2 is widely used, many people find it easier to see patterns in data if the reference group is drawn as the baseline or "target" level of QoL and the patient-means are plotted as differences about this baseline. An advantage of this format, shown in Figure 16.3, is that it discourages casual readers from comparing absolute values of the different scales with each other. When reading Figure 16.2, for example, there might be the temptation to think that patients have lower role functioning than social functioning, since the mean scores are 61 and 70 respectively. This would be an unfounded statement as there is no evidence that a particular score on one scale is equivalent to the same score on other scales.

Example

In Figure 16.3 it is easy to see that role functioning of patients is about 25 units below that of the general population, although it is visually more difficult to read this value from Figure 16.2. Pain appears slightly reduced by the third assessment, which may be attributable to better pain medication by this stage.

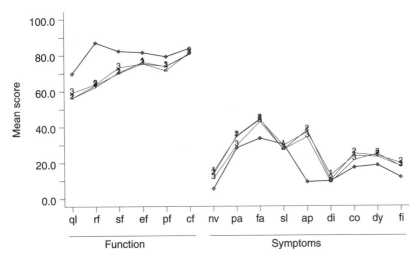

Figure 16.2 EORTC QLQ-C30 scale scores at months 1, 2 and 3 during treatment, for 287 patients with head and neck cancer. The bold line shows age- and sex-matched reference values from the general Norwegian population (Based on Bjordal *et al.*, 1999, and Hjermstad *et al.*, 1998b)

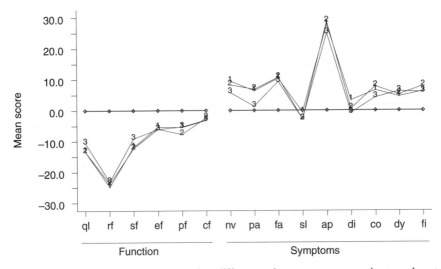

Figure 16.3 Data of Figure 16.2, showing differences between cancer patients and matched reference values of the general population (Based on Bjordal *et al.*, 1999, and Hjermstad *et al.*, 1998b)

Caution should be used when contrasting the differences from different scales. Although it appears convincing from Figure 16.3 that role functioning is more severely affected than, say, social functioning, there is no guarantee that intervals on the different scales are equivalent. It is possible that a change of 5 units may be important on one scale, whilst changes less than 10 may be unimportant on another. An alternative method, which may be preferable when comparing scales, is to plot effect sizes, as described in Section 16.8.

SELECTIVE REPORTING AND RESPONSE SHIFT

Patients may tend to ignore or discount those problems they believe are unrelated to their illness. For example, a patient with bladder cancer who has also previously been incontinent for many years might respond to a question on this topic by reporting no problem. However, patients who have experienced a recent change or who believe they have illness-related problems are more likely to make accurate responses. This *selective reporting bias* can distort the analyses and interpretation of results. To some extent it can be controlled by suitable "framing" of the question-naire, which consists of instructions telling the patient whether to report *all* symptoms and problems, irrespective of origin or cause.

When a questionnaire is given to the general population, however, one might expect no such discounting of problems. As a consequence, QoL levels for patients may appear to be more favourable than those expected from population-based reference values. Sometimes this effect can be quite marked, even to the extent of making patients appear to have better QoL than the general population.

Example from the literature

Fayers *et al.* (1991) reported QoL assessments in a randomised trial comparing maintenance versus no maintenance chemotherapy for small-cell lung cancer patients. Because this chemotherapy was likely to induce vomiting, the patient questionnaire asked about nausea and vomiting, and these too were recorded by the clinicians.

In a total of 956 patient-visits (Table 16.3), patients reported 626 (65%) episodes of vomiting, compared with 245 (26%) reports by physicians. Patients reported 371 episodes of vomiting where physicians recorded no problems with nausea and vomiting. Curiously, in 49 instances physicians reported vomiting when patients indicated no problems.

The authors suggested that if patients' reported vomiting, it was likely to be true. Thus there was a high degree of selective reporting by clinicians, who perhaps ignored and under-reported mild vomiting because they expected this to occur in nearly all patients.

Table 16.3 Small-cell lung cancer patients' and their physicians' assessments of nausea and vomiting (Based on Fayers *et al.*, 1991)

Physicians' assessments	Patients' assessments			
	None	Nausea	Vomiting	Totals
Not reported	125	78	371	574
Nausea	27	31	79	137
Vomiting	49	20	176	245
Totals	201	129	626	956

Many patients adapt over time, and their perceptions of QoL may change. Learning to cope with problems is a well-recognised feature in the chronically ill.

For example, patients who experience a constant level of pain for a long period may come to cope with it, and hence report diminishing levels over time. Also, patients may meet others whose condition is better or worse than their own, and this can also lead to a recalibration of their own internal standards and values. Such subjective changes in patients' perceptions are known as *response shift* (Schwartz and Sprangers, 1999). It may be argued that, when assessing QoL, all that matters is the patients' current perception. Hence if pain is perceived as diminishing, then we can regard it as becoming less important to the patient even though the pain receptor cells are receiving the same signals as previously. However, many clinicians would argue that it remains just as important to address the pain, even though patients may claim that they can cope and that it is becoming less of a problem.

Response shift can work in both directions. Patients may find that continuing symptoms cause increasing distress, and may therefore report them as becoming more severe.

Example from the literature

Groenvold *et al.* (1999) investigated anxiety and depression in newly diagnosed breast cancer patients, using the HADS. A sample of 466 Danish breast cancer patients at low risk of recurrence was recruited within seven weeks following their surgery. Their level of anxiety and depression was compared with that of 609 women randomly selected from the Danish general population.

Contrary to expectations, the HADS scores of breast cancer patients were significantly lower than those of the general population sample, indicating less anxiety and depression. The respective patient and population mean scores were 5.3 and 6.0 ($p = 0.02$) for anxiety, and 2.8 and 3.4 ($p = 0.001$) for depression. The differences were consistent across all five age groups examined.

The authors were sceptical regarding the results, and questioned the validity of comparing HADS scores of breast cancer patients against those obtained from the general population. Firstly, the HADS was developed and validated in hospital patients, and has not been validated in the general population. Secondly, there might be selective reporting. Since the patients knew they were in a cancer study, they might have excluded complaints that they attributed to non-cancer causes. This might lead to an underestimate of anxiety and depression for the breast cancer patients. Thirdly, there may have been response shift. The cancer patients may have changed their internal standards as a result of their experiences. The authors concluded: "The results of the HADS applied in the general population are probably not directly comparable with the results from the breast cancer patients."

Selective reporting and response shift may result in both subjective and supposedly objective symptoms being reported differently by patients and the general population. Selective reporting can clearly present a serious bias problem when using normative data, although response shift is arguably less important if perceptions are considered to matter more than reality. In QoL studies it is rarely possible to quantify the overall bias, and these two effects cannot be separated.

Both forms of bias are usually of less importance for treatment comparisons in a clinical trial, since they apply equally to all treatment arms. However, it is important to bear in mind their potential impact on particular studies. We have already seen that clinicians may under-report symptoms such as vomiting, which they regard as the inevitable consequence of chemotherapy for cancer. Similarly, selective reporting bias could occur in a trial of long-term chemotherapy versus "no treatment" if the treatment-group gradually regarded some symptoms as inevitable and stopped reporting them. Thus selective reporting might lead to serious under-estimation of QoL differences between the chemotherapy and control groups.

16.6   MINIMAL CLINICALLY IMPORTANT DIFFERENCE

Whereas norms are based upon surveys of the prevailing QoL states in reference populations, the minimal clinically important difference takes into account the opinions and values of patients. The minimal clinically important difference is the smallest difference in score in the domain of interest that patients perceive as beneficial and which would cause clinicians to consider a change in the patient's management (assuming no side-effects or major cost considerations).

In order to determine the size of this difference, patients can be asked whether they have noticed a change in their condition and how important they regard that change. Most QoL questionnaires relate to present or recent QoL status; for example: "During the past week, did you feel depressed?" Therefore, the strategy is to ask the patient to complete a questionnaire at their first visit, and then again at the second visit. Immediately following this, they are asked whether they perceived any change and whether this has been an important change. Questions regarding the change in level are sometimes called "transition questions". The number of categories in the transition questions, and their descriptive wording, may influence the value obtained for the minimal clinically important difference. Most investigators have used at least seven categories, with the central one being "no change" and the extreme categories being something like "very much better" (or worse) or "a great deal better" (or worse).

Example from the literature

The Chronic Respiratory Questionnaire and Chronic Heart Failure were investigated by Jaeschke, Singer and Guyatt (1989) to determine the minimal clinically important differences. Initial discussion with staff experienced in administering the questionnaires suggested that a mean change of 0.5 on the seven-point scales would represent a change that patients felt was important to their daily life. In a subsequent study, 75 patients completed QoL questionnaires at baseline and at 2, 6, 12 and 24 weeks. After completing the second and subsequent assessments, they also scored themselves on "global rating scales" according to whether their condition was "a very great deal worse" (−7) through to "a very great deal better" (+7).

Small changes of "somewhat worse" were defined as those between −3 and −1, moderate changes were −5 and −4 ("moderately or a good deal worse"), and large were −7 and −6 ("a great deal or a very great deal worse"). Corresponding positive values were defined for getting better.

Table 16.4 shows the mean change in reported levels of dyspnoea, fatigue and emotional function, divided according to whether patients thought that the overall change was none, small, moderate or large. In this table, positive and negative changes have been combined. For example, the recorded levels of dyspnoea changed by an average of 0.96 in those patients who reported a moderate overall change, with a decrease in dyspnoea for those reporting benefit and a corresponding increase for those improving.

Thus Jaeschke *et al.* (1989) confirmed their preliminary estimates that a small change on the seven-point scales would correspond to a change in score of approximately 0.5, since the mean of the observed values 0.43, 0.64 and 0.49 is 0.52.

Table 16.4 Mean change scores for dyspnoea, fatigue and emotional function, by size of global rating of the change (Based on Jaeschke *et al.*, 1989)

| | Global rating of change | | | |
	None	Small	Moderate	Large
Dyspnoea	0.10	0.43	0.96	1.47
Fatigue	0.12	0.64	0.87	0.94
Emotion	0.02	0.49	0.81	0.86

Example from the literature

A later study by Juniper *et al.* (1994) used the same global rating of change with the Asthma Quality of Life Questionnaire (AQLQ). Thirty-nine patients were evaluated, and the results confirmed that 0.5 represents small, 1.0 was moderate, and that differences greater than 1.5 appear to be large. Juniper *et al.* (1994) also examined the direction of the change, and found that the relationship between "better" and "worse" appeared to be symmetrical.

Example from the literature

Osoba *et al.* (1998) applied a similar approach, and examined the "subjective significance" of the EORTC QLQ-C30 scales for physical, emotional and social functioning and global health/QoL. Seven-category scales were used for the transition questions, ranging from "very much worse" through "no change" to "very much better." For each of the four scales, the patients were asked about change since the last assessment. The question for physical functioning was "Since the last time I filled out a questionnaire, my *physical condition* is: . . .", and similar questions were used for the other scales. In total 246 patients in a breast cancer trial and 111 in a small-cell lung cancer trial were evaluated.

In general, on the 100-point scales, for those who reported "a little" change to the transition question, the mean score change was between 5 and 10 points. For "moderate" change it was 10 to 20, and for "very much" change it was more than 20 points.

Transition questions use the patient as their own control, and seek to determine whether any changes that occur are large enough to be of importance to the patient. They can therefore be described as "within-person" methods. An alternative "between-person" approach, in which patients are asked to compare their present state relative to that of others who have the same condition, has been explored by Redelmeier, Guyatt and Goldstein (1996). Reassuringly, they found it resulted in broadly similar estimates for the minimal clinically important difference.

16.7 IMPACT OF STATE OF QUALITY OF LIFE

The extent to which reduced QoL affects daily living may sometimes serve as an indicator of its importance. This is likely to be particularly true for causal scales. An example is pain: patients can be asked both about levels of pain, and its *impact* upon various activities.

Thus the Brief Pain Inventory (BPI) asks patients to rate their pain at the time of completing the questionnaire (pain now), and also its worst, least and average over the previous week. One form of scoring the BPI is to use the "pain-worst" scale as the primary response variable. To calibrate the pain-worst scale in terms of the impact of pain, patients can additionally be asked to rate how much their pain interferes with various activities and states.

Example from the literature

Table 16.5, from Cleeland (1991), shows the levels at which specific functions begin to be impaired by "pain worst" recorded on the BPI. For example, patients were asked to rate how much pain interferes with their "enjoyment of life", with 0 being "no interference" and 10 being "interferes completely". Using an interference rating of 4 to mean "impaired function", Table 16.5 shows that enjoyment of life becomes impaired when "pain worst" reaches a level of 3. Most of the items became impaired when pain reached a level of 5. This is consistent with other studies, where the midpoint of pain rating scales has been found to represent a critical value beyond which patients report disproportionate impairment of functional status. Because of these findings, Cleeland suggests, it is possible to define "significant pain" as pain that is rated at the midpoint or higher on pain intensity scales.

Table 16.5 Pain severity levels reported as impairing function (Based on Cleeland *et al.*, 1991)

Impaired function	Rating of worst pain
Enjoyment of life	3
Work	4
Mood	5
Sleep	5
General activity	5
Walking	7
Relations with others	8

16.8   CHANGES IN RELATION TO LIFE EVENTS

Since QoL scales involve unfamiliar measures, studies that relate the observed changes to changes in more familiar or objective measures can be easier to interpret. One such method is to compare changes in QoL in patients with the size of change that is expected to occur in persons who experience various major life events such as family illness, loss of a job, or bereavement.

Example from the literature

Testa and Simonson (1996), in two randomised clinical trials of antihypertensive therapy, used the General Perceived Health (GPH) scale and the Life Events Index, as well as several other QoL scales. The GPH scale contains 11 items relating to vitality, general health status including bodily disorders, and sleep disturbance. The changes from baseline were expressed using standardised response means as in equation (16.1), with the change-scores being divided by the SD of the changes observed during a period whilst the patients were stable.

The Life Events Index consists of 42 scales for major life events rated from 0 to 100 according to their level of stress. For example, a minor violation of the law was associated with a change in Life Events Index score of 11 points. Columns one and two of Table 16.6 summarise the changes relating to various life events. The authors then used linear regression to calibrate the GPH scale in terms of the Life Events Index (column three in Table 16.6).

They found that a change of 0.1 SD in the GPH scale corresponded to approximately 37 points on the Life Events Index. This corresponds to the impact that might be expected from the death of a close friend (37 points), or from sexual difficulties (39 points). A change of 0.15 SD in General Perceived Health similarly corresponds to a 55-point life events change, and this is equivalent to the impact on QoL that a major personal illness (53 points) or the

Table 16.6   Changes in QoL score, measured by the Life Events Index, that are associated with various life events (Based on Testa and Simonson, 1996)

Stressful life event	Life Events Index: change in score	General Perceived Health (GPH)	
		SD units	Corresponding change in Life Events Index
Minor violation of the law	−11		
Major change in sleeping habits	−16		
Major change in working conditions	−20	0.05	−19
Change in residence	−20		
Trouble with boss	−23		
Death of a close friend	−37	0.10	−37
Sexual difficulties	−39		
Being fired from work	−47		
Major personal injury or illness	−53	0.15	−55
Death of a close family member	−63		
Divorce	−73	0.20	−73
Death of a spouse	−100		

death of a close family member (63 points) might have. It was concluded that although there was broad variability in responses from person to person, values between 0.1 and 0.2 *SD* units can be considered clinically meaningful and represent the lower bound of what constitutes a minimally important response to treatment.

In this study, overall QoL scores shifted positively by 0.11 for treatment with captopril, and negatively by 0.11 for enalapril, an overall difference of 0.22. Testa *et al.* comment: "Our findings indicate that drug-induced changes in the QoL can be substantial and clinically meaningful even when they involve drugs in the same pharmacological class."

16.9   EFFECT SIZE

The methods discussed so far to estimate the magnitude of important changes make use of information collected from surveys of the population or from studies that investigate QoL changes in patients. When such information is unavailable, "effect sizes" may be useful. These are based solely upon the distribution of the observed data, and in particular the variability of the measurements. These measures were initially proposed for use in sample size estimation, and have been mentioned in that context in Chapter 14. Methods based upon effect size have the advantage of simplicity. Their limitation is that they do not consider the values and opinions of patients. Despite this, many investigators have found that effect sizes often seem to produce values that correspond very roughly to those obtained using patient-orientated methods.

Suppose changes in a patient's QoL are assessed using several different instruments. Some instruments may use a scale that is scored, say, 1 to 7, whilst others might score the patient from 0 to 100. Thus changes will appear to be larger on some instruments than others. One way to standardise the measurements is to divide the observed changes by the *SD*. A particular change is likely to be of greater clinical significance and of more importance to patients if it occurs on a scale that has a narrow range of values and therefore shows little variation as indicated by a small *SD*. Having scaled for the variability in this way, the standardised changes should then be of comparable magnitude to each other, despite the scales having different ranges of values.

Considering the patient-perspective, too, it can be sensible to allow for different *SD*s. The levels of QoL will vary within a patient, day-to-day. If there is a high degree of variability in QoL levels implying a large *SD*, a small improvement due to therapy may not even be noticed by the patient and would not be considered useful.

Cohen (1969, 1988) proposed this form of standardisation in order to simplify the estimation of sample sizes. He noted that to calculate a sample size, one must first specify the size of the effect that it is wished to detect. Sometimes the investigator will have knowledge or beliefs about likely, important, treatment effects, and will be able to base estimates upon that. Frequently, there will be no such prior information upon which to base decisions. Thus Cohen proposed that the mean change divided by the *SD* would serve as an "effect size index" that is suitable for sample size estimation. Based upon his experience in the social sciences, he suggested that effect sizes of 0.2 to 0.5 have generally been regarded by investigators as being "small", 0.5 to 0.8 are "moderate", and those 0.8 or above are "large".

These apparently arbitrary thresholds have stood the test of time very well. Perhaps surprisingly, the values 0.2, 0.5 and 0.8 have since been found to be broadly applicable in many fields of research as well as in social sciences from where Cohen had drawn his experience.

The name "effect size" has become used to cover a wide range of standardised measures of change, and so there is some confusion sometimes over what is intended. Two in particular stand out in QoL research. The first, the *standardised response mean*, is perhaps closest to the "effect size" of Cohen. The second method, often simply called the *effect size*, uses a different *SD*.

STANDARDIZED RESPONSE MEAN (*SRM*)

The standardised response mean (*SRM*) is the mean of the changes in the QoL scores recorded at assessments of the same subjects at two different times, divided by the *SD* of these changes in scores. Thus:

$$SRM = \frac{\bar{x}_{Time2} - \bar{x}_{Time1}}{SD_{Differrence}}. \tag{16.1}$$

A large *SRM* indicates that the change is large relative to the background variability in the measurements. Thus the *SRM* is a form of Cohen's effect-size index, and is the most widely used measure of the size of effects. The $SD_{Difference}$ should in principle be estimated from stable patients whose overall level of QoL is not expected to be changing. For example, if untreated patients under observation are expected to have a stable QoL, they might provide an estimate of the background variability. Sometimes $SD_{Difference}$ may be available from previous test–retest reliability studies conducted when developing the QoL instrument itself, since those studies also require stable patients. In practice, data on stable patients are often unavailable and the $SD_{Difference}$ of the study patients themselves is most frequently used.

EFFECT SIZE (*ES*)

The effect size (*ES*) is the mean change in scores, divided by the *SD* of the QoL scores recorded on the first occasion. The "baseline" measurement, at *Time1*, is usually chosen to be either immediately prior to starting active treatment or pre-randomisation in a clinical trial:

$$ES = \frac{\bar{x}_{Time2} - \bar{x}_{Time1}}{SD_{Time1}}. \tag{16.2}$$

Whereas the *SRM* used the $SD_{Difference}$, the *ES* uses the *SD* of the between-patient baseline scores. Thus, in support of the *ES* it may be argued that we want to consider patient baseline values and variability in order to decide what magnitude of QoL change would be important. In general, the *SD* of the baseline scores is usually larger than $SD_{Difference}$, and so *ES* is often smaller than *SRM*, although the differences are usually minor and the same thresholds of 0.2, 0.5 and 0.8 are commonly interpreted as indicating small, moderate and large effect sizes.

Example from the literature

Kazis, Anderson and Meenan (1989) describe a follow-up study involving 299 patients with rheumatoid arthritis in which the Arthritis Impact Measurement Scale (AIMS) was completed at the beginning and end of a five-year period. The AIMS is a patient self-administered questionnaire that includes 64 items, of which 45 are health status questions. These items are grouped into nine scales that are scored from 0 to 10, with higher scores indicating worse health status.

Effect-size calculations were used as a standard for determining a clinically meaningful change. Thus Table 16.7 gives the results for the nine scales, and shows both the change scores and the *SRM* values that were observed. The scales are scored so that the maximum possible worsening is −10 and the maximum improvement is +10.

The effect sizes for the changes, as measured by *SRM*, were all less than small (as defined by Cohen) except for the improvement in pain, which at 0.42 was small to moderate. Using a paired *t*-test, five of the changes reached statistical significance at $p < 0.05$. Thus these changes are statistically significant but not clinically meaningful.

Table 16.7 Change scores and effect sizes that were observed in a five-year follow-up study of 299 rheumatoid arthritis patients (Based on Kazis *et al.*, 1989)

Scale	Change score				Effect size
	$\bar{x}_5 - \bar{x}_1$	$SD_{Difference}$	t	p-value	SRM
Mobility	0.07	2.80	0.43	0.6	+0.02
Physical activity	0.41	2.57	2.76	0.006	+0.17
Dexterity	0.42	3.63	2.00	0.046	+0.12
Activities of daily living	0.02	1.76	0.20	0.8	+0.01
Household activities	0.05	1.61	0.54	0.6	−0.03
Anxiety	0.19	2.01	1.63	0.1	+0.09
Depression	0.25	1.71	2.53	0.012	+0.14
Pain	0.96	2.49	6.67	0.001	+0.42
Social activity	0.36	2.11	2.95	0.003	+0.17

Example from the literature

In the study of Osoba *et al.* (1998) described above, the results obtained using the approach of minimal clinically important difference were contrasted with the values for *ES*, and the two methods were broadly consistent. In most cases, the *ES* was 0.5 or greater ("moderate to large") when the transition questions indicated moderate or greater change. The *ES* was mostly between 0.2 and 0.5 ("small") when the transition question indicated little change, and was mostly less than 0.2 when no change was reported.

Example

> Figure 16.3 can be redrawn using the principle of effect sizes. The differences
> between the values of patients and the reference population have been divided
> by the pre-treatment between patient *SD*s, leading to the *ES* values in Figure
> 16.4. The dotted lines correspond to small, moderate and large *ES* of 0.2, 0.5
> and 0.8. Since some of the scales had approximately similar *SD*s of around 30
> points, the plot is superficially similar to that of Figure 16.3 apart from a
> scaling factor. However, role functioning is pulled towards the centre since it
> has a larger *SD* = 40, whilst emotional and cognitive functioning are accentu-
> ated since their *SD*s are 24 and 23 respectively. The effect sizes are in the region
> between small to moderate for most of the scales, but the change in appetite is
> large, and the role functioning and overall QoL show moderate reductions.

16.10   EFFECT SIZES AND META-ANALYSIS

Effect sizes are a form of standardisation, and provide a "dimensionless" number
that summarises the results. For example, if a mean treatment difference were
measured in millimetres, dividing by the *SD* which is also expressed in millimetres
would result in a number that has no measurement units. Thus the *ES* provides a
useful method for comparing results across a number of clinical trials, even when
several different instruments have been used. It therefore enables *meta-analyses* to
be carried out with QoL data.

Example from the literature

> Sheard and Maguire (1999) used *ES* to examine the effect of psychological
> intervention for anxiety and depression. Between 1976 and 1992, 19 randomised
> trials had reported results of intervention for anxiety in cancer patients, using a
> number of different instruments. The majority of trials had not detected any
> statistically significant effect, possibly sometimes because their sample sizes were
> inadequate. However, the meta-analysis, summarised in Figure 16.5, indicates
> that preventive psychological interventions may have a moderate clinical effect
> upon anxiety.
>   In Figure 16.5, the mean *ES* observed in each study is represented by a
> square, with a horizontal line indicating the 95% confidence intervals. The
> dashed vertical line represents the mean *ES* of 0.42, calculated across all 19
> studies, and the horizontal limits of the diamond show the 95% *CI* of this mean
> estimate, that is, 0.08 to 0.74.

16.11   PATIENT VARIABILITY

Most of the methods described make use of comparisons of means, and therefore
inherently assume that all patients will derive the same benefit or deterioration in
QoL according to their treatment. That is, all patients are assumed to change by the

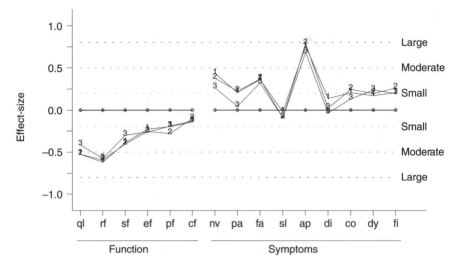

Figure 16.4 Using effect sizes, instead of absolute differences as in Figure 16.3 (Based on Bjordal *et al.*, 1999, and Hjermstad *et al.*, 1998b)

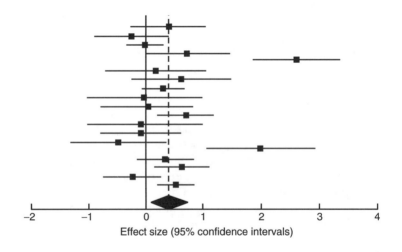

Figure 16.5 Meta-analysis of 19 trials that examined the effect of psychological intervention for anxiety in cancer patients (Based on Sheard and Maguire, 1999)

same average amount. It is also assumed that QoL scores may be sensibly aggregated by averaging—and that, for example, two patients scoring say 50% of maximum are equivalent to one patient scoring 75% and another scoring 25%.

Clearly there is variability in patient-to-patient responses. If QoL improves, on average, by 15%, most patients will experience changes that are either smaller or larger than this value and few if any will experience exactly this change. Thus even a small average benefit might allow some patients to obtain a major and very worthwhile improvement. Although it is important to know the overall mean changes, it is also important to consider the potential advantage (or disadvantage) to those patients who benefit (or suffer) most from the treatment. The *normal range* is the estimated range of values that includes a specified percentage of the observations. For example, the 95% normal range for the change in QoL would be the range of values that is expected to include 95% of patients from the relevant patient population. The limits of the normal range would indicate the magnitude of the likely benefit to those patients with the best 21/2% (upper limit of range) and worst 21/2% (lower limit of range) of responses, and also show the degree of variability in the observations. If the observations have a Normal distribution, the following formula estimates the normal range (for further details, see Campbell and Machin, 1999):

$$\text{Normal range} = \bar{x} - z_{1-\alpha/2} \times SD \text{ to } \bar{x} + z_{1-\alpha/2} \times SD. \qquad (16.3)$$

z_α is the value from Appendix Table T1 that corresponds to the proportion of patients outside the normal range (e.g. $1 - \alpha/2 = 0.975$ for 95% normal range, in which case $z_{1-\alpha/2} = 1.96$), $\bar{x}$ is the mean value, and SD is the standard deviation.

Example

> For the pain score of Table 16.7, the mean change was 0.96 and the corresponding $SD_{Difference}$ was 2.49. Assuming a Normal distribution for mean change, the 95% normal range would be $0.96 - (1.96 \times 2.49)$ to $0.96 + (1.96 \times 2.49)$ or -3.9 to $+5.8$. Therefore, we expect 95% of patients to lie within this range, but 2½% are expected to have more extreme deterioration and 2½% a more marked improvement. This is a range of 9.7 or nearly 10 points on the pain scale, and is approximately half the total range (-10 to $+10$) possible for the scale. Thus, although the mean change in pain score was 0.96, which corresponded to a small effect size, many patients could experience large and clinically important increases or decreases in pain.

16.12 NUMBER NEEDED TO TREAT

An alternative way to allow for the variation in treatment effect upon QoL is known as the *number needed to treat (NNT)*. This is an estimate of the number of patients who need to be treated with the new treatment in order for one additional patient to benefit. The *NNT* can be estimated whenever a clinical trial has a binary outcome. When evaluating QoL, one possible binary outcome might be the proportion of patients with a "moderate improvement" in QoL, where moderate improvement could be defined as an improvement greater than some specified value. Similarly, the number of psychiatric "cases", such as cases of depression, could be used.

The proportion of patients with "moderate deterioration" or "cases" can be estimated for each treatment group. If the proportions are p_T and p_C for the test and control treatments, the difference $p_T - p_C$ is called the *absolute risk reduction (ARR)*. The *NNT* is simply

$$NNT = \frac{1}{ARR} = \frac{1}{p_T - p_C}. \qquad (16.4)$$

When p_T and p_C are the proportions improving, $p_T - p_C$ is called the *absolute benefit increase* (*ABI*), and $NNT = 1/ABI$.

Example from the literature

Guyatt *et al.* (1998) describe a cross-over trial of treatment for asthma. The multi-centre double-blind randomised trial recruited 140 patients. During the three periods in this cross-over study, each patient received salmeterol, salbutamol or placebo in random sequence. Patients completed the asthma-specific AQLQ.

Two AQLQ scales were examined, asthma symptoms and activity limitations. Table 16.8 shows that the mean differences between salmeterol and the other two treatments were all statistically highly significant, but are "small" for AQLQ scores according to the classification of minimal clinically important difference in Section 16.5. The *NNT* is calculated from the proportion of patients who had obtained benefit from salmeterol, where "better" was defined as an improvement of 0.5, minus the proportion of patients who obtained a similar sized benefit from the alternative treatment. Thus in the first row of Table 16.8, these proportions are 0.42 and 0.12 for salmeterol versus salbutamol, giving *ABI* = 0.30, and hence *NNT* = 1/0.30 = 3.3. Therefore 33 patients would need to be treated for 10 to gain an important benefit in symptom reduction.

Table 16.8 Differences between groups given different treatments for asthma, showing the number needed to treat for a single patient to benefit from salmeterol (Based on Guyatt *et al.*, 1998)

AQLQ domains	Difference between treatments		Proportion better on salmeterol	Proportion better on salbutamol or placebo	Proportion who benefited	*NNT*
	Mean	*p*-value				
Salmeterol vs. salbutamol						
Asthma symptoms	0.5	<0.0001	0.42	0.12	0.30	3.3
Activity limitations	0.3	<0.0001	0.32	0.10	0.22	4.5
Salmeterol vs. placebo						
Asthma symptoms	0.7	<0.0001	0.50	0.09	0.41	2.4
Activity limitations	0.4	<0.0001	0.42	0.08	0.34	2.9

The above example related to a cross-over trial in which patients received all three treatments. Consequently the proportion of patients better on one treatment or the other could be estimated directly. In a majority of randomised trials each patient only receives one of the treatments, say C or T. Therefore we must estimate how many patients benefit from C and how many from T. Let us suppose that for the N_C controls the proportions improved, unchanged, and deteriorated are $i_C\%$, $u_C\%$ and $d_C\%$. Although $i_T\%$ of the N_T patients in the T-group improved, we might expect that some of these patients would have improved even if they had received the C instead. Assuming independence between the two groups, we can estimate that i_C of the $i_T\%$ patients would have improved anyway. Therefore, of the improved patients in the T-group, we estimate the proportion who truly benefited from T as $i_T - (i_C \times i_T) = (u_C + d_C) \times i_T$. In addition, $d_C\%$ of the T-group patients who were unchanged might have been expected to have deteriorated if they were in the C-group, giving another $d_C \times u_T$ who benefited from T. Hence, after allowing for those patients expected to benefit from C, the total proportion of the N_T patients who really benefited from T is estimated as

$$[(u_C + d_C) \times i_T] + (d_C \times u_T).$$

Similar calculations for the C-group give the proportion of the C patients that might be expected to have benefited from C, and as before $ARR = p_C - p_T$.

Example from the literature

> Guyatt *et al.* (1998) describe a parallel group trial involving 78 patients with chronic airflow limitation. In the control group, the proportions of patients whose dyspnoea was improved, unchanged and deteriorated were $i_C = 0.28$, $u_C = 0.49$ and $d_C = 0.23$. The comparable proportions for the treatment group were $i_T = 0.48$, $u_T = 0.42$ and $d_T = 0.10$. Therefore the estimated proportion who were better in the treatment group is $(0.49 + 0.23) \times 0.48 + (0.23 \times 0.42) = 0.44$. Similar calculation for the estimated proportion who are better in the control group gives $0.28 \times (0.42 + 0.10) + (0.49 \times 0.10) = 0.20$. Hence $ARR = 0.44 - 0.20 = 0.24$, and $NNT = 1/0.24 = 4.2$.
>
> Thus for every 42 patients treated it may be expected that 10 patients would have an important improvement in dyspnoea reduction as a consequence of therapy.

16.13 CONCLUSIONS

This chapter has described a variety of ways of approaching clinical significance and interpretation of results. Some methods aim to provide a better feel for the interpretation and meaning of scale scores, for example by estimating the values that may be expected in patients and in other groups such as healthy people. Other methods place greater emphasis upon the patients' perspective and clinical significance.

The interpretation of QoL results remains essentially qualitative. Clinical significance is subjective, and is a matter of opinion. The values and opinions of individual patients will differ, as will the opinions of the treating clinician and those of society in general. Thus, for a QoL measurement scale, it is unlikely that a single threshold value will be universally accepted as a cut-point that separates clinically important changes from trivial and unimportant ones. It is also likely that patients may consider changes in some aspects of QoL to be more important than others, and a change of, say, 5 points on one scale may be as clinically important as a change of 20 on another. However, many investigators are finding that, for a variety of scales assessing overall QoL and some of its dimensions, changes of between 5% and 10% (or 5 to 10 points on a 100-point scale) are noticed by patients and are regarded by them as "significant" changes.

Appendix Examples of Instruments

Contents

APPENDIX E1   SICKNESS IMPACT PROFILE (SIP)   *Page 1 of 2*
                 [EXTRACT ONLY]

PLEASE RESPOND TO (CHECK) <u>ONLY</u> THOSE STATEMENTS THAT YOU ARE <u>SURE</u>
DESCRIBE YOU TODAY AND ARE RELATED TO YOUR STATE OF HEALTH.

---

1. I am confused and start several actions at a time   ___

2. I have more minor accidents, for example, drop things, trip and fall,
    bump into things   ___

3. I react slowly to things that are said or done   ___

4. I do not finish things I start   ___

5. I have difficulty reasoning and solving problems, for example,
    making plans, making decisions, learning new things   ___

6. I sometimes behave as if I were confused or disorientated in place
    or time, for example, where I am, who is around, directions, what day it is   ___

7. I forget a lot, for example, things that happened recently, where I put
    things, appointments   ___

8. I do not keep my attention on any activity for long   ___

9. I make more mistakes than usual   ___

10. I have difficulty doing activities involving concentration and thinking   ___

CHECK HERE WHEN YOU HAVE READ ALL STATEMENTS ON THIS PAGE   ☐

© Johns Hopkins University

For permission to use contact: Health Services Research & Development Center, Johns
Hopkins School of Hygiene and Public Health, 624 North Broadway, Baltimore, MD 21205-
1901, USA

APPENDIX E1   SICKNESS IMPACT PROFILE (SIP)   *Page 2 of 2*
                [EXTRACT ONLY]

PLEASE RESPOND TO (CHECK) <u>ONLY</u> THOSE STATEMENTS THAT YOU ARE <u>SURE</u> DESCRIBE YOU TODAY AND ARE RELATED TO YOUR STATE OF HEALTH.

1. I am having trouble writing or typing   ___

2. I communicate mostly by gestures, for example, moving head, pointing,
   sign language   ___

3. My speech is understood only by a few people who know me well   ___

4. I often lose control of my voice when I talk, for example, my voice
   gets louder or softer, trembles, changes unexpectedly   ___

5. I don't write except to sign my name   ___

6. I carry on a conversation only when very close to the other person
   or looking at him   ___

7. I have difficulty speaking, for example, get stuck, stutter, stammer,
   slur my words   ___

8. I am understood with difficulty   ___

9. I do not speak clearly when I am under stress   ___

CHECK HERE WHEN YOU HAVE READ ALL STATEMENTS ON THIS PAGE   ☐

| At the end of the SIP, a reminder: |

NOW, PLEASE REVIEW THE QUESTIONNAIRE TO BE CERTAIN YOU HAVE FILLED OUT ALL THE INFORMATION. LOOK OVER THE BOXES ON EACH PAGE TO MAKE SURE EACH ONE IS CHECKED SHOWING THAT YOU HAVE READ ALL OF THE STATEMENTS. IF YOU FIND A BOX WITHOUT A CHECK, THEN READ THE STATEMENTS ON THAT PAGE.

For permission to use contact: Health Services Research & Development Center, Johns Hopkins School of Hygiene and Public Health, 624 North Broadway, Baltimore, MD 21205-1901, USA

APPENDIX E2   NOTTINGHAM HEALTH PROFILE (NHP) [EXTRACT ONLY]

Nottingham Health Profile

Please do
not write in
this margin

LISTED BELOW ARE SOME PROBLEMS PEOPLE MIGHT HAVE IN THEIR
DAILY LIVES.
READ THE LIST CAREFULLY AND PUT A TICK IN THE BOX ☐ UNDER
<u>YES</u> FOR ANY PROBLEM THAT APPLIES TO YOU <u>AT THE MOMENT</u>. TICK
THE BOX ☐ UNDER <u>NO</u> FOR ANY PROBLEM THAT DOES NOT APPLY
TO YOU. <u>PLEASE ANSWER EVERY QUESTION</u>. IF YOU ARE NOT SURE
WHETHER TO ANSWER YES OR NO, TICK WHICHEVER ANSWER YOU THINK
IS <u>MOST</u> TRUE AT THE MOMENT.

	YES	NO
I'm tired all the time	☐	☐
I have pain at night	☑	☐
Things are getting me down	☐	☑

	YES	NO
I have unbearable pain	☐	☐
I take tablets to help me sleep	☐	☐
I've forgotten what it's like to enjoy myself	☐	☐

	YES	NO
I'm feeling on edge	☐	☐
I find it painful to change position	☐	☐
I feel lonely	☐	☐

Please turn over the page

For permission to use contact: Dr Stephen McKenna, Galen Research, Enterprise
House, Manchester Science Park, Lloyd Street North, Manchester M15 6SU, UK

The SF-36™ Health Survey

Instructions for Completing the Questionnaire

Please answer every question. Some questions may look like others, but each one is different. Please take the time to read and answer each question carefully by filling in the bubble that best represents your response.

EXAMPLE

This is for your review. Do not answer this question. The questionnaire begins with the section *Your Health in General* below.

For each question you will be asked to fill in a bubble in each line.

1.   How strongly do you agree or disagree with each of the following statements?

	Strongly agree	Agree	Uncertain	Disagree	Strongly disagree
a) I enjoy listening to music.	○	●	○	○	○
b) I enjoy reading magazines.	●	○	○	○	○

Please begin answering the questions now.

Your Health in General

1.   In general, would you say your health is:

Excellent	Very good	Good	Fair	Poor
○	○	○	○	○

2.   **Compared to one year ago**, how would you rate your health <u>now</u>?

Much better now than one year ago	Somewhat better now than one year ago	About the same as one year ago	Somewhat worse now than one year ago	Much worse now than one year ago
○	○	○	○	○

Please turn the page and continue

For permission to use contact: Dr John Ware, Medical Outcomes Trust, 20 Park Plaza, Suite 1014, Boston, MA 02116-4313, USA

APPENDIX E3 MEDICAL OUTCOMES STUDY (SF-36) *Page 2 of 3*

3. The following items are about activities you might do during a typical day. **Does your health now limit you** in these activities? If so, how much?

	Yes, limited a lot	Yes, limited a little	No, not limited at all
a) **Vigorous activities**, such as running, lifting heavy objects, participating in strenuous sports	○	○	○
b) **Moderate activities**, such as moving a table, pushing a vacuum cleaner, bowling, or playing golf	○	○	○
c) Lifting or carrying groceries	○	○	○
d) Climbing **several** flights of stairs	○	○	○
e) Climbing **one** flight of stairs	○	○	○
f) Bending, kneeling, or stooping	○	○	○
g) Walking **more than a mile**	○	○	○
h) Walking **several blocks**	○	○	○
i) Walking **one block**	○	○	○
j) Bathing or dressing yourself	○	○	○

4. During the **past 4 weeks**, have you had any of the following problems with your work or other regular daily activities as a result of your physical health?

	Yes	No
a) Cut down on the **amount of time** you spent on work or other activities	○	○
b) **Accomplished less** than you would like	○	○
c) Were limited in the **kind** of work or other activities	○	○
d) Had **difficulty** performing the work or other activities (for example, it took extra time)	○	○

5. During the **past 4 weeks**, have you had any of the following problems with your work or other regular daily activities as a result of any emotional problems (such as feeling depressed or anxious)?

	Yes	No
a) Cut down on the **amount of time** you spent on work or other activities	○	○
b) **Accomplished less** than you would like	○	○
c) Didn't do work or other activities as **carefully** as usual	○	○

Please turn the page to continue

For permission to use contact: Dr John Ware, Medical Outcomes Trust, 20 Park Plaza, Suite 1014, Boston, MA 02116-4313, USA

APPENDIX E3   MEDICAL OUTCOMES STUDY (SF-36)   *Page 3 of 3*

6. During the **past 4 weeks**, to what extent has your physical health or emotional problems interfered with your normal social activities with family, friends, neighbors, or groups?

Not at all	Slightly	Moderately	Quite a bit	Extremely
○	○	○	○	○

7. How much <u>bodily</u> pain have you had during the **past 4 weeks**?

None	Very mild	Mild	Moderate	Severe	Very severe
○	○	○	○	○	○

8. During the **past 4 weeks**, how much did <u>pain</u> interfere with your normal work (including both work outside the home and housework)?

Not at all	A little bit	Moderately	Quite a bit	Extremely
○	○	○	○	○

9. These questions are about how you feel things have been with you during the **past 4 weeks**. For each question, please give the one answer that comes closest to the way you have been feeling. How much of the time during the **past 4 weeks** . . .

	All of the time	Most of the time	A good bit of the time	Some of the time	A little of the time	None of the time
a) Did you feel full of pep?	○	○	○	○	○	○
b) Have you been a very nervous person?	○	○	○	○	○	○
c) Have you felt so down in the dumps nothing could cheer you up?	○	○	○	○	○	○
d) Have you felt calm and peaceful?	○	○	○	○	○	○
e) Did you have a lot of energy?	○	○	○	○	○	○
f) Have you felt downhearted and blue?	○	○	○	○	○	○
g) Did you feel worn out?	○	○	○	○	○	○
h) Have you been a happy person?	○	○	○	○	○	○
i) Did you feel tired?	○	○	○	○	○	○

10. During the **past 4 weeks**, how much of the time has your <u>physical health or emotional problems</u> interfered with your social activities (like visiting friends, relatives, etc.)?

All of the time	Most of the time	Some of the time	A little of the time	None of the time
○	○	○	○	○

11. How TRUE or FALSE is <u>each</u> of the following statements for you?

	Definitely true	Mostly true	Don't know	Mostly false	Definitely false
a) I seem to get sick a little easier than other people	○	○	○	○	○
b) I am as healthy as anybody I know	○	○	○	○	○
c) I expect my health to get worse	○	○	○	○	○
d) My health is excellent	○	○	○	○	○

THANK YOU FOR COMPLETING THIS QUESTIONNAIRE!

For permission to use contact: Dr John Ware, Medical Outcomes Trust, 20 Park Plaza, Suite 1014, Boston, MA 02116-4313, USA

By placing a tick in one box in each group below, please indicate which
statements best describe your own health state today.

Mobility

I have no problems in walking about ☐

I have some problems in walking about ☑

I am confined to bed ☐

Self-Care

I have no problems with self-care ☑

I have some problems washing or dressing myself ☐

I am unable to wash or dress myself ☐

Usual activities *(e.g. work, study, housework, family or
leisure activities)*

I have no problems with performing my usual activities ☐

I have some problems with performing my usual activities ☐

I am unable to perform my usual activities ☐

Pain/Discomfort

I have no pain or discomfort ☐

I have moderate pain or discomfort ☐

I have extreme pain or discomfort ☐

Anxiety/Depression

I am not anxious or depressed ☐

I am moderately anxious or depressed ☐

I am extremely anxious or depressed ☐

For permission to use contact: Dr Frank de Charro, EuroQoL Group Business Manager,
PO Box 4443, 3006 AK Rotterdam, The Netherlands

APPENDIX E4   EURoQol (EQ-5D)   *Page 2 of 2*

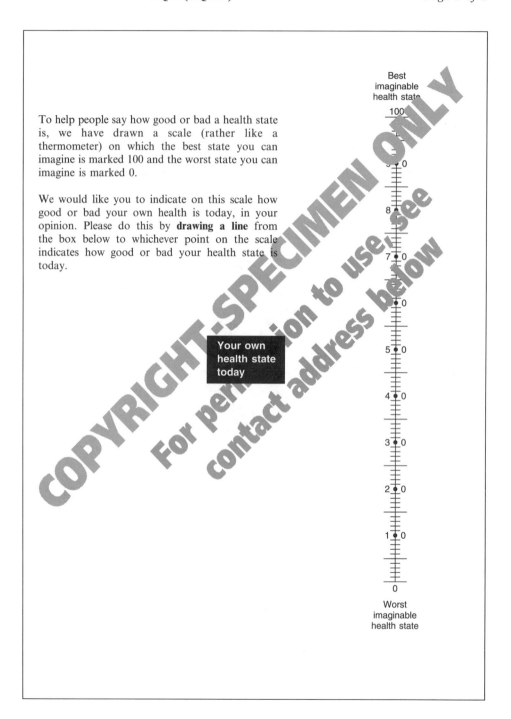

To help people say how good or bad a health state is, we have drawn a scale (rather like a thermometer) on which the best state you can imagine is marked 100 and the worst state you can imagine is marked 0.

We would like you to indicate on this scale how good or bad your own health is today, in your opinion. Please do this by **drawing a line** from the box below to whichever point on the scale indicates how good or bad your health state is today.

Your own health state today

APPENDIX E5 A PATIENT GENERATED INDEX© OF QUALITY OF LIFE (PGI)

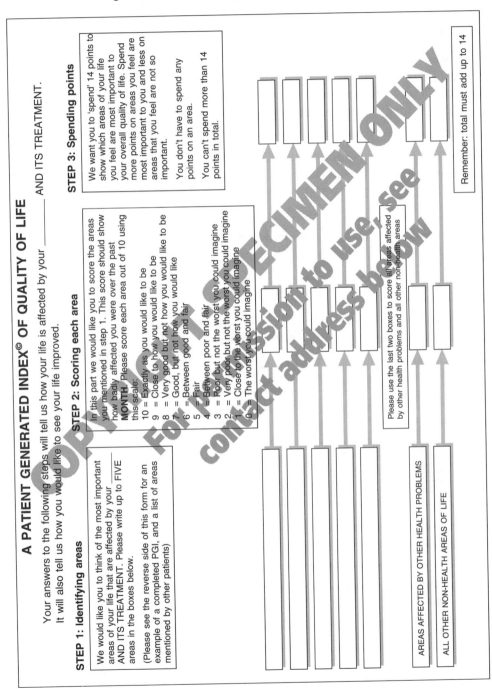

A PATIENT GENERATED INDEX© OF QUALITY OF LIFE

Your answers to the following steps will tell us how your life is affected by your _____ AND ITS TREATMENT.
It will also tell us how you would like to see your life improved.

STEP 1: Identifying areas

We would like you to think of the most important areas of your life that are affected by your _____ AND ITS TREATMENT. Please write up to FIVE areas in the boxes below.

(Please see the reverse side of this form for an example of a completed PGI, and a list of areas mentioned by other patients)

STEP 2: Scoring each area

In this part we would like you to score the areas you mentioned in step 1. This score should show how badly affected you were over the past MONTH. Please score each area out of 10 using this scale:

10 = Exactly as you would like to be
9 = Close to how you would like to be
8 = Very good but not how you would like to be
7 = Good, but not how you would like
6 = Between good and fair
5 = Fair
4 = Between poor and fair
3 = Poor but not the worst you could imagine
2 = Very poor but not the worst you could imagine
1 = Close to the worst you could imagine
0 = The worst you could imagine

STEP 3: Spending points

We want you to 'spend' 14 points to show which areas of your life you feel are most important to your overall quality of life. Spend more points on areas you feel are most important to you and less on areas that you feel are not so important.

You don't have to spend any points on an area.

You can't spend more than 14 points in total.

Please use the last two boxes to score all areas affected by other health problems and all other non-health areas.

AREAS AFFECTED BY OTHER HEALTH PROBLEMS

ALL OTHER NON-HEALTH AREAS OF LIFE

Remember: total must add up to 14

For permission to use contact: Dr Danny Ruta, Department of Epidemiology & Public Health, Ninewells Hospital & Medical School, Dundee DD1 9SY, Scotland

EORTC QLQ-C30 (version 3)

We are interested in some things about you and your health. Please answer all of the questions yourself by circling the number that best applies to you. There are no "right" or "wrong" answers. The information that you provide will remain strictly confidential.

Please fill in your initials: ⊔⌷⌷⌷⌷

Your birthdate (Day, Month, Year): ⊔⌷⌷⌷⌷⌷⌷

Today's date (Day, Month, Year): ⊔⌷⌷⌷⌷⌷⌷

		Not at all	A little	Quite a bit	Very much
1.	Do you have any trouble doing strenuous activities, like carrying a heavy shopping bag or a suitcase?	1	2	3	4
2.	Do you have any trouble taking a long walk?	1	2	3	4
3.	Do you have any trouble taking a short walk outside of the house?	1	2	3	4
4.	Do you need to stay in bed or a chair during the day?	1	2	3	4
5.	Do you need help with eating, dressing, washing yourself or using the toilet?	1	2	3	4

During the past week:		Not at all	A little	Quite a bit	Very much
6.	Were you limited in doing either your work or other daily activities?	1	2	3	4
7.	Were you limited in pursuing your hobbies or other leisure time activities?	1	2	3	4
8.	Were you short of breath?	1	2	3	4
9.	Have you had pain?	1	2	3	4
10.	Did you need to rest?	1	2	3	4
11.	Have you had trouble sleeping?	1	2	3	4
12.	Have you felt weak?	1	2	3	4
13.	Have you lacked appetite?	1	2	3	4
14.	Have you felt nauseated?	1	2	3	4
15.	Have you vomited?	1	2	3	4

Please go on to the next page

For permission to use contact: Quality of Life Unit, EORTC Data Centre, Avenue E Mounier 83-B11, 1200 Brussels, Belgium

During the past week:	Not at all	A little	Quite a bit	Very much
16. Have you been constipated?	1	2	3	4
17. Have you had diarrhea?	1	2	3	4
18. Were you tired?	1	2	3	4
19. Did pain interfere with your daily activities?	1	2	3	4
20. Have you had difficulty in concentrating on things, like reading a newspaper or watching television?	1	2	3	4
21. Did you feel tense?	1	2	3	4
22. Did you worry?	1	2	3	4
23. Did you feel irritable?	1	2	3	4
24. Did you feel depressed?	1	2	3	4
25. Have you had difficulty remembering things?	1	2	3	4
26. Has your physical condition or medical treatment interfered with your <u>family</u> life?	1	2	3	4
27. Has your physical condition or medical treatment interfered with your <u>social</u> activities?	1	2	3	4
28. Has your physical condition or medical treatment caused you financial difficulties?	1	2	3	4

For the following questions please circle the number between 1 and 7 that best applies to you

29. How would you rate your overall <u>health</u> during the past week?

1	2	3	4	5	6	7
Very poor						Excellent

30. How would you rate your overall <u>quality of life</u> during the past week?

1	2	3	4	5	6	7
Very poor						Excellent

For permission to use contact: Quality of Life Unit, EORTC Data Centre, Avenue E Mounier 83-B11, 1200 Brussels, Belgium

APPENDIX E7   EORTC HEAD AND NECK MODULE *Page 1 of 2*
(EORTC QLQ-H&N35)

EORTC QLQ-H&N35

Patients sometimes report that they have the following symptoms or problems. Please indicate the extent to which you have experienced these symptoms or problems <u>during the past week</u>. Please answer by circling the number that best applies to you.

During the past week:	Not at all	A little	Quite a bit	Very much
1. Have you had pain in your mouth?	1	2	3	4
2. Have you had pain in your jaw?	1	2	3	4
3. Have you had soreness in your mouth?	1	2	3	4
4. Have you had a painful throat?	1	2	3	4
5. Have you had problems swallowing liquids?	1	2	3	4
6. Have you had problems swallowing pureed food?	1	2	3	4
7. Have you had problems swallowing solid food?	1	2	3	4
8. Have you choked when swallowing?	1	2	3	4
9. Have you had problems with your teeth?	1	2	3	4
10. Have you had problems opening your mouth wide?	1	2	3	4
11. Have you had a dry mouth?	1	2	3	4
12. Have you had sticky saliva?	1	2	3	4
13. Have you had problems with your sense of smell?	1	2	3	4
14. Have you had problems with your sense of taste?	1	2	3	4
15. Have you coughed?	1	2	3	4
16. Have you been hoarse?	1	2	3	4
17. Have you felt ill?	1	2	3	4
18. Has your appearance bothered you?	1	2	3	4

<u>Please go on to the next page</u>

For permission to use contact: Quality of Life Unit, EORTC Data Centre, Avenue E Mounier 83-B11, 1200 Brussels, Belgium

APPENDIX E7 EORTC HEAD AND NECK MODULE (EORTC QLQ-H&N35) *Page 2 of 2*

During the past week:	Not at all	A little	Quite a bit	Very much
19. Have you had trouble eating?	1	2	3	4
20. Have you had trouble eating in front of your family?	1	2	3	4
21. Have you had trouble eating in front of other people?	1	2	3	4
22. Have you had trouble enjoying your meals?	1	2	3	4
23. Have you had trouble talking to other people?	1	2	3	4
24. Have you had trouble talking on the telephone?	1	2	3	4
25. Have you had trouble having social contact with your family?	1	2	3	4
26. Have you had trouble having social contact with friends?	1	2	3	4
27. Have you had trouble going out in public?	1	2	3	4
28. Have you had trouble having physical contact with family or friends?	1	2	3	4
29. Have you felt less interest in sex?	1	2	3	4
30. Have you felt less sexual enjoyment?	1	2	3	4

During the past week:	No	Yes
31. Have you used pain-killers?	1	2
32. Have you taken any nutritional supplements (excluding vitamins)?	1	2
33. Have you used a feeding tube?	1	2
34. Have you lost weight?	1	2
35. Have you gained weight?	1	2

For permission to use contact: Quality of Life Unit, EORTC Data Centre, Avenue E Mounier 83-B11, 1200 Brussels, Belgium

APPENDIX E8 FUNCTIONAL ASSESSMENT OF   *Page 1 of 2*
                     CANCER—GENERAL VERSION (FACT-G)

FACT-G (Version 4)

Below is a list of statements that other people with your illness have said are important. **By circling one (1) number per line, please indicate how true each statement has been for you during the past 7 days**.

	PHYSICAL WELL-BEING	Not at all	A little bit	Some-what	Quite a bit	Very much
GP 1	I have a lack of energy.........................	0	1	2	3	4
GP 2	I have nausea	0	1	2	3	4
GP 3	Because of my physical condition, I have trouble meeting the needs of my family.................	0	1	2	3	4
GP 4	I have pain	0	1	2	3	4
GP 5	I am bothered by the side effects of treatment	0	1	2	3	4
GP 6	I feel ill	0	1	2	3	4
GP 7	I am forced to spend time in bed.................	0	1	2	3	4

	SOCIAL/FAMILY WELL-BEING	Not at all	A little bit	Some-what	Quite a bit	Very much
GS 1	I feel close to my friends........................	0	1	2	3	4
GS 2	I get emotional support from my family...........	0	1	2	3	4
GS 3	I get support from my friends	0	1	2	3	4
GS 4	My family has accepted my illness	0	1	2	3	4
GS 5	I am satisfied with family communication about my illness	0	1	2	3	4
GS 6	I feel close to my partner (or the person who is my main support).................................	0	1	2	3	4
Q1	*Regardless of your current level of sexual activity, please answer the following question. If you prefer not to answer it, please check this box* ☐ *and go to the next section.*					
GS 7	I am satisfied with my sex life	0	1	2	3	4

For permission to use contact: Dr David F. Cella, Center on Outcomes, Research & Education, Evanston Northwestern Healthcare, 1000 Central Street, Suite 101, Evanston, IL 60201, USA

FACT-G (Version 4)

By circling one (1) number per line, please indicate how true each statement has been for you during the past 7 days.

EMOTIONAL WELL-BEING	Not at all	A little bit	Some-what	Quite a bit	Very much
GE 1 I feel sad...	0	1	2	3	4
GE 2 I am satisfied with how I am coping with my illness .	0	1	2	3	4
GE 3 I am losing hope in the fight against my illness......	0	1	2	3	4
GE 4 I feel nervous...................................	0	1	2	3	4
GE 5 I worry about dying	0	1	2	3	4
GE 6 I worry that my condition will get worse............	0	1	2	3	4

FUNCTIONAL WELL-BEING	Not at all	A little bit	Some-what	Quite a bit	Very much
GF 1 I am able to work (include work at home).........	0	1	2	3	4
GF 2 My work (include work at home) is fulfilling.......	0	1	2	3	4
GF 3 I am able to enjoy life	0	1	2	3	4
GF 4 I have accepted my illness.....................	0	1	2	3	4
GF 5 I am sleeping well	0	1	2	3	4
GF 6 I am enjoying the things I usually do for fun	0	1	2	3	4
GF 7 I am content with the quality of my life right now...	0	1	2	3	4

Rotterdam Symptom Checklist　　　　　　　　　**Confidential**

date of completion _____ 19 _____

In this questionnaire you will be asked about your symptoms. Would you please, for all symptoms mentioned, indicate to what extent you have been bothered by it, by circling the answer most applicable to you. The questions are related to the past week.

Example: *Have you been bothered, during the past week, by*

headaches	not at all	(a little)	quite a bit	very much

Have you, during the past week, been bothered by

lack of appetite	not at all	a little	quite a bit	very much
irritability	not at all	a little	quite a bit	very much
tiredness	not at all	a little	quite a bit	very much
worrying	not at all	a little	quite a bit	very much
sore muscles	not at all	a little	quite a bit	very much
depressed mood	not at all	a little	quite a bit	very much
lack of energy	not at all	a little	quite a bit	very much
low back pain	not at all	a little	quite a bit	very much
nervousness	not at all	a little	quite a bit	very much
nausea	not at all	a little	quite a bit	very much
despairing about the future	not at all	a little	quite a bit	very much
difficulty sleeping	not at all	a little	quite a bit	very much
headaches	not at all	a little	quite a bit	very much
vomiting	not at all	a little	quite a bit	very much
dizziness	not at all	a little	quite a bit	very much
decreased sexual interest	not at all	a little	quite a bit	very much
tension	not at all	a little	quite a bit	very much
abdominal (stomach) aches	not at all	a little	quite a bit	very much
anxiety	not at all	a little	quite a bit	very much
constipation	not at all	a little	quite a bit	very much

For permission to use contact: Professor J.C.J.M. de Haes, Academisch Medisch Centrum, Universiteit van Amsterdam, Meibergdreef 9 Postbus 22660, 1100 DD Amsterdam, The Netherlands

APPENDIX E9 ROTTERDAM SYMPTOM CHECKLIST© (RSCL)

diarrhoea	not at all	a little	quite a bit	very much
acid indigestion	not at all	a little	quite a bit	very much
shivering	not at all	a little	quite a bit	very much
tingling hands or feet	not at all	a little	quite a bit	very much
difficulty concentrating	not at all	a little	quite a bit	very much
sore mouth/pain when swallowing	not at all	a little	quite a bit	very much
loss of hair	not at all	a little	quite a bit	very much
burning/sore eyes	not at all	a little	quite a bit	very much
shortness of breath	not at all	a little	quite a bit	very much
dry mouth	not at all	a little	quite a bit	very much

A number of activities is listed below. *We do not want to know whether you actually do these, but only whether you are able to perform them presently. Would you please mark the answer that applies most to your condition of the past week.*

	unable	only with help	without help, with difficulty	without help
care for myself (wash etc)	○	○	○	○
walk about the house	○	○	○	○
light housework/household jobs	○	○	○	○
climb stairs	○	○	○	○
heavy housework/household jobs	○	○	○	○
walk out of doors	○	○	○	○
go shopping	○	○	○	○
go to work	○	○	○	○

All things considered, how would you describe your quality of life during the past week?

- ○ excellent
- ○ good
- ○ moderately good
- ○ neither good nor bad
- ○ rather poor
- ○ poor
- ○ extremely poor

Would you please check whether you answered all questions?

Thank you for your help. patient number _____

For permission to use contact: Professor J.C.J.M. de Haes, Academisch Medisch Centrum, Universiteit van Amsterdam, Meibergdreef 9 Postbus 22660, 1100 DD Amsterdam, The Netherlands

APPENDIX E10   QUALITY OF LIFE IN EPILEPSY (QOLIE-89) *Page 1 of 4*
[EXTRACT ONLY]

QUALITY OF LIFE IN EPILEPSY QUOLIE-89 (*Version 1.0*)

*Do Not
Write in
This Space*

Patient Inventory

Today's date __/__/__

Patient's name _____

Patient's ID# _____

Gender: ☐ Male ☐ Female   Birthdate __/__/__

INSTRUCTIONS

This survey asks you about your health and daily activities. **Answer every question** by circling the appropriate number (1, 2, . . .).

If you are unsure about how to answer a question, please give the best answer you can and write a comment or explanation in the margin.

Please feel free to ask someone to assist you if you need help reading or marking the form.

1.   In general, would you say your health is: (Circle one number)

Excellent	1
Very good	2
Good	3
Fair	4
Poor	5

2.   Overall, how would you rate your quality of life?

(Circle one number on the scale below)

10 9   8 7   6 5   4 3   2 1   0
Best Possible   Worst Possible
Quality of Life   Quality of Life
                                           (as bad as or worse
                                           than being dead)

For permission to use contact: Dr O. Devinsky, Office of Contract and Grant Services, RAND, 1700 Main Street, PO Box 2138, Santa Monica, CA 90407-2138, USA

APPENDIX E10 QUALITY OF LIFE IN EPILEPSY (QOLIE-89) *Page 2 of 4*
[EXTRACT ONLY]

---

3. **Compared to 1 year ago**, how would you rate your health in general **now**? | *Do Not Write in This Space*

(Circle one number)

Much better now than 1 year ago	1
Somewhat better now than 1 year ago	2
About the same as 1 year ago	3
Somewhat worse now than 1 year ago	4
Much worse now than 1 year ago	5

4–13: The following questions are about activities you might do during a typical day. Does **your health** limit you in these activities? If so, **how much**?

(Circle 1, 2, or 3 on each line)

		Yes, limited a lot	Yes, limited a little	No, not limited at all
4.	*Vigorous activities*, such as running, lifting heavy objects, participating in strenuous sports	1	2	3
5.	*Moderate activities*, such as moving a table, pushing a vacuum cleaner, bowling, or playing golf	1	2	3
6.	Lifting or carrying groceries	1	2	3
7.	Climbing *several* flights of stairs	1	2	3
8.	Climbing *one* flight of stairs	1	2	3
9.	Bending, kneeling, or stooping	1	2	3
10.	Walking *more than one mile*	1	2	3
11.	Walking *several* blocks	1	2	3
12.	Walking *one block*	1	2	3
13.	Bathing or dressing yourself	1	2	3

For permission to use contact: Dr O. Devinsky, Office of Contract and Grant Services, RAND, 1700 Main Street, PO Box 2138, Santa Monica, CA 90407-2138, USA

APPENDIX E10   QUALITY OF LIFE IN EPILEPSY (QOLIE-89) *Page 3 of 4*
[EXTRACT ONLY]

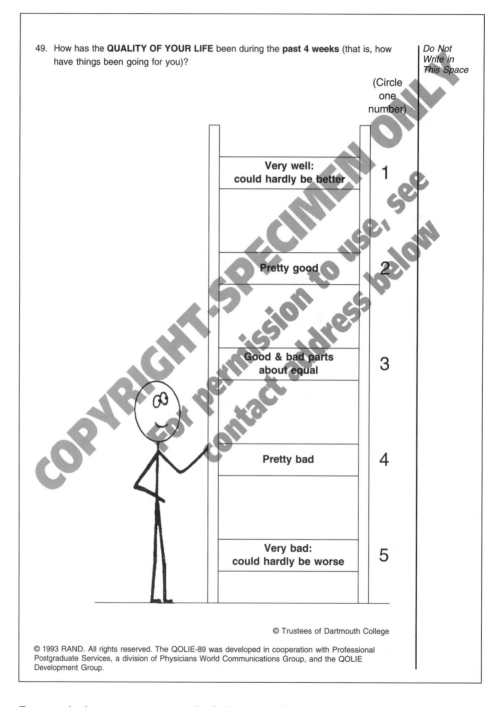

49. How has the **QUALITY OF YOUR LIFE** been during the **past 4 weeks** (that is, how have things been going for you)?

Do Not Write in This Space

(Circle one number)

Very well: could hardly be better	1
Pretty good	2
Good & bad parts about equal	3
Pretty bad	4
Very bad: could hardly be worse	5

© Trustees of Dartmouth College

For permission to use contact: Dr O. Devinsky, Office of Contract and Grant Services, RAND, 1700 Main Street, PO Box 2138, Santa Monica, CA 90407-2138, USA

APPENDIX E10   QUALITY OF LIFE IN EPILEPSY (QOLIE-89) *Page 4 of 4*
                 [EXTRACT ONLY]

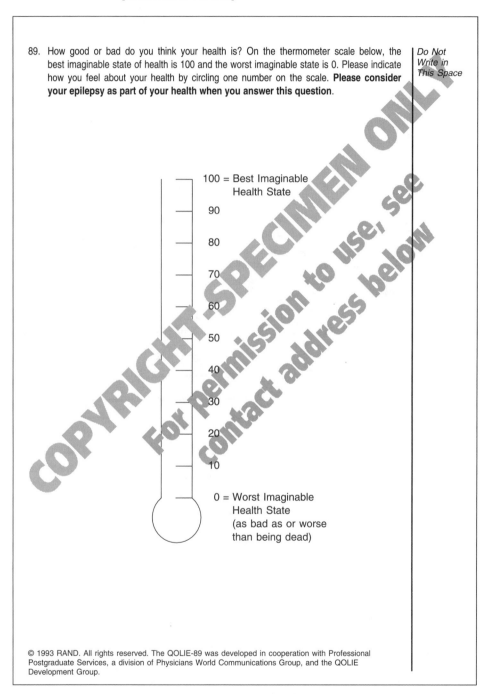

89. How good or bad do you think your health is? On the thermometer scale below, the *Do Not Write in This Space* best imaginable state of health is 100 and the worst imaginable state is 0. Please indicate how you feel about your health by circling one number on the scale. **Please consider your epilepsy as part of your health when you answer this question**.

100 = Best Imaginable
       Health State

90

80

70

60

50

40

30

20

10

0 = Worst Imaginable
    Health State
    (as bad as or worse
    than being dead)

For permission to use contact: Dr O. Devinsky, Office of Contract and Grant Services, RAND, 1700 Main Street, PO Box 2138, Santa Monica, CA 90407-2138, USA

APPENDIX E11   PAEDIATRIC ASTHMA QUALITY OF LIFE *Page 1 of 2*
QUESTIONNAIRE (PAQLQ)
[EXTRACT ONLY]

PAEDIATRIC ASTHMA QUALITY OF LIFE QUESTIONNAIRE

PATIENT ID _____

SELF-ADMINISTERED   DATE _____

Page 1 of 5

ACTIVITIES

Because you have asthma, you may have found some of the things you like doing difficult or not much fun.

We want you to think about all the things that you do in which you have been bothered by your asthma.

Some people are bothered by asthma when doing some of the following activities. Please read through the list. Think about how your asthma has bothered you during the last week.

On the next page, write down the **three** (3) things in which you have been bothered **most** by your asthma during the last week. These activities must be activities that you will be doing regularly during the study. The three activities you choose can be from this list or you can think of other activities as long as you do them regularly.

1. BALL HOCKEY	19. WALKING UPSTAIRS
2. BASEBALL	20. LAUGHING
3. BASKETBALL	21. STUDYING
4. DANCING (BALLET/JAZZ)	22. DOING HOUSEHOLD CHORES
5. FOOTBALL	23. SINGING
6. PLAYING AT RECESS	24. DOING CRAFTS OR HOBBIES
7. PLAYING WITH PETS	25. SHOUTING
8. PLAYING WITH FRIENDS	26. GYMNASTICS
9. RIDING A BICYCLE	27. ROLLERBLADING/ROLLERSKATING
10. RUNNING	28. SKATEBOARDING
11. SKIPPING ROPE	29. TRACK AND FIELD
12. SHOPPING	30. TOBOGGANING
13. SLEEPING	31. SKIING
14. SOCCER	32. ICE SKATING
15. SWIMMING	33. CLIMBING
16. VOLLEYBALL	34. GETTING UP IN THE MORNING
17. WALKING	35. TALKING
18. WALKING UPHILL	

Write your 3 activities on the next page.

For permission to use contact: Professor E. Juniper, Department of Clinical Epidemiology & Biostatistics, McMaster University Medical Centre, Room 2C10, 1200 Main Street West, Hamilton, Ontario, Canada L8N 3Z5

APPENDIX E11   PAEDIATRIC ASTHMA QUALITY OF LIFE *Page 2 of 2*
QUESTIONNAIRE (PAQLQ)
[EXTRACT ONLY]

On the lines below, please write down the 3 activities in which you have been bothered **most** by your asthma. We then want you to tell us how much you have been bothered doing these things **during the last week because of your asthma**.

Put an x in the box that best describes how bothered you have been.

HOW **BOTHERED** HAVE YOU BEEN DURING THE LAST WEEK?

	Extremely bothered	Very bothered	Quite bothered	Somewhat bothered	Bothered a bit	Hardly bothered at all	Not bothered	Activity not done
	1	2	3	4	5	6	7	
1. _____	☐	☐	☐	☐	☐	☐	☐	☐
2. _____	☐	☐	☐	☐	☐	☐	☐	☐
3. _____	☐	☐	☐	☐	☐	☐	☐	☐
4. COUGHING	☐	☐	☐	☐	☐	☐	☐	☐

IN GENERAL, **HOW OFTEN** DURING THE LAST WEEK DID YOU:

	All of the time	Most of the time	Quite often	Some of the time	Once in a while	Hardly any of the time	None of the time
	1	2	3	4	5	6	7
5. Feel FRUSTRATED because of your asthma?	☐	☐	☐	☐	☐	☐	☐
6. Feel TIRED because of your asthma?	☐	☐	☐	☐	☐	☐	☐
7. Feel WORRIED, CONCERNED OR TROUBLED because of your asthma?	☐	☐	☐	☐	☐	☐	☐

-------------- **Example of a later question** --------------
↓   ↓

THINK ABOUT ALL THE ACTIVITIES THAT YOU DID IN THE PAST WEEK:

	Extremely bothered	Very bothered	Quite bothered	Somewhat bothered	Bothered a bit	Hardly bothered at all	Not bothered
	1	2	3	4	5	6	7
22. How much were you bothered by your asthma during these activities?	☐	☐	☐	☐	☐	☐	☐

For permission to use contact: Professor E. Juniper, Department of Clinical Epidemiology & Biostatistics, McMaster University Medical Centre, Room 2C10, 1200 Main Street West, Hamilton, Ontario, Canada L8N 3Z5

APPENDIX E12   HOSPITAL ANXIETY AND   *Page 1 of 1*
                 DEPRESSION SCALE (HADS)
                 [EXTRACT ONLY]

Hospital Anxiety and Depression (HAD) Scale

Name: _____   Trial No: ☐☐☐

Hospital: _____   Date of Completion: ☐☐ ☐☐ ☐☐
                                                               d   m   y

Doctors are aware that emotions play an important part in most illnesses. If your doctor knows about these feelings he will be able to help you more.

This questionnaire is designed to help your doctor to know how you feel. Read each item and place a firm tick in the box opposite the reply which comes closest to how you have been feeling in the past week.

Don't take too long over your replies: your immediate reaction to each item will probably be more accurate than a long thought-out response.

Tick only one box in each section

I feel tense or 'wound up':
Most of the time .... ☐
A lot of the time .... ☐
Time to time, occasionally .... ☐
Not at all .... ☐

I feel as if I am slowed down:
Nearly all the time .... ☐
Very often .... ☐
Sometimes .... ☐
Not at all .... ☐

I still enjoy the things I used to enjoy:
Definitely as much .... ☐
Not quite as much .... ☐
Only a little .... ☐
Hardly at all .... ☐

I get a sort of frightened feeling like 'butterflies' in the stomach:
Not at all .... ☐
Occasionally .... ☐
Quite often .... ☐
Very often .... ☐

For permission to use contact: NFER-NELSON, Darville House, 2 Oxford Road East, Windsor, Berkshire SL4 1DF, UK

SHORT-FORM McGILL PAIN QUESTIONNAIRE
RONALD MELZACK

PATIENT'S NAME: _____   DATE: _____

	NONE	MILD	MODERATE	SEVERE
THROBBING	0) ____	1) ____	2) ____	3) ____
SHOOTING	0) ____	1) ____	2) ____	3) ____
STABBING	0) ____	1) ____	2) ____	3) ____
SHARP	0) ____	1) ____	2) ____	3) ____
CRAMPING	0) ____	1) ____	2) ____	3) ____
GNAWING	0) ____	1) ____	2) ____	3) ____
HOT-BURNING	0) ____	1) ____	2) ____	3) ____
ACHING	0) ____	1) ____	2) ____	3) ____
HEAVY	0) ____	1) ____	2) ____	3) ____
TENDER	0) ____	1) ____	2) ____	3) ____
SPLITTING	0) ____	1) ____	2) ____	3) ____
TIRING-EXHAUSTING	0) ____	1) ____	2) ____	3) ____
SICKENING	0) ____	1) ____	2) ____	3) ____
FEARFUL	0) ____	1) ____	2) ____	3) ____
PUNISHING-CRUEL	0) ____	1) ____	2) ____	3) ____

```
NO
PAIN |---------------------------------------------| WORST
                                                     POSSIBLE
                                                     PAIN
```

PPI

0	NO PAIN	_____
1	MILD	_____
2	DISCOMFORTING	_____
3	DISTRESSING	_____
4	HORRIBLE	_____
5	EXCRUCIATING	_____

For permission to use contact: Dr Ronald Melzack, Department of Psychology, McGill University, 1205 Dr Penfield Avenue, Montreal, Quebec, Canada H3A 1B1

APPENDIX E14 MULTIDIMENSIONAL FATIGUE INVENTORY (MFI-20)

MULTIDIMENSIONAL FATIGUE INVENTORY
MFI-20

Instructions:

By means of the following statements we would like to get an idea of how you have been feeling <u>lately</u>. There is, for example, the statement:

"I FEEL RELAXED"

If you think that this is <u>entirely true</u>, that indeed you have been feeling relaxed lately, please place an X in the extreme left box; like this:

yes, that is true **X**   no, that is not true

The more you <u>disagree</u> with the statement, the more you can place an X in the direction of "no, that is not true". Please, do not miss out a statement, and place one X next to each statement.

1. I feel fit   yes, that is true   no, that is not true

2. Physically I feel only able to do a little   yes, that is true   no, that is not true

3. I feel very active   yes, that is true   no, that is not true

4. I feel like doing all sorts of nice things   yes, that is true   no, that is not true

5. I feel tired   yes, that is true   no, that is not true

6. I think I do a lot in a day   yes, that is true   no, that is not true

7. When I am doing something, I can keep my
   thoughts on it   yes, that is true   no, that is not true

8. Physically I can take on a lot   yes, that is true   no, that is not true

9. I dread having to do things   yes, that is true   no, that is not true

For permission to use contact: Dr Ellen Smets, Academisch Medisch Centrum, Universiteit van Amsterdam, Meibergdreef 9, Postbus 22660, 1100 DD Amsterdam, The Netherlands

APPENDIX E14   MULTIDIMENSIONAL FATIGUE INVENTORY (MFI-20)

Page 2 of 2

10. I think I do very little in a day

yes, that is true ☐☐☐☐☐ no, that is not true

11. I can concentrate well

yes, that is true ☐☐☐☐☐ no, that is not true

12. I am rested

yes, that is true ☐☐☐☐☐ no, that is not true

13. It takes a lot of effort to concentrate on things

yes, that is true ☐☐☐☐☐ no, that is not true

14. Physically I feel I am in a bad condition

yes, that is true ☐☐☐☐☐ no, that is not true

15. I have a lot of plans

yes, that is true ☐☐☐☐☐ no, that is not true

16. I tire easily

yes, that is true ☐☐☐☐☐ no, that is not true

17. I get little done

yes, that is true ☐☐☐☐☐ no, that is not true

18. I don't feel like doing anything

yes, that is true ☐☐☐☐☐ no, that is not true

19. My thoughts easily wander

yes, that is true ☐☐☐☐☐ no, that is not true

20. Physically I feel I am in an excellent condition

yes, that is true ☐☐☐☐☐ no, that is not true

Thank you very much for your cooperation

For permission to use contact: Dr Ellen Smets, Academisch Medisch Centrum, Universiteit van Amsterdam, Meibergdreef 9, Postbus 22660, 1100 DD Amsterdam, The Netherlands

APPENDIX E15   BARTHEL INDEX OF DISABILITY
(MODIFIED) (BI)

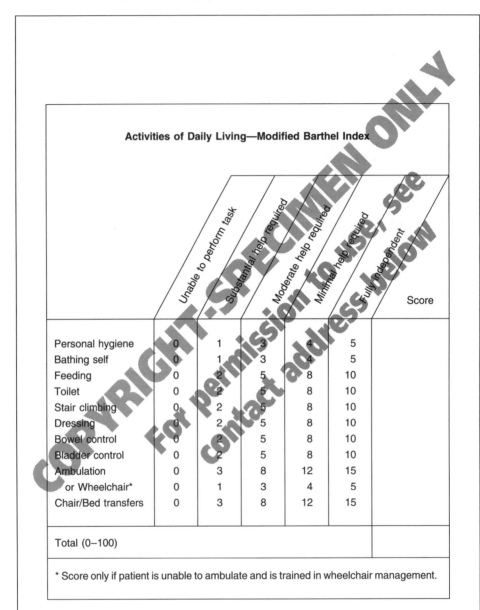

Activities of Daily Living—Modified Barthel Index

	Unable to perform task	Substantial help required	Moderate help required	Minimal help required	Fully independent	Score
Personal hygiene	0	1	3	4	5	
Bathing self	0	1	3	4	5	
Feeding	0	2	5	8	10	
Toilet	0	2	5	8	10	
Stair climbing	0	2	5	8	10	
Dressing	0	2	5	8	10	
Bowel control	0	2	5	8	10	
Bladder control	0	2	5	8	10	
Ambulation	0	3	8	12	15	
or Wheelchair*	0	1	3	4	5	
Chair/Bed transfers	0	3	8	12	15	
Total (0–100)						

* Score only if patient is unable to ambulate and is trained in wheelchair management.

For permission to use contact: Dr Surya Shah, School of Health Sciences, University of Teesside, Middlesbrough TS1 3BA, UK

Statistical Tables

TABLE T1   NORMAL DISTRIBUTION

The value tabulated is the probability, α, that a random variable, Normally distributed with mean zero and standard deviation one, will be greater than z or less than $-z$. The tabulated values are also known as two-tailed or two-sided p-values.

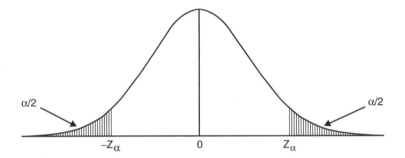

Example: The two-tailed p-value corresponding to $z = 1.96$ is 0.0500.

z	α	z	α	z	α	z	α
0.00	1.0000	0.30	0.7642	0.60	0.5485	0.90	0.3681
0.01	0.9920	0.31	0.7566	0.61	0.5419	0.91	0.3628
0.02	0.9840	0.32	0.7490	0.62	0.5353	0.92	0.3576
0.03	0.9761	0.33	0.7414	0.63	0.5287	0.93	0.3524
0.04	0.9681	0.34	0.7339	0.64	0.5222	0.94	0.3472
0.05	0.9601	0.35	0.7263	0.65	0.5157	0.95	0.3421
0.06	0.9522	0.36	0.7188	0.66	0.5093	0.96	0.3371
0.07	0.9442	0.37	0.7114	0.67	0.5029	0.97	0.3320
0.08	0.9362	0.38	0.7039	0.68	0.4965	0.98	0.3271
0.09	0.9283	0.39	0.6965	0.69	0.4902	0.99	0.3222
0.10	0.9203	0.40	0.6892	0.70	0.4839	1.00	0.3173
0.11	0.9124	0.41	0.6818	0.71	0.4777	1.01	0.3125
0.12	0.9045	0.42	0.6745	0.72	0.4715	1.02	0.3077
0.13	0.8966	0.43	0.6672	0.73	0.4654	1.03	0.3030
0.14	0.8887	0.44	0.6599	0.74	0.4593	1.04	0.2983
0.15	0.8808	0.45	0.6527	0.75	0.4533	1.05	0.2937
0.16	0.8729	0.46	0.6455	0.76	0.4473	1.06	0.2891
0.17	0.8650	0.47	0.6384	0.77	0.4413	1.07	0.2846
0.18	0.8572	0.48	0.6312	0.78	0.4354	1.08	0.2801
0.19	0.8493	0.49	0.6241	0.79	0.4295	1.09	0.2757
0.20	0.8415	0.50	0.6171	0.80	0.4237	1.10	0.2713
0.21	0.8337	0.51	0.6101	0.81	0.4179	1.11	0.2670
0.22	0.8259	0.52	0.6031	0.82	0.4122	1.12	0.2627
0.23	0.8181	0.53	0.5961	0.83	0.4065	1.13	0.2585
0.24	0.8103	0.54	0.5892	0.84	0.4009	1.14	0.2543
0.25	0.8026	0.55	0.5823	0.85	0.3953	1.15	0.2501
0.26	0.7949	0.56	0.5755	0.86	0.3898	1.16	0.2460
0.27	0.7872	0.57	0.5687	0.87	0.3843	1.17	0.2420
0.28	0.7795	0.58	0.5619	0.88	0.3789	1.18	0.2380
0.29	0.7718	0.59	0.5552	0.89	0.3735	1.19	0.2340

z	α	z	α	z	α	z	α
1.20	0.2301	1.70	0.0891	2.20	0.0278	2.70	0.0069
1.21	0.2263	1.71	0.0873	2.21	0.0271	2.71	0.0067
1.22	0.2225	1.72	0.0854	2.22	0.0264	2.72	0.0065
1.23	0.2187	1.73	0.0836	2.23	0.0257	2.73	0.0063
1.24	0.2150	1.74	0.0819	2.24	0.0251	2.74	0.0061
1.25	0.2113	1.75	0.0801	2.25	0.0244	2.75	0.0060
1.26	0.2077	1.76	0.0784	2.26	0.0238	2.76	0.0058
1.27	0.2041	1.77	0.0767	2.27	0.0232	2.77	0.0056
1.28	0.2005	1.78	0.0751	2.28	0.0226	2.78	0.0054
1.29	0.1971	1.79	0.0735	2.29	0.0220	2.79	0.0053
1.30	0.1936	1.80	0.0719	2.30	0.0214	2.80	0.0051
1.31	0.1902	1.81	0.0703	2.31	0.0209	2.81	0.0050
1.32	0.1868	1.82	0.0688	2.32	0.0203	2.82	0.0048
1.33	0.1835	1.83	0.0672	2.33	0.0198	2.83	0.0047
1.34	0.1802	1.84	0.0658	2.34	0.0193	2.84	0.0045
1.35	0.1770	1.85	0.0643	2.35	0.0188	2.85	0.0044
1.36	0.1738	1.86	0.0629	2.36	0.0183	2.86	0.0042
1.37	0.1707	1.87	0.0615	2.37	0.0178	2.87	0.0041
1.38	0.1676	1.88	0.0601	2.38	0.0173	2.88	0.0040
1.39	0.1645	1.89	0.0588	2.39	0.0168	2.89	0.0039
1.40	0.1615	1.90	0.0574	2.40	0.0164	2.90	0.0037
1.41	0.1585	1.91	0.0561	2.41	0.0160	2.91	0.0036
1.42	0.1556	1.92	0.0549	2.42	0.0155	2.92	0.0035
1.43	0.1527	1.93	0.0536	2.43	0.0151	2.93	0.0034
1.44	0.1499	1.94	0.0524	2.44	0.0147	2.94	0.0033
1.45	0.1471	1.95	0.0512	2.45	0.0143	2.95	0.0032
1.46	0.1443	1.96	0.0500	2.46	0.0139	2.96	0.0031
1.47	0.1416	1.97	0.0488	2.47	0.0135	2.97	0.0030
1.48	0.1389	1.98	0.0477	2.48	0.0131	2.98	0.0029
1.49	0.1362	1.99	0.0466	2.49	0.0128	2.99	0.0028
1.50	0.1336	2.00	0.0455	2.50	0.0124	3.00	0.00270
1.51	0.1310	2.01	0.0444	2.51	0.0121	3.10	0.00194
1.52	0.1285	2.02	0.0434	2.52	0.0117	3.20	0.00137
1.53	0.1260	2.03	0.0424	2.53	0.0114	3.30	0.00097
1.54	0.1236	2.04	0.0414	2.54	0.0111	3.40	0.00067
1.55	0.1211	2.05	0.0404	2.55	0.0108	3.50	0.00047
1.56	0.1188	2.06	0.0394	2.56	0.0105	3.60	0.00032
1.57	0.1164	2.07	0.0385	2.57	0.0102	3.70	0.00022
1.58	0.1141	2.08	0.0375	2.58	0.0099	3.80	0.00014
1.59	0.1118	2.09	0.0366	2.59	0.0096	3.90	0.00010
1.60	0.1096	2.10	0.0357	2.60	0.0093	4.00	0.00006
1.61	0.1074	2.11	0.0349	2.61	0.0091		
1.62	0.1052	2.12	0.0340	2.62	0.0088		
1.63	0.1031	2.13	0.0332	2.63	0.0085		
1.64	0.1010	2.14	0.0324	2.64	0.0083		
1.65	0.0989	2.15	0.0316	2.65	0.0080		
1.66	0.0969	2.16	0.0308	2.66	0.0078		
1.67	0.0949	2.17	0.0300	2.67	0.0076		
1.68	0.0930	2.18	0.0293	2.68	0.0074		
1.69	0.0910	2.19	0.0285	2.69	0.0071		

TABLE T2   PROBABILITY POINTS OF THE NORMAL DISTRIBUTION

The value z in Table T1 is called the standard Normal deviate. This table tabulates the value of z corresponding to the probabilities, α, for one and two-sided p-values.

Example: For an observed test statistic of $z = 2.4$, the two-sided p-value is < 0.02.

One-sided α	z	Two-sided α
0.0001	3.891	0.0002
0.0005	3.291	0.0010
0.0025	2.807	0.0050
0.0050	2.576	0.0100
0.0100	2.326	0.0200
0.0125	2.241	0.0250
0.0250	1.960	0.0500
0.0500	1.645	0.1000
0.1000	1.282	0.2000
0.1500	1.036	0.3000
0.2000	0.842	0.4000
0.2500	0.674	0.5000
0.3000	0.524	0.6000
0.3500	0.385	0.7000
0.4000	0.253	0.8000

TABLE T3   STUDENT'S *t*-DISTRIBUTION

The value tabulated is t_α, such that if X is distributed as Student's *t*-distribution with *df* degrees of freedom, then α is the probability that $X \le -t_\alpha$ or $X \ge t_\alpha$.

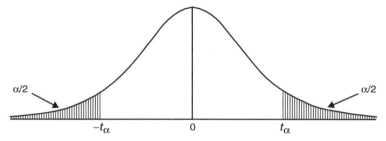

Example: The value of t_α corresponding to a two-tailed *p*-value of 0.05 is 1.960 if there are infinite degrees of freedom, but this increases to 2.228 if there are only 10 degrees of freedom.

				α				
Degrees of freedom (d)	0.2	0.1	0.05	0.04	0.03	0.02	0.01	0.001
1	3.078	6.314	12.706	15.894	21.205	31.821	63.656	636.578
2	1.886	2.920	4.303	4.849	5.643	6.965	9.925	31.600
3	1.638	2.353	3.182	3.482	3.896	4.541	5.841	12.924
4	1.533	2.132	2.776	2.999	3.298	3.747	4.604	8.610
5	1.476	2.015	2.571	2.757	3.003	3.365	4.032	6.869
6	1.440	1.943	2.447	2.612	2.829	3.143	3.707	5.959
7	1.415	1.895	2.365	2.517	2.715	2.998	3.499	5.408
8	1.397	1.860	2.306	2.449	2.634	2.896	3.355	5.041
9	1.383	1.833	2.262	2.398	2.574	2.821	3.250	4.781
10	1.372	1.812	2.228	2.359	2.527	2.764	3.169	4.587
11	1.363	1.796	2.201	2.328	2.491	2.718	3.106	4.437
12	1.356	1.782	2.179	2.303	2.461	2.681	3.055	4.318
13	1.350	1.771	2.160	2.282	2.436	2.650	3.012	4.221
14	1.345	1.761	2.145	2.264	2.415	2.624	2.977	4.140
15	1.341	1.753	2.131	2.249	2.397	2.602	2.947	4.073
16	1.337	1.746	2.120	2.235	2.382	2.583	2.921	4.015
17	1.333	1.740	2.110	2.224	2.368	2.567	2.898	3.965
18	1.330	1.734	2.101	2.214	2.356	2.552	2.878	3.922
19	1.328	1.729	2.093	2.205	2.346	2.539	2.861	3.883
20	1.325	1.725	2.086	2.197	2.336	2.528	2.845	3.850
21	1.323	1.721	2.080	2.189	2.328	2.518	2.831	3.819
22	1.321	1.717	2.074	2.183	2.320	2.508	2.819	3.792
23	1.319	1.714	2.069	2.177	2.313	2.500	2.807	3.768
24	1.318	1.711	2.064	2.172	2.307	2.492	2.797	3.745
25	1.316	1.708	2.060	2.167	2.301	2.485	2.787	3.725
30	1.310	1.697	2.042	2.147	2.278	2.457	2.750	3.646
40	1.303	1.684	2.021	2.123	2.250	2.423	2.704	3.551
50	1.299	1.676	2.009	2.109	2.234	2.403	2.678	3.496
60	1.296	1.671	2.000	2.099	2.223	2.390	2.660	3.460
∞	1.282	1.645	1.960	2.054	2.170	2.327	2.576	3.291

TABLE T4   THE χ^2 DISTRIBUTION

The value tabulated is $\chi^2(\alpha)$, such that if X is distributed as χ^2 with df degrees of freedom, then α is the probability that $X \geq \chi^2$.

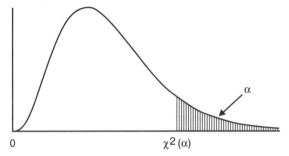

Example: If the observed test statistic, X, has a value of 7.1 with one degree of freedom, the p-value lies between 0.01 and 0.001.

Degrees of freedom (d)	α							
	0.2	0.1	0.05	0.04	0.03	0.02	0.01	0.001
1	1.64	2.71	3.84	4.22	4.71	5.41	6.63	10.83
2	3.22	4.61	5.99	6.44	7.01	7.82	9.21	13.82
3	4.64	6.25	7.81	8.31	8.95	9.84	11.34	16.27
4	5.99	7.78	9.49	10.03	10.71	11.67	13.28	18.47
5	7.29	9.24	11.07	11.64	12.37	13.39	15.09	20.51
6	8.56	10.64	12.59	13.20	13.97	15.03	16.81	22.46
7	9.80	12.02	14.07	14.70	15.51	16.62	18.48	24.32
8	11.03	13.36	15.51	16.17	17.01	18.17	20.09	26.12
9	12.24	14.68	16.92	17.61	18.48	19.68	21.67	27.88
10	13.44	15.99	18.31	19.02	19.92	21.16	23.21	29.59
11	14.63	17.28	19.68	20.41	21.34	22.62	24.73	31.26
12	15.81	18.55	21.03	21.79	22.74	24.05	26.22	32.91
13	16.98	19.81	22.36	23.14	24.12	25.47	27.69	34.53
14	18.15	21.06	23.68	24.49	25.49	26.87	29.14	36.12
15	19.31	22.31	25.00	25.82	26.85	28.26	30.58	37.70
16	20.47	23.54	26.30	27.14	28.19	29.63	32.00	39.25
17	21.61	24.77	27.59	28.44	29.52	31.00	33.41	40.79
18	22.76	25.99	28.87	29.75	30.84	32.35	34.81	42.31
19	23.90	27.20	30.14	31.04	32.16	33.69	36.19	43.82
20	25.04	28.41	31.41	32.32	33.46	35.02	37.57	45.31
21	26.17	29.62	32.67	33.60	34.76	36.34	38.93	46.80
22	27.30	30.81	33.92	34.87	36.05	37.66	40.29	48.27
23	28.43	32.01	35.17	36.13	37.33	38.97	41.64	49.73
24	29.55	33.20	36.42	37.39	38.61	40.27	42.98	51.18
25	30.68	34.38	37.65	38.64	39.88	41.57	44.31	52.62
26	31.79	35.56	38.89	39.89	41.15	42.86	45.64	54.05
27	32.91	36.74	40.11	41.13	42.41	44.14	46.96	55.48
28	34.03	37.92	41.34	42.37	43.66	45.42	48.28	56.89
29	35.14	39.09	42.56	43.60	44.91	46.69	49.59	58.30
30	36.25	40.26	43.77	44.83	46.16	47.96	50.89	59.70

TABLE 5   THE *F*-DISTRIBUTION

The value tabulated is $F(\alpha,v_1,v_2)$, such that if X has an F-distribution with v_1 and v_2 degrees of freedom, then α is the probability that $X \geq F(\alpha,v_1,v_2)$.

Example: For an observed test statistic of $X = 5.1$ with three and four degrees of freedom, $0.10 > \alpha > 0.05$.

		v_1											
v_2	α	1	2	3	4	5	6	7	8	9	10	20	∞
1	0.10	39.86	49.50	53.59	55.83	57.24	58.20	58.91	59.44	59.86	60.19	61.74	63.30
1	0.05	161.45	199.50	215.71	224.58	230.16	233.99	236.77	238.88	240.54	241.88	248.02	254.19
1	0.01	4052.18	4999.34	5403.53	5624.26	5763.96	5858.95	5928.33	5980.95	6022.40	6055.93	6208.66	6362.80
2	0.10	8.53	9.00	9.16	9.24	9.29	9.33	9.35	9.37	9.38	9.39	9.44	9.49
2	0.05	18.51	19.00	19.16	19.25	19.30	19.33	19.35	19.37	19.38	19.40	19.45	19.49
2	0.01	98.50	99.00	99.16	99.25	99.30	99.33	99.36	99.38	99.39	99.40	99.45	99.50
3	0.10	5.54	5.46	5.39	5.34	5.31	5.28	5.27	5.25	5.24	5.23	5.18	5.13
3	0.05	10.13	9.55	9.28	9.12	9.01	8.94	8.89	8.85	8.81	8.79	8.66	8.53
3	0.01	34.12	30.82	29.46	28.71	28.24	27.91	27.67	27.49	27.34	27.23	26.69	26.14
4	0.10	4.54	4.32	4.19	4.11	4.05	4.01	3.98	3.95	3.94	3.92	3.84	3.76
4	0.05	7.71	6.94	6.59	6.39	6.26	6.16	6.09	6.04	6.00	5.96	5.80	5.63
4	0.01	21.20	18.00	16.69	15.98	15.52	15.21	14.98	14.80	14.66	14.55	14.02	13.47
5	0.10	4.06	3.78	3.62	3.52	3.45	3.40	3.37	3.34	3.32	3.30	3.21	3.11
5	0.05	6.61	5.79	5.41	5.19	5.05	4.95	4.88	4.82	4.77	4.74	4.56	4.37
5	0.01	16.26	13.27	12.06	11.39	10.97	10.67	10.46	10.29	10.16	10.05	9.55	9.03
6	0.10	3.78	3.46	3.29	3.18	3.11	3.05	3.01	2.98	2.96	2.94	2.84	2.72
6	0.05	5.99	5.14	4.76	4.53	4.39	4.28	4.21	4.15	4.10	4.06	3.87	3.67
6	0.01	13.75	10.92	9.78	9.15	8.75	8.47	8.26	8.10	7.98	7.87	7.40	6.89
7	0.10	3.59	3.26	3.07	2.96	2.88	2.83	2.78	2.75	2.72	2.70	2.59	2.47
7	0.05	5.59	4.74	4.35	4.12	3.97	3.87	3.79	3.73	3.68	3.64	3.44	3.23
7	0.01	12.25	9.55	8.45	7.85	7.46	7.19	6.99	6.84	6.72	6.62	6.16	5.66
8	0.10	3.46	3.11	2.92	2.81	2.73	2.67	2.62	2.59	2.56	2.54	2.42	2.30
8	0.05	5.32	4.46	4.07	3.84	3.69	3.58	3.50	3.44	3.39	3.35	3.15	2.93
8	0.01	11.26	8.65	7.59	7.01	6.63	6.37	6.18	6.03	5.91	5.81	5.36	4.87
9	0.10	3.36	3.01	2.81	2.69	2.61	2.55	2.51	2.47	2.44	2.42	2.30	2.16
9	0.05	5.12	4.26	3.86	3.63	3.48	3.37	3.29	3.23	3.18	3.14	2.94	2.71
9	0.01	10.56	8.02	6.99	6.42	6.06	5.80	5.61	5.47	5.35	5.26	4.81	4.32
10	0.10	3.29	2.92	2.73	2.61	2.52	2.46	2.41	2.38	2.35	2.32	2.20	2.06
10	0.05	4.96	4.10	3.71	3.48	3.33	3.22	3.14	3.07	3.02	2.98	2.77	2.54
10	0.01	10.04	7.56	6.55	5.99	5.64	5.39	5.20	5.06	4.94	4.85	4.41	3.92
20	0.10	2.97	2.59	2.38	2.25	2.16	2.09	2.04	2.00	1.96	1.94	1.79	1.61
20	0.05	4.35	3.49	3.10	2.87	2.71	2.60	2.51	2.45	2.39	2.35	2.12	1.85
20	0.01	8.10	5.85	4.94	4.43	4.10	3.87	3.70	3.56	3.46	3.37	2.94	2.43
30	0.10	2.88	2.49	2.28	2.14	2.05	1.98	1.93	1.88	1.85	1.82	1.67	1.46
30	0.05	4.17	3.32	2.92	2.69	2.53	2.42	2.33	2.27	2.21	2.16	1.93	1.63
30	0.01	7.56	5.39	4.51	4.02	3.70	3.47	3.30	3.17	3.07	2.98	2.55	2.02

v_2	α	1	2	3	4	5	6	7	8	9	10	20	∞
												v_1	
40	0.10	2.84	2.44	2.23	2.09	2.00	1.93	1.87	1.83	1.79	1.76	1.61	1.38
40	0.05	4.08	3.23	2.84	2.61	2.45	2.34	2.25	2.18	2.12	2.08	1.84	1.52
40	0.01	7.31	5.18	4.31	3.83	3.51	3.29	3.12	2.99	2.89	2.80	2.37	1.82
50	0.10	2.81	2.41	2.20	2.06	1.97	1.90	1.84	1.80	1.76	1.73	1.57	1.33
50	0.05	4.03	3.18	2.79	2.56	2.40	2.29	2.20	2.13	2.07	2.03	1.78	1.45
50	0.01	7.17	5.06	4.20	3.72	3.41	3.19	3.02	2.89	2.78	2.70	2.27	1.70
100	0.10	2.76	2.36	2.14	2.00	1.91	1.83	1.78	1.73	1.69	1.66	1.49	1.22
100	0.05	3.94	3.09	2.70	2.46	2.31	2.19	2.10	2.03	1.97	1.93	1.68	1.30
100	0.01	6.90	4.82	3.98	3.51	3.21	2.99	2.82	2.69	2.59	2.50	2.07	1.45
∞	0.10	2.71	2.31	2.09	1.95	1.85	1.78	1.72	1.68	1.64	1.61	1.43	1.08
∞	0.05	3.85	3.00	2.61	2.38	2.22	2.11	2.02	1.95	1.89	1.84	1.58	1.11
∞	0.01	6.66	4.63	3.80	3.34	3.04	2.82	2.66	2.53	2.43	2.34	1.90	1.16

References

Aaronson NK, Ahmedzai S, Bergman B, Bullinger M, Cull A, Duez NJ, Filiberti A, Flechtner H, Fleishman SB, de Haes JCJM, Kaasa S, Klee MC, Osoba D, Razavi D, Rofe PB, Schraub S, Sneeuw KCA, Sullivan M and Takeda F (1993). The European Organization for Research and Treatment of Cancer QLQ-C30: A quality-of-life instrument for use in international clinical trials in oncology. *Journal of the National Cancer Institute*, **85**, 365–376.

Altman DG (1991). *Practical Statistics for Medical Research*. Chapman & Hall, London.

Altman DG, Machin D, Bryant TN and Gardner MJ (2000). *Statistics with Confidence*. British Medical Association, London.

Anderson RT, Aaronson NK and Wilkin D (1993). Critical review of the international assessments of health-related quality of life. *Quality of Life Research*, **2**, 369–395.

Andrich D (1988). *Rasch Models for Measurement*. Sage Publications, London.

Apajasalo M, Sintonen H, Holmberg C, Sinkkonen J, Aalberg V, Pihko H, Siimes MA, Kaitila I, Makela A, Rantakari K, Anttila R and Rautonen J (1996). Quality of life in early adolescence: a sixteen-dimensional health-related measure (16D). *Quality of Life Research*, **5**, 205–211.

Apgar V (1953). A proposal for a new method of evaluation of the newborn infant. *Anesthetics and Analgesics*, **32**, 260–267.

Arbuckle JL (1997). *Amos Users' Guide Version 3.6*. SmallWaters Corporation, Chicago.

Aristotle 384–322 BC (1926). *Nichomachean Ethics, Book 1 (iv)* translated by H. Rackham. W. Heinemann, London.

Bailey AJ, Parmar MKB and Stephens RJ (1998). Patients-reported short-term and long-term physical and psychologic symptoms: results of the continuous hyperfractionated accelerated radiotherapy (CHART) randomized trial in non-small-cell lung cancer. *Journal of Clinical Oncology*, **16**, 3082–3093.

Baker F and Intagliata J (1982). Quality of life in the evaluation of community support systems. *Evaluation and Program Planning*, **5**, 69–79.

Bartholomew DJ (1987). *Latent Variable Models and Factor Analysis*. Charles Griffin & Co., London.

Beaton DE, Hogg-Johnson S and Bombardier C (1997). Evaluating change in health status: reliability and responsiveness of five generic health status measures in workers with musculoskeletal disorders. *Journal of Clinical Epidemiology*, **50**, 79–93.

Beck AT, Ward CH, Mendelson M, Mock J and Erbaugh J (1961). An inventory for measuring depression. *Archives of General Psychiatry*, **4**, 561–571.

Begg C, Cho M, Eastwood S, Horton R, Moher D, Olkin I, Pitkin R, Rennie D, Schulz KF, Simel D and Stroup DF (1996). Improving the quality of reporting of randomized controlled trials: the CONSORT statement. *Journal of American Medical Association*, **276**, 637–639.

Beller E, Tattersall M, Lumley T, Levi J, Dalley D, Olver I, Page J, Abdi E, Wynne C, Friedlander M, Boadle D, Wheeler H, Margrie S and Simes RJ (1997). Improved quality of life with megestrol acetate in patients with endocrine-insensitive advanced cancer: a randomised placebo-controlled trial. *Annals of Oncology*, **8**, 277–283.

Bentler PM (1995). *EQS Structural Equations Program Manual*. Multivariate Software, Inc., Encino, CA.

Bergner M, Bobbit RA, Carter WB and Gilson BS (1981). The Sickness Impact Profile: development and final revision of a health status measure. *Medical Care*, **19**, 787–805.

Bernhard J and Gelber RD (1998). Workshop on missing data in quality of life research in cancer clinical trials. *Statistics in Medicine*, **17**, 511–796.

Bjordal K and Kaasa S (1995). Psychological distress in head and neck cancer patients 7–11 years after curative treatment. *British Journal of Cancer*, **71**, 592–597.

Bjordal K, Ahlner-Elmqvist M, Tollesson E, Jensen AB, Razavi D, Maher EJ and Kaasa S (1994a). Development of a European Organization for Research and Treatment of Cancer (EORTC) questionnaire module to be used in quality of life assessments in head and neck cancer patients. *Acta Oncologica*, **33**, 879–885.

Bjordal K, Kaasa S and Mastekaasa A (1994b). Quality of life in patients treated for head and neck cancer: a follow-up study 7 to 11 years after radiotherapy. *International Journal of Radiation Oncology, Biology, Physics*, **28**, 847–856.

Bjordal K, Hammerlid E, Ahlner-Elmqvist M, de Graeff A, Boysen M, Evensen JF, Biörklund A, de Leeuw RJ, Fayers PM, Jannert M, Westin T and Kaasa S (1999). Quality of life in head and neck cancer patients: validation of the European Organization for Research and Treatment of Cancer Quality of Life Questionnaire-H&N35. *Journal of Clinical Oncology*, **17**, 1008–1019.

Blalock HM (1982). *Conceptualization and Measurement in the Social Sciences*. Sage Publications, Beverly Hills.

Bland JM and Altman DG (1986). Statistical methods for assessing agreement between two methods of clinical measurement. *Lancet*, **1**, 307–310.

Bland JM and Altman DG (1996). Logarithms. *British Medical Journal*, **312**, 700.

Bollen KA (1989). *Structural Equations with Latent Variables*. J Wiley & Sons, New York.

Bonkovsky HL, Woolley JM and the Consensus Interferon Study Group (1999). Reduction of health-related quality of life in chronic hepatitis C and improvement with interferon therapy. *Hepatology*, **29**, 264–270.

Bowling A (1995). *Measuring Disease: A Review of Disease-Specific Quality of Life Measurement Scales*. Open University Press, Milton Keynes.

Bowling A (1997). *Measuring Health: A Review of Quality of Life Measurement Scales*. Open University Press, Milton Keynes.

British Medical Journal (1996). Advice to authors. *British Medical Journal*, **312**, 41–44.

Brooks R and with the EuroQol group (1996). EuroQol: the current state of play. *Health Policy*, **37**, 53–72.

Bryk AS, Raudenbush S and Congdon R (1996). *Hierarchical Linear and Nonlinear Modeling with the HLM/2L and HLM/3L Programs*. Scientific Software International, Chicago.

Buccheri GF, Ferrigno D, Curcio A, Vola F and Rosso A (1989). Continuation of chemotherapy versus supportive care alone in patients with inoperable non-small-cell lung cancer and stable disease after two or three cycles of MACC: results of a randomized prospective study. *Cancer*, **63**, 428–432.

Burton P, Gurrin L and Sly P (1998). Extending the simple linear regression model to account for correlated responses: an introduction to generalized estimating equations and multi-level modelling. *Statistics in Medicine*, **17**, 1261–1291.

Calman KC (1984). Quality of life in cancer patients: an hypothesis. *Journal of Medical Ethics*, **10**, 124–127.

Camilli G and Shepard LA (1994). *Methods for Identifying Biased Test Items*. Sage Publications, Thousand Oaks, California.

Campbell MJ and Machin D (1999). *Medical Statistics: A Commonsense Approach* (3rd edn). John Wiley & Sons, Chichester.

Campbell MJ, Julious SA and Altman DG (1995). Estimating sample sizes for binary, ordered categorical, and continuous outcomes in two group comparisons. *British Medical Journal*, **311**, 1145–1147.

Cella DF, Tulsky DS, Gray G, Sarafian B, Linn E, Bonomi AE, Silberman M, Yellen SB, Winicour P, Brannon J, Eckberg K, Lloyd S, Purl S, Blendowski C, Goodman M, Barnicle M, Stewart I, McHale M, Bonomi P, Kaplan E, Taylor S, Thomas CR and Harris J (1993). The Functional Assessment of Cancer Therapy scale: development and validation of the general measure. *Journal of Clinical Oncology*, **11**, 570–579.

Cleeland CS (1991). Pain assessment in cancer. *In*: Osoba D (ed.) *Effect of Cancer on Quality of Life*. CRC Press, Boca Raton: 293–304.

Cnaan A, Laird NM and Slasor P (1997). Using the general linear mixed model to analyse unbalanced repeated measures and longitudinal data. *Statistics in Medicine*, **16**, 2349–2380.

Coates A, Gebski V, Bishop JF, Jeal PN, Woods RL, Snyder R, Tattersall MH, Byrne M, Harvey V and Gill G *et al.* (1987). Improving the quality of life during chemotherapy for advanced breast cancer: a comparison of intermittent and continuous treatment strategies. *New England Journal of Medicine*, **317**, 1490–1495.

Coates A, Thomson D, McLeod GR, Hersey P, Gill PG, Olver IN, Kefford R, Lowenthal RM, Beadle G and Walpole E (1993). Prognostic value of quality of life scores in a trial of chemotherapy with or without interferon in patients with metastatic malignant melanoma. *European Journal of Cancer*, **29A**, 1731–1734.

Coates A, Porzsolt F and Osoba D (1997). Quality of life in oncology practice: prognostic value of EORTC QLQ-C30 scores in patients with advanced malignancy. *European Journal of Cancer*, **33**, 1025–1030.

Cohen J (1969). *Statistical Power Analysis for the Behavioral Sciences* (1st edn). Lawrence Erlbaum, Hillsdale, NJ.

Cohen J (1988). *Statistical Power Analysis for the Behavioral Sciences* (2nd edn). Lawrence Erlbaum, Hillsdale, NJ.

Cole BF, Gelber RD, Anderson KM and for the IBCSG (1994). Parametric approaches to quality-adjusted survival analysis. *Biometrics*, **50**, 621–631.

Conover WJ (1998). *Practical Nonparametric Statistics*. John Wiley & Sons, New York.

Cook DJ, Guyatt GH, Juniper EF, Griffith L, McIlroy W, Willan A, Jaeschke R and Epstein R (1993). Interviewer versus self-administered questionnaires in developing a disease-specific, health-related quality of life instrument for asthma. *Journal of Clinical Epidemiology*, **46**, 529–534.

Cox DR, Fitzpatrick R, Fletcher AE, Gore SM, Spiegelhalter DJ and Jones DR (1992). Quality-of-life assessment: can we keep it simple? *Journal of the Royal Statistical Society, Series A*, **155**, 353–393.

CPMP Working Party on Efficacy of Medicinal Products (1995). Biostatistical methodology in clinical trials in applications for marketing authorizations for medicinal products. *Statistics in Medicine*, **14**, 1659–1682.

Cronbach LJ (1951). Coefficient alpha and the internal structure of tests. *Psychometrika*, **16**, 297–334.

Croog SH, Levine S, Testa MA, Brown B, Bulpitt CJ, Jenkins CD, Klerman GL and Williams GH (1986). The effects of antihypertensive therapy on the quality of life. *New England Journal of Medicine*, **314**, 1657–1664.

Curran D, Fayers PM, Molenberghs G and Machin D (1998a). Analysis of incomplete quality of life data in clinical trials. In: Staquet MJ, Hays RD and Fayers PM (eds) *Quality of Life Assessment in Clinical Trials*. Oxford University Press, Oxford.

Curran D, Molenberghs G, Fayers PM and Machin D (1998b). Incomplete quality of life data in randomized trials: missing forms. *Statistics in Medicine*, **17**, 697–709.

de Haes JCJM and Stiggelbout AM (1996). Assessment of values, utilities and preferences in cancer patients. *Cancer Treatment Reviews*, **22**, Suppl A, 13–26.

de Haes JCJM, Olschewski M, Fayers PM, Visser MRM, Cull A, Hopwood P and Sanderman R (1996). *Measuring the Quality of Life of Cancer Patients: The Rotterdam Symptom Checklist (RSCL): A Manual*. Northern Centre for Healthcare Research, Groningen.

Devinsky O, Vickrey BG, Cramer J, Perrine K, Hermann B, Meador K and Hays RD (1995). Development of the quality of life in epilepsy inventory. *Epilepsia*, **36**, 1089–1104.

Diggle PJ, Liang K-Y and Zeger SL (1994). *Analysis of Longitudinal Data*. Oxford University Press, Oxford.

Fairclough DL and Cella DF (1996). Functional Assessment of Cancer Therapy (FACT-G): non-response to individual questions. *Quality of Life Research*, **5**, 321–329.

Fayers PM and Hand DJ (1997a). Factor analysis, causal indicators, and quality of life. *Quality of Life Research*, **6**, 139–150.

Fayers P and Hand DJ (1997b). Generalisation from phase III clinical trials: survival, quality of life, and health economics. *Lancet*, **350**, 1025–1027.

Fayers PM, Bleehen NM, Girling DJ and Stephens RJ (1991). Assessment of quality of life in small-cell lung cancer using a Daily Diary Card developed by the Medical Research Council Lung Cancer Working Party. *British Journal of Cancer*, **64**, 299–306.

Fayers PM, Hand DJ, Bjordal K and Groenvold M (1997a). Causal Indicators in quality of life research. *Quality of Life Research*, **6**, 393–406.

Fayers PM, Hopwood P, Harvey A, Girling DJ, Machin D and Stephens R (1997b). Quality of life assessment in clinical trials: guidelines and a checklist for protocol writers. The UK Medical Research Council experience. *European Journal of Cancer Part A*, **33**, 20–28.

Fayers PM, Curran D and Machin D (1998a). Incomplete quality of life data in randomized trials: missing items. *Statistics in Medicine*, **17**, 679–696.

Fayers PM, Weeden S, Curran D and on behalf of the EORTC Quality of Life Study Group (1998b). *EORTC QLQ-C30 Reference Values*. EORTC, Brussels.

Fayers PM, Aaronson NK, Bjordal K, Curran D, Groenvold M on behalf of the EORTC Quality of Life Study Group (1999). *EORTC QLQ-C30 Scoring Manual* (2nd edn). EORTC, Brussels.

Feeny D, Furlong W, Boyle M and Torrance GW (1995). Multi-attribute health-status classification systems: Health Utilities Index. *PharmacoEconomics*, **7**, 490–502.

Feinstein AR (1987). *Clinimetrics*. Yale University Press, New Haven.

Fisher AG (1993). The assessment of IADL motor-skills: an application of many-faceted Rasch analysis. *American Journal of Occupational Therapy*, **47**, 319–329.

Frost NA, Sparrow JM, Durant JS, Donovan JL, Peters TJ and Brookes ST (1998). Development of a questionnaire for measurement of vision-related quality of life. *Ophthalmic Epidemiology*, **5**, 185–210.

Ganz PA, Haskell CM, Figlin RA, La SN and Siau J (1988). Estimating the quality of life in a clinical trial of patients with metastatic lung cancer using the Karnofsky performance status and the Functional Living Index–Cancer. *Cancer*, **61**, 849–856.

Geddes DM, Dones L, Hill E, Law K, Harper PG, Spiro SG, Tobias JS and Souhami RL (1990). Quality of life during chemotherapy for small-cell lung cancer: assessment and use of a daily diary card in a randomized trial. *European Journal of Cancer*, **26**, 484–492.

Gelber RD, Cole BF, Gelber S and Goldhirsch A (1995). Comparing treatments using quality-adjusted survival: the Q-TWIST method. *American Statistician*, **49**, 161–169.

Gill TM (1995). Quality of life assessment: values and pitfalls. *Journal of Royal Society of Medicine*, **88**, 680–682.

Gill TM and Feinstein AR (1994). A critical appraisal of the quality of quality-of-life measurements. *Journal of American Medical Association*, **272**, 619–626.

Glaser AW, Nik Abdul Rashid NF, U CL and Walker DA (1997). School behaviour and health status after central nervous system tumours in childhood. *British Journal of Cancer*, **76**, 643–650.

Goldstein H, Rasbash L, Plewis I, Draper D, Browne W, Yang M, Woodhouse G and Healy M (1998). *A User's Guide to MLwiN*. Institute of Education, London.

Gorsuch RL (1983). *Factor Analysis* (2nd edn). Lawrence Erlbaum, Hillsdale, NJ.

Gotay CC and Moore TD (1992). Assessing quality of life in head and neck cancer. *Quality of Life Research*, **1**, 5–17.

Greenwald HP (1987). The specificity of quality-of-life measures among the seriously ill. *Medical Care*, **25**, 642–651.

Greimel ER, Padilla GV and Grant MM (1997). Physical and psychosocial outcomes in cancer patients: a comparison of different age groups. *British Journal of Cancer*, **76**, 251–255.

Groenvold M, Bjørner JB, Klee MC and Kreiner S (1995). Test for item bias in a quality of life questionnaire. *Journal of Clinical Epidemiology*, **48**, 805–816.

Groenvold M, Fayers PM, Sprangers MAG, Bjørner JB, Klee MC, Aaronson NK, Bech P and Mouridsen HT (1999). Anxiety and depression in breast cancer patients at low risk of recurrence compared with the general population: a valid comparison? *Journal of Clinical Epidemiology*, **52**, 523–530.

Guyatt GH, Feeny DH and Patrick DL (1993). Measuring health-related quality of life. *Annals of Internal Medicine*, **118**, 622–629.

Guyatt GH, Juniper EF, Walter SD, Griffith LE and Goldstein RS (1998). Interpreting treatment effects in randomised trials. *British Medical Journal*, **316**, 690–693.

Haley SM, McHorney CA and Ware JE (1994). Evaluation of the MOS SF-36 physical functioning scale (PF-10): 1. Unidimensionality and reproducibility of the Rasch item scale. *Journal of Clinical Epidemiology*, **47**, 671–684.

Hambleton RK, Swaminathan H and Rogers HJ (1991). *Fundamentals of Item Response Theory*. Sage Publications, Thousand Oaks, CA.

Hart O, Mullee MA, Lewith G and Miller J (1997). Double-blind, placebo controlled, randomized trial of homeopathic arnica C30 for pain and infection after total abdominal hysterectomy. *Journal of Royal Society of Medicine*, **90**, 73–78.

Hickey AM, Bury G, O'Boyle CA, Bradley F, O'Kelly FD and Shannon W (1996). A new short-form individual quality of life measure (SEIQoL-DW): application in a cohort of individuals with HIV/AIDS. *British Medical Journal*, **313**, 29–33.

Hillner BE, Smith TJ and Desch CE (1992). Efficacy and cost-effectiveness of autologous bone marrow transplantation in metastatic breast cancer: estimates using decision analysis while awaiting clinical trial results. *Journal of American Medical Association*, **267**, 2055–2061.

Hjermstad MJ, Fayers PM, Bjordal K and Kaasa S (1998a). Health-related quality of life in the general Norwegian population assessed by the European Organization for Research and Treatment of Cancer Core Quality-of-Life Questionnaire: the QLQ-C30 (+3). *Journal of Clinical Oncology*, **16**, 1188–1196.

Hjermstad MJ, Fayers PM, Bjordal K and Kaasa S (1998b). Using reference data on quality of life: the importance of adjusting for age and gender, exemplified by the EORTC QLQ-C30 (+3). *European Journal of Cancer*, **34**, 1381–1389.

Hopwood P, Stephens RJ, Machin D and for the Medical Research Council Lung Cancer Working Party (1994). Approaches to the analysis of quality of life data: experiences gained from a Medical Research Council Lung Cancer Working Party palliative chemotherapy trial. *Quality of Life Research*, **3**, 339–352.

Hunt SM and McKenna SP (1992). The QLDS: a scale for the measurement of quality of life in depression. *Health Policy*, **22**, 307–319.

Hunt SM, McKenna SP, McEwen J, Williams J and Papp E (1981). The Nottingham Health Profile: subjective health status and medical consultations. *Social Science & Medicine*, **15A**, 221–229.

Hürny C, Bernhard J, Joss R, Willems Y, Cavalli F, Kiser J, Brunner K, Favre S, Alberto P, Glaus A, *et al.* (1992). Feasibility of quality of life assessment in a randomized phase III trial of small-cell lung cancer: lesson from the real world. The Swiss Group for Clinical Cancer Research SAKK. *Annals of Oncology*, **3**, 825–831.

Hürny C, Bernhard J, Bacchi M, Vanwegberg B, Tomamichel M, Spek U, Coates A, Castiglione M, Goldhirsch A and Senn HJ (1993). The perceived adjustment to chronic illness scale (PACIS): a global indicator of coping for operable breast-cancer patients in clinical trials. *Supportive Care in Cancer*, **1**, 200–208.

Jachuk SJ, Brierly H, Jachuk S and Willcox PM (1982). The effect of hypotensive drugs on quality of life. *Journal of the Royal College of General Practitioners*, **32**, 103–105.

Jaeschke R, Singer J and Guyatt GH (1989). Measurement of health status: ascertaining the minimally clinically important difference. *Controlled Clinical Trials*, **10**, 407–415.

Jenkins CD (1992). Quality-of-life assessment in heart surgery. *Theoretical Surgery*, **7**, 14–17.

Jöreskog KG and Sörbom D (1996). *LISREL 8: User's Reference Guide*. Scientific Software International, Chicago.

Jones DA and West RR (1996). Psychological rehabilitation after myocardial infarction: multicentre randomised controlled trial. *British Medical Journal*, **313**, 1517–1521.

Julious SA and Campbell MJ (1996). Sample size calculations for ordered categorical data. *Statistics in Medicine*, **15**, 1065–1066.

Julious SA, George S, Machin D and Stephens RJ (1997). Sample sizes for randomized trials measuring quality of life in cancer patients. *Quality of Life Research*, **6**, 109–117.

Juniper EF, Guyatt GH, Ferrie PJ and Griffith LE (1993). Measuring quality of life in asthma. *American Review of Respiratory Disease*, **147**, 832–838.

Juniper EF, Guyatt GH, Willan A and Griffith LE (1994). Determining a minimal important change in a disease-specific quality of life questionnaire. *Journal of Clinical Epidemiology*, **47**, 81–87.

Juniper EF, Guyatt GH, Feeny DH, Ferrie PJ, Griffith LE and Townsend M (1996). Measuring quality of life in children with asthma. *Quality of Life Research*, **5**, 35–46.

Kaiser HF (1960). The application of electronic computers to factor analysis. *Educational and Psychological Measurement*, **20**, 141–151.

Kaplan RM, Bush JW and Berry CC (1979). Health status index category rating versus magnitude estimation for measuring levels of well-being. *Medical Care*, **17**, 501–525.

Karnofsky DA and Burchenal JH (1947). The clinical evaluation of chemotherapeutic agents in cancer. *In*: Maclead CM (ed.) *Evaluation of Chemotherapeutic Agents*. Columbia University Press, New York.

Katz LA, Ford AB, Moskowitz RW, Jackson BA and Jaffe MW (1963). Studies of illness in the aged: the index of ADL, a standardized measure of biological and psychosocial function. *Journal of American Medical Association*, **185**, 914–919.

Kazis LE, Anderson JJ and Meenan RF (1989). Effect sizes for interpreting changes in health-status. *Medical Care*, **27**, S178–S189.

King MT, Dobson AJ and Harnett PR (1996). A comparison of two quality-of-life questionnaires for cancer clinical trials: the Functional Living Index–Cancer (FLIC) and the Quality of Life Questionnaire Core Module (QLQ-C30). *Journal of Clinical Epidemiology*, **49**, 21–29.

Langfitt JT (1995). Comparison of the psychometric characteristics of three quality of life measures in intractable epilepsy. *Quality of Life Research*, **4**, 101–114.

Lee SY, Poon WY and Bentler PM (1995). A two-stage estimation of structural equation models with continuous and polytomous variables. *British Journal of Mathematical and Statistical Psychology*, **48**, 339–358.

Lenderking WR, Gelber RD, Cotton DL, Cole BE, Goldhirsch A, Volderding PA and Testa MA (1994). Evaluation of quality-of-life assessment in asymptomatic human immunodeficiency virus infection. *New England Journal of Medicine*, **330**, 738–743.

Liddell A and Locker D (1997). Gender and age differences in attitudes to dental pain and dental control. *Community Dentistry and Oral Epidemiology*, **25**, 314–318.

Likert RA (1932). A technique for the measurement of attitudes. *Archives of Psychology*, **140**, 1–55.

Likert RA (1952). A technique for the development of attitude scales. *Educational and Psychological Measurement*, **12**, 313–315.

Lindley C, Vasa S, Sawyer WT and Winer EP (1998). Quality of life and preferences for treatment following systemic therapy for early-stage breast cancer. *Journal of Clinical Oncology*, **16**, 1380–1387.

Loge JH, Abrahamsen AF, Ekeberg O and Kaasa S (1999). Hodgkin's disease survivors more fatigued than the general population. *Journal of Clinical Oncology*, **17**, 253–261.

Lord FM and Novick MR (1968). *Statistical Theories of Mental Test Scores*. Addison-Wesley, Reading, MA.

Lydick E, Epstein RS, Himmelberger DU and White CJ (1995). Area under the curve: a metric for patient subjective responses in episodic diseases. *Quality of Life Research*, **4**, 41–45.

Machin D and Weeden S (1998). Suggestions for the presentation of quality of life data from clinical trials. *Statistics in Medicine*, **17**, 711–724.

Machin D, Campbell MJ, Fayers PM and Pinol APY (1997). *Sample Size Tables for Clinical Studies* (2nd edn). Blackwell Science, Oxford.

Mahoney FI and Barthel DW (1965). Functional evaluation: the Barthel Index. *Maryland State Medical Journal*, **14**, 61–65.

Marx RG, Bombardier C, Hogg-Johnson S and Wright JG (1999). Clinimetric and psychometric strategies for development of a health measurement scale. *Journal of Clinical Epidemiology*, **52**, 105–111.

Matthews JNS, Altman DG, Campbell MJ and Royston P (1990). Analysis of serial measurements in medical research. *British Medical Journal*, **300**, 230–235.

McCormack HM, Horne DJ and Sheather S (1988). Clinical applications of visual analogue scales: a critical review. *Psychological Medicine*, **18**, 1007–1019.

McHorney CA, Ware JE, Lu JFR and Sherbourne CD (1994). The MOS 36–item short-form health survey (SF-36). 3: Tests of data quality, scaling assumptions, and reliability across diverse patient groups. *Medical Care*, **32**, 40–66.

Medical Research Council Lung Cancer Working Party (1992). A Medical Research Council (MRC) randomized trial of palliative radiotherapy with 2 fractions or a single fraction in patients with inoperable non-small-cell lung cancer and poor performance status. *British Journal of Cancer*, **65**, 934–941.

Medical Research Council Lung Cancer Working Party (1996). Randomised trial of four-drug vs. less intensive two-drug chemotherapy in the palliative treatment of patients with small-cell lung cancer (SCLC) and poor prognosis. *British Journal of Cancer*, **73**, 406–413.

Melzack R (1975). The McGill Pain Questionnaire: major properties and scoring methods. *Pain*, **1**, 277–299.

Melzack R (1987). The short-form McGill Pain Questionnaire. *Pain*, **30**, 191–197.

Morton AP and Dobson AJ (1990). Analyzing ordered categorical-data from two independent samples. *British Medical Journal*, **301**, 971–973.

Moum T (1988). Yea-saying and mood-of-the-day effects in self-reported quality of life. *Social Indicators Research*, **20**, 117–139.

Muthén BO and Kaplan D (1992). A comparison of some methodologies for the factor-analysis of non-normal Likert variables: a note on the size of the model. *British Journal of Mathematical and Statistical Psychology*, **45**, 19–30.

Nelson EC, Landgraf JM, Hays RD, Wasson JH and Kirk JW (1990). The functional status of patients: how can it be measured in physicians' offices? *Medical Care*, **28**, 1111–1126.

Nordic Myeloma Study Group (1996). Interferon-alpha2b added to melphalan-prednisone for initial and maintenance therapy in multiple myeloma. *Annals of Internal Medicine*, **124**, 212–222.

Norusis MJ and SPSS Inc. (1997). *SPSS Professional Statistics 7.5*. SPSS Inc., Chicago.

Nunnally JC and Bernstein IH (1994). *Psychometric Theory* (3rd edn). McGraw-Hill, New York.

Osoba D, Aaronson NK, Zee B, Sprangers MAG and te Velde A (1997). Modification of the EORTC QLQ-C30 (version 2.0) based upon content validity and reliability testing in large samples of patients with cancer. *Quality of Life Research*, **6**, 103–108.

Osoba D, Rodrigues G, Myles J, Zee B and Pater J (1998). Interpreting the significance of changes in health-related quality-of-life scores. *Journal of Clinical Oncology*, **16**, 139–144.

Osterlind SJ (1983). *Test Item Bias*. Sage Publications, London.

Parmar MKB and Machin D (1995). *Survival Analysis: A Practical Approach*. John Wiley & Sons, Chichester.

Pernegger TV (1998). What's wrong with Bonferroni adjustments. *British Medical Journal*, **316**, 1236–1238.

Pfeffer RI, Kurosaki TT, Harrah CH Jr, Chance JM and Filos S (1982). Measurement of functional activities in older adults in the community. *Journal of Gerontology*, **37**, 323–329.

Priestman TJ and Baum M (1976). Evaluation of quality of life in patients receiving treatment for advanced breast cancer. *Lancet*, **1**, 899–901.

Rasch G (1960). *Probabilistic Models for Some Intelligence and Attainment Tests*. Danish Institute for Educational Research, Copenhagen.

Redelmeier DA, Guyatt GH and Goldstein RS (1996). Assessing the minimal important difference in symptoms: a comparison of two techniques. *Journal of Clinical Epidemiology*, **49**, 1215–1219.

Regidor E, Barrio G, de la Fuente L, Domingo A, Rodriguez C and Alonso J (1999). Association between educational level and health related quality of life in Spanish adults. *Journal of Epidemiology & Community Health*, **53**, 75–82.

Rosenberg M (1965). *Society and the Adolescent Self Image*. Princeton University Press, Princeton, NJ.

Rosenberg R (1995). Health-related quality of life between naturalism and hermeneutics. *Social Science & Medicine*, **41**, 1411–1415.

Rothman KJ (1976). Causes. *American Journal of Epidemiology*, **104**, 587–592.

Rubin DB (1987). *Multiple Imputation for Nonresponse in Surveys*. John Wiley & Sons, New York.

Ruta DA, Garratt AM, Leng M, Russell IT and Macdonald LM (1994). A new approach to the measurement of quality-of-life: the Patient Generated Index. *Medical Care*, **32**, 1109–1126.

Ryan M (1999). Using conjoint analysis to take account of patient preferences and go beyond health outcomes: an application to *in vitro* fertilisation. *Social Science & Medicine*, **48**, 535–546.

Sadura A, Pater J, Osoba D, Levine M, Palmer M and Bennett K (1992). Quality-of-life assessment: patient compliance with questionnaire completion. *Journal of the National Cancer Institute*, **84**, 1023–1026.

Salek S (1998). *Compendium of Quality of Life Instruments*. John Wiley & Sons, Chichester.

Salmon P, Manzi F and Valori RM (1996). Measuring the meaning of life for patients with incurable cancer: the Life Evaluation Questionnaire (LEQ). *European Journal of Cancer*, **32A**, 755–760.

SAS Institute Inc. (1996). *SAS/STAT User's Guide, Version 6, Volumes 1 and 2*. SAS Inst. Inc., Cary, NC.

Schag CA, Ganz PA, Kahn B and Petersen L (1992). Assessing the needs and quality of life of patients with HIV infection: development of the HIV Overview of Problems–Evaluation System (HOPES). *Quality of Life Research*, **1**, 397–413.

Schipper H, Clinch J, McMurray A and Levitt M (1984). Measuring the quality of life of cancer patients: the Functional Living Index–Cancer: development and validation. *Journal of Clinical Oncology*, **2**, 472–483.

Schwartz CE and Sprangers MAG (1999). Methodological approaches for assessing response shift in longitudinal health-related quality-of-life research. *Social Science & Medicine*, **48**, 1531–1548.

Selby PJ, Chapman JA, Etazadi-Amoli J, Dalley D and Boyd NF (1984). The development of a method for assessing the quality of life in cancer patients. *British Journal of Cancer*, **50**, 13–22.

Shah S, Vanclay F and Cooper B (1989). Improving the sensitivity of the Barthel Index for stroke rehabilitation. *Journal of Clinical Epidemiology*, **42**, 703–709.

Shaw GB (1900). *In: Collected Letters Vol. 2: (1898–1910)*. Max Reinhart, London, 1972.

Sheard T and Maguire P (1999). The effect of psychologic interventions on anxiety and depression in cancer patients: results of two meta-analyses. *British Journal of Cancer*, **80**, 1770–1780.

Slade GD (1998). Assessing change in quality of life using the Oral Health Impact Profile. *Community Dentistry and Oral Epidemiology*, **26**, 52–61.

Slevin ML, Stubbs L, Plant HJ, Wilson P, Gregory WM, Armes PJ and Downer SM (1990). Attitudes to chemotherapy: comparing views of patients with cancer with those of doctors, nurses, and general public. *British Medical Journal*, **300**, 1458–1460.

Smets EMA, Garssen B, Bonke B and de Haes JCJM (1995). The Multidimensional Fatigue Inventory (MFI): psychometric qualities of an instrument to assess fatigue. *Journal of Psychosomatic Research*, **39**, 315–325.

Smets EM, Visser MR, Willems-Groot AF, Garssen B, Schuster-Uitterhoeve AL and de Haes JCJM (1998). Fatigue and radiotherapy: (B) experience in patients 9 months following treatment. *British Journal of Cancer*, **78**, 907–912.

Sneeuw KCA, Aaronson NK, de Haan RJ and Limburg M (1997). Assessing quality of life after stroke: the value and limitations of proxy ratings. *Stroke*, **28**, 1541–1549.

Spearman C (1904). General intelligence objectively determined and measured. *American Journal of Psychology*, **15**, 201–293.

Spector PE (1992). *Summated Rating Scale Construction: An Introduction*. Sage Publications, London.

Spiegelhalter DJ, Thomas A, Best NG and Gilks WR (1996). *BUGS Version 0.5: Bayesian Inference Using Gibbs Sampling: Manual Version ii*. MRC Biostatistics Unit, Cambridge.

Sprangers M, Cull A, Groenvold M on behalf of the EORTC Quality of Life Study Group (1998). *EORTC Quality of Life Study Group Guidelines for Developing Questionnaire Modules*. EORTC, Brussels.

Staquet M, Berzon R, Osoba D and Machin D (1996). Guidelines for reporting results of quality of life assessments in clinical trials. *Quality of Life Research*, **5**, 496–502.

StataCorp (1999). *STATA Statistical Software: Release 6.0*. Stata Corporation, College Station, TX.

Stiggelbout AM, de Haes JCJM, Vree R, van de Velde CJH, Bruijninckx CMA, van Groningen K and Kievit J (1997). Follow-up of colorectal cancer patients; quality of life and attitudes towards follow-up. *British Journal of Cancer*, **75**, 914–920.

Stucki G, Daltroy L, Katz JN, Johannesson M and Liang MH (1996). Interpretation of change scores in ordinal clinical scales and health status measures: the whole may not equal the sum of the parts. *Journal of Clinical Epidemiology*, **49**, 711–717.

Sudman S and Bradburn N (1982). *Asking Questions: A Practical Guide to Questionnaire Design*. Jossey-Bass, San Francisco.

Testa MA and Simonson DC (1996). Assessment of quality-of-life outcomes. *New England Journal of Medicine*, **334**, 835–840.

Testa MA, Anderson RB, Nackley JF and Hollenberg NK (1993). Quality of life and antihypertensive therapy in men: a comparison of captopril with enalapril. The Quality-of-Life Hypertension Study Group. *New England Journal of Medicine*, **328**, 907–913.

Torrance GW, Feeny DH, Furlong WJ, Barr RD, Zhang Y and Wang Q (1996). Multi-attribute utility function for a comprehensive health status classification system. Health Utilities Index Mark 2. *Medical Care*, **34**, 702–722.

Vickrey BG, Hays RD, Genovese BJ, Myers LW and Ellison GW (1997). Comparison of a generic to disease-targeted health-related quality-of-life measures for multiple sclerosis. *Journal of Clinical Epidemiology*, **50**, 557–569.

Walter SD, Eliasziw M and Donner A (1998). Sample size and optimal designs for reliability studies. *Statistics in Medicine*, **17**, 101–110.

Ware JE Jr, Snow KK, Kosinski M and Gandek B (1993). *SF-36 Health Survey Manual and Interpretation Guide*. New England Medical Centre, Boston, MA.

Ware JE, Harris WJ, Gandek B, Rogers BW and Reese PR (1998). *MAP-R Multitrait/Multi-Item Analysis Program: Revised, for Windows; User's Guide*. Health Assessment Lab, Boston, MA.

Whitehead J (1993). Sample-size calculations for ordered categorical-data. *Statistics in Medicine*, **12**, 2257–2271.

Wisløff F, Hjorth M, Kaasa S and Westin J (1996). Effect of interferon on the health-related quality of life of multiple myeloma patients: results of a Nordic randomized trial comparing melphalan-prednisone to melphalan-prednisone + alpha-interferon. The Nordic Myeloma Study Group. *British Journal of Haematology*, **94**, 324–332.

World Health Organization (1948). *Constitution of the World Health Organization*. WHO Basic Documents, Geneva.

Wright JG and Young NL (1997). A comparison of different indices of responsiveness. *Journal of Clinical Epidemiology*, **50**, 239–246.

Young T, de Haes JCJM, Curran D, Fayers PM, Brandberg Y on behalf of the EORTC Quality of Life Study Group (1999). *Guidelines for Assessing Quality of Life in EORTC Clinical Trials*. EORTC, Brussels.

Youngblut JM and Casper GR (1993). Focus on psychometrics: single-item indicators in nursing research. *Research in Nursing & Health*, **16**, 459–465.

Zigmond AS and Snaith RP (1983). The Hospital Anxiety and Depression Scale. *Acta Psychiatrica Scandinavica*, **67**, 361–370.

Zung WWK (1983). A self-rating Pain and Distress Scale. *Psychosomatics*, **24**, 887–894.

Index

Index compiled by A.C. Purton